T0093624

PHYSIC

PHYSIC
A Primer in Herbal Medicine

Julian Barker

AEON

First published in 2024 by
Aeon Books

British Library Cataloguing in Publication Data

A C.I.P. for this book is available from the British Library

ISBN-13: 978-1-80152-135-2

Typeset by Medlar Publishing Solutions Pvt Ltd, India

www.aeonbooks.co.uk

Dedicated to fellow apprentices

PLANT NAMES

In the text, medicinal plants are referred to either by their common name or, more often, by the shorthand therapeutic name (usually the traditional genus name alone) typically employed by herbalists conversationally.

Full botanic nomenclature for plants mentioned in the texts will be found at the end of the text, before appendices.

Full publication details of authors cited in footnotes will be found in the bibliography.

CONTENTS

PART THREE:
PHYSIC FROM THE ELEMENTS OF WATER, SUN, AIR
AND EARTH—NATURE IS OUR NURTURE

PREFACE

How to be concise when faced with such a large and intricate subject? While writing my previous book, I had felt the scornful presence of the Duke of Gloucester peering over my shoulder. He had accosted Edward Gibbon when *Decline and Fall of the Roman Empire* was published with "Another damned, thick, square book! Always, scribble, scribble, scribble! Eh, Mr Gibbon?".[1] Another glutton—like Gibbon more quoted than read these days—had the line "In every fat man a thin man is striving to get out". This was Cyril Connolly, the author of the by no means slim *Enemies of Promise* a quotation wonderfully reworked by Jennifer Saunders in the television sitcom *AbFab* to which her apparently sweet old mother replies acerbically "Just the one, dear?". Like all comedy, it needs to be seen and not heard at second hand as I am doing.

Out of my previous fat book, then, this slim volume has wanted to emerge. It is a primer in the physiology that I think herbalists need in order to provide physic to their patients. It is a condensation of themes explored in *Human Health*[2] but I hope that its new material comes across as less a précis and more a development of ideas in succinct form. Besides, I have changed my mind or at least have modified my attitudes to a number of observations I made in the previous work.

The world is all movement, ceaselessly interconverting matter and energy. This remains my core physiological idea—that all biological health is energetic—and only our capacitance allows us to flourish. Capacitance construed as an ability to maintain an adaptive ratio that I call *poise*.

Quite apart from any immediate therapeutic actions they may have, edible and medicinal plants possess a unique and necessary property of promoting our capacity for health

---

[1] Alternatively attributed to the Duke of Cumberland and George III. As for Gibbon's fat book itself, I can warmly recommend DM Low's slimmer single volume version for Chatto, reprinted by Pelican in 1965.

[2] *Human Health and its Maintenance with the Aid of Medicinal Plants* Aeon Books 2020.

and maintaining our poise. This property—ecological as much as biological—involves slight and subtle adjustments in the way our own personal physiology calibrates our present, our own historical past, and our inheritances. These, in turn, abut onto our psychosocial and psychosexual lives. Plants can provide—with irresistible constancy—encouragements with constraints that enable energetic health throughout a lifetime.

As any visitor to the Chelsea Garden of that name will know, *physic* is the old word for medicine, a plant given to alter the physicality of someone and the physical enterprise of their lives.[3] I use the word not to appear antiquated but to remind myself that life is ancient and precious as expressed in *phusiké*, the Greek for nature. The practice of physic is neither antiquated nor modern, but perennial.

Herbal medicine, like any other social enterprise, cannot be separated from its cultural milieu. The medical herbalist needs to pay as much attention to the patient and the arena where the interactions take place as to the actions expressed in the *materia medica*, which forms the third part of this book. *Bios* (the stuff and organisation of life in contrast to *Zoë* and *Pneuma* its spark and breath) provides the platform on which our social and linguistic psyche operates. These make up Part One with its wide take on inner physiology and Part Two with the physical human in motion and interaction. Part Three features the influence of plants on people. It was my intention to have the three parts porous to one another because order depends upon flow more than on borders and divides. Everything is connecting and mutually informing. Separating the physical world from body and mind has too long been a bizarre fiction. Life flits about like a bee seeking nectar, so it can be healthy to interrupt a narrative from its linearity.

As this is meant to be a primer, I ought to begin by drawing some markers and make my intentions clear. I want this work to supply a parallel reading to foundational sciences, of which there are so many excellent texts, to serve as a pointer to the physiology and other disciplines that will encourage the student and apprentice towards the broad and deep potential that herbal medicine can offer in the hands of a therapist with a broad and deep knowledge base. I believe strongly that a deep understanding of formative sciences better equips us as herbalists than does the memorisation of a detailed repertoire of strictly physiological pathways, pharmacodynamics, and pharmacokinetics, to say nothing of the 'actions' and 'uses' we ascribe to plants. To pan out, in other words, to a very wide horizon.

That is why I ask the reader to wait until Part Three for much mention of herbs at all. This is not a herbal. You can look for all the information on any plant of interest among the many herbal pharmacopoeias and herbals of all sorts derived from many levels of competence and experience. All I can add to them is the benefit of my experience, such as it is. Experience converts information into knowledge. What I hope to offer is a comprehensive approach to the problems the herbalist may encounter and may realistically be able to help. You can combine the plants you know with the schedule of plants I happen to have used. For all your own reasons you may choose others, but if you learn botany well and become grounded in plant systematics, you will begin to see relationships,

---

[3] The Regius Professorship of Physic at the University of Cambridge was founded by Henry VIII in 1540. "Physic" provided the root of the word physician; physics came later.

similarities, and contrasts between groups of the many thousands of flowering plants open to you, to say nothing of gymnosperms and medicinal fungi.

Text books have to make sure of the comprehensive and reliable details of their subject and may assume (perhaps unrealistically) that there will be plenty of time for the student and apprentice to discuss and consider foundational truths. This primer outlines a synopsis of the broad needs of the human patient and the practitioner who looks after them. In presenting at least some of the necessary themes, it becomes a reader: it makes the assumption that after study comes practice but also the enjoyment of further reading, thinking for oneself, and discovering that some questions just can't be answered by finding out more facts.

It is not a question of repudiating facts but keeping all that is known in mind, of expanding knowledge so that one can move comfortably from the general to the particular, a need of the general practitioner who wants to practise personalised medicine.

I want to suggest that the herbalist aspires to be first a biologist, because the medicine we practise is biological, second, a therapist-physician, and third, the type of humanist each of us wants to be.

If you are as committed as I am to lifelong learning, I would list the importance of these broader areas of knowledge as follows:

- Contemporary physiology
- An understanding of basic thermodynamics and of the core biochemical pathways
- Human embryology, especially implantation, gastrulation and the events of the first trimester[4]
- Systems biology
  (and a nodding acquaintance with the controversies of evolutionary biology)
- Human developmental biology and psychology
- Plant physiology and ecology

These have kept me fully occupied throughout my years in practice and continue to fascinate and engage my attention. It is not a question of 'mastering' these bodies of knowledge, which one person could only hope to engage in the most general way. Rather a way of concentrating your thinking, keep you interested and learning. Thinking as a form of meditation guarantees that you and your practice flourish.[5]

I want to persuade my fellow herbalists that continuous study, being at least on nodding acquaintance with core ideas will make flexible and adaptable physicians of us all. Most of us of forget much of the detail of the core pathology we learnt studying medicine, but one can always look them up. Thinking, like imagination—turning over ideas in your mind and meditating on their consequences—is something you do on your own terms, allowing feeling to be a guide.[6]

---

[4] It is well documented that child nutritional status is a direct outcome of the maternal environment during gestation. The child is the parent of its adulthood.

[5] Slow thinking (Type 2) in the sense explored by Kahneman (2011).

[6] 'Reflective practice', in short. Learning as you go along.

Practice evolves with experience but also needs turning over ideas from the world. In writing this primer, I have aspired to do more than interpret a syllabus that wants to match 'actions' of phytochemicals with 'conditions' that our patients may exhibit. Witnessing the entirety of the life of the patient—not just the expression of their illness—helps us match them with medicinal plants. You may become privileged to help with the health of their extended family from more than one generation.

Personalised medicine requires very broad generalised knowledge but also an intensity of detail. In the therapeutic arena, all detail is meaningful, not to be weeded out.

Generalisations found in the materia medica are correct and adequate in the broad sense (*sensu latu* as plant taxonomists say): by modifying them in accordance with the particularities you uncover in personalised practice, you will be led to a fuller understanding of the diffuse and long-lasting effects that plants can have upon people, benefits not shared by many other pharmacons.[7] The modern herbalist becomes a specialist physician with a very broad set of understandings. We cannot rest upon our *Laurus nobilis*!

Then, there is another focus of study. The science of human consciousness—otherwise known as poetry and literature—that explores (in parallel with medicine) the range and richness of experience. Literary imagination has parallels with medicine in allowing a self to be seen in the third person. The literary and dramatic arts, complementary to the scientific literature, offer the practitioner the richest and most fertile repertoire towards an understanding of the personalities and histories of individual patients. They do so much more universally than academic psychology.

I want also to draw attention to the different modes and planes of interaction between plants and the human body as follows:

1. Dietary
2. Direct sensory and cumulative sensorial effects, mostly smell and taste, reinforced by personal experience and cultural feedback
3. Rapid direct effects upon intestinal epithelial tissues, other mucosal surfaces, and skin
4. Cumulative effects of complex plant constituents—polyphenols, for example—and many other compounds upon endothelial tissues, on blood viscosity and laminar flow within vessels
5. Synergistic effects of polyphenols and other compounds derived from dietary fibre on the healthy diversity of the microbiome
6. Direct effects of aromatic, astringent and emollient plants (via olfactory, tactile and gustatory routes) and their indirect, diffuse and cumulative effects (via limbic systems) upon neurotransmitters (probably more modulatory than synaptic) and upon other endocrine agents and signalling pathways
7. Sparing, supporting and draining effects that plant compounds exert upon organs and cavities of the axial skeleton
8. Direct pharmacological activity where small clusters of compounds in relatively dilute concentrations generate signals that produce downstream effects out of proportion to

---

[7] *Pharmacons* denote any drug in the everyday meaning of pharmacology, including toxicology. *Pharmakon* as remedy has the further sense according to the Liddell-Scott-Jones *Greek-English Lexicon* as "a means of producing something".

their concentration; although these effects may be transient, they may also by repetition become long-lasting and cumulative; probably they achieve this by up-regulating signal pathways and by augmenting hormone receptor density

And then there is, in direct contrast to our work, for better for worse, depending upon the circumstances:

9. Direct pharmacological activity according to contemporary understandings of pharmaceutical science where single standardised purified substances, can be tested for reproducible effects and monitored for safety.

The ninth item on this list belongs properly only with pharmaceutical drugs and with drug-plants, such as *Ephedra*, foxglove or the opium poppy. These may be slightly preferable to the standardised drug given the ballasting effect that plant tissue materials may provide on absorption and distribution of the therapeutic compound.[8] These may confer some real advantages especially when the more potent plant is buffered by the admixture of other plants. As useful as this effect can be, it does not justify placing drug plants in an entirely different category of pharmakon from drugs.

I want to suggest that those drug plants we are permitted to use should feature last on a herbalist's intentions for the patient just as they might come first on a doctor's.

A pharmaceutical chemist would probably cite the first eight items on the list as evidence of weak, transient effects. I would agree: the weakness is precisely their strength: they do not overwhelm an already stressed terrain, especially one depleted by poor or inappropriate diet.[9] [Hormesis may play a part; see §3.3]

Much study may be necessary to understand the deep biology of our patients but herbal medicine is an eminently practical undertaking, so, I am sure that anyone drawn to it probably already has been taken with the following principles and suggested activities …

> First know your plants directly:
> primary knowledge by experience is always
> better than secondary knowledge from books.
>
> Explore natural ecosystems…
> acquaint yourself with all the plants you can,
> whether or not they are supposed to be
> medicinal
> and…
>
> get your hands into the earth

---

[8] These effects sometimes work in reverse: the isolated alkaloid colchicine is usually better tolerated than seed or corm of *Colchicum autumnale* from which it is derived.

[9] "Constitution" sounds like a solid and settled affair in contrast to "terrain" with which it is often used interchangeably. As the term appears so soon I had better point to Section 1.1, where I try to define it more precisely.

An extraordinary prejudice within orthodox circles considers the whole matter of pharmacons settled since William Withering discarded the presence of "impurities" in crude drugs as detrimental compared to the purified and single compound. He was talking about a mixture of wild plants that included foxglove, a potent and dangerous plant[10] and so was right in only a crude reductive sense; the "impurities" modify the action of the drug, making it less standardised but less toxic.

Pharmaceutical chemistry—with its remarkable biochemical insights—has given us products which—on balance—have provided great boons to human wellbeing so for herbalists to entertain a similar prejudice against the whole enterprise serves no one. But neither should we slavishly endorse its exclusionary reach nor its totalising social influence. As we recognise the strengths but also limitations of a pervasive culture of drug therapy, we offer an approach in parallel. [See Parallel Medicine in Section 3.1]

I had the good fortune to be taught phytochemistry by Peter Hylands, whose research drew attention to the phenomenon of plant compounds that did not on their own demonstrate physiological activity but were necessary for the "active constituents" to have their effect.[11] He presented his latest findings (with reference to traditional Chinese medicine as practised in the UK) to a meeting of the Society of Apothecaries in January 2016 and then to their joint meeting hosted by the Royal College of Physicians also in London on 11th September 2017 within the precincts of their herb garden.

Before talking about professional herbal medicine, let us—by way of *Introduction*— talk about the way all of us humans self-medicate with common types of plant physic…

---

[10] See The Foxglove Saga, Chapter 13 in *Green Pharmacy* by Barbara Griggs 2nd Edition.

[11] Sorely missed by colleagues; at his death in 2019, he was Head of the Institute of Pharmaceutical Science and Head of Pharmacy Department at King's College, London. He would remind us herbal students that all chemicals are chemicals and would make no distinction between molecules inside and outside living organisms. Even so, his later research showed how the presence of 'inactive' compounds permits the actives. He conducted trials on Feverfew, findings published in BMJ 291, 569 Efficacy of Feverfew on prophylactic treatment of migraine.

INTRODUCTION: MEDICINAL HUMANS

All humans come to ingest substances, mostly from plants and fungi, that are not essential nutriments but affect the way we feel. The way we feel is the primary index of our health: the way we might truthfully answer the universally posed question "how are you today"? We take these substances, often beverages, even when we feel well, perhaps to feel even better, to normalise. We may take them in a routine way, as if to mark the day. I don't want to labour the point with a deal of anthropological reading but speak from my own cultural practices, narrowly averting a lengthy footnote. When we feel not so well or unsure about how we feel, we may imbibe more of these potent substances to which we have become habituated or, banning them from our diet temporarily, switch to other beverages. *The implication is that we sense what is good for us.*

When we are decidedly unwell, we may seek advice from others about what to do and what to ingest, sometimes paying them for their services. So much is platitudinous but the rather obvious point I want to make is that what conjoins the taking of beverages routinely (to make us feel different even when perfectly "well") and prescribing for ourselves or seeking prescription from others when feeling *unwell*, is the conscious *feeling*. This is the state that provokes the primary impulse, a long way down the road before blood tests or a physical examination by a physician of any sort. If we recover within a short time, we attribute our changed state to an infection (a 'virus' doing the rounds) or have such an attribution made upon us. Other states, not attributed to infection, resolve also within time, such as migraines or mild mood alterations.

Lurking behind all such questions we pose ourselves (or ask advice about) looms the threat of disease. Disease implies some alteration in structure. The practice of medicine is taken up with diagnosing and treating disease or determining that, according to current understanding, disease is not present. In that case, what *is* present, then? For this anomaly practitioners of medicine tend to invent explanations, some offering reassurance, others haughty dismissal, and some genuine expressions of unknowingness.

Deferring the question of herbal medicine and disease, I want to stay with the state that prompts the universal daily "self-medication" which gives way on occasion to medication proper. Both are devices to change how we feel but one is what we fancy and the other what might return us to a former fanciable state.

Consciousness conjoins all us social animals but, in its intractable non-communicability, makes every person an island, an isolation that mothers and lovers want to penetrate. When ordinarily conscious, we locate our bodies and selves in time and place, depending on our level of focus and attention, and the activity we are engaged in. As banal as this description is, the question "how are you?" may be answered automatically without undue attention paid. Either we have barely enough enthusiasm to investigate ourselves or, if we know only too well, may conceal our emotional condition.[12] Our state of consciousness will reflect our current physiological situation but also our history and personality. Whatever we ingest, for whatever purpose (though 'purpose' as an input may alter the outcome), will inevitably influence our current physiological state. For this must reflect all our intakes from outside as well as inputs and outputs from inside. The taste, smell, and texture of an ingested plant, will produce some effect, however transient and subtle. Taking something to make you feel good without obvious detriment must confer benefit without having to blather on about efficacy and what studies are deemed to show. Opponents of herbal medicine (who tend to make a categorical distinction between food and medicament) may rather mean that most plants have no lasting therapeutic effect. A less biased question concerns the persistence of effects and their incorporation into the limbic repertoire. This raises the question of how you came by the plant and what you wanted to achieve by ingesting it. Plants are native to every ecosystem and are imbibed by every culture. Being at one with others provides untold benefits for us as social animals.

These are the subjects over which I want to range in this book. If herbal medicine is as inevitable as the daily ingestion of beverages, its adherents only need practise as well as they can, responding to change with the measured pace of trees rather than with the enthusiasm of passing fashion, maintaining their Hippocratic oath all the while. Reflecting and revising convivially with peers, learning from them and from patients as well as from reasonable critics. The opposition of the latter will be more useful than indifference or ignorance. In our culture, as in many others, social power is exercised by priests, scientists, lawyers and doctors. Status anxiety can make people strident or timid. Neither is useful. We do not need to be shrill. Best to gain what approbation we can by our own efforts and from the respect of our patients. If that is not enough, perhaps journey along a different path.

Humans will always self-medicate, usually with plants. I want to persuade the reader that the earlier these plants enter the infant's diet, primed for health, the less she or he will need a herbalist later in life. I will go on to argue that, when consulted, after placing her-himself at their disposal, the first thing a herbalist should enquire about concerns the person's nurture. In emergencies, we are duty bound to attend to the crisis, but in the

---

[12] Most of us accept that the question does not, outside a therapeutic context, invite a lengthy or even authentic disquisition. Undue attention given to the question may indicate some level of eccentricity, self-absorption, or just a deeply analytical temperament. Among many competitors, I rate highly a story about the great mathematician Paul Dirac which I hope is true. When asked out of conversational politeness, he took forty-five minutes before replying: "Why do you want to know"?

treatment of chronic illness, I offer the following approach: the place of plant medication comes third in a sequence of priorities, thus:

"first the witness, then the nurture, only then the herb"

If this sounds almost familiar it was the sequence of priorities offered by the physician, philosopher and surgeon we call Avicenna:[13] *"first the word, then the herb, only then the knife"*.

I need to elaborate on what I mean by these three terms with their implied sequence and to explain how they are interdependent, and how herbs—when used to obtain change in a person's metabolic life—are themselves as much nurture as medication. But, just as we train first in medical sciences before our clinical training, those three components of herbal medical practice need to await an exploration of physiology: the physics, chemistry and biology of our ecosphere.

But let me reiterate why the *materia medica* comes mainly into the third part of this book:

Craft is complementary to Art. In medicine,
as everywhere, we need both. The craft of the
apothecary is a gift to the art of the physician.
Our professional history has elected us to
perform both,
    so…
The art of the physician, and I suggest your
primary and most important task:
    is *to ensu*re that the patient leaves your consulting space
feeling better than when they entered. They should feel enriched,
    never diminished and pleased that they had booked the
    appointment with you
This is not a technical affair but one of affect.
But you want of course to build upon this
meeting and to help them further. The
diagnostic and strategic thinking for each case
depends upon your knowledge and
understanding of physiology, which has
graduated from data via information to
knowledge. Experience will translate this
knowledge into wisdom.
You develop the crafts of the apothecary in
training and as you practice and merge them
with the arts of prescribing. These crafts will
then graduate from information (which can be
complex enough) to integrated knowledge.

---

[13] From Ibn-Sina (980–1037), a Jewish Iranian muslim, who is more fully styled Abu Ali al-Husayn ibn Abd Allah ibn Sina to which al-Balkhi al-Bukhari might be appended. Bertrand Russell gave him a sympathetic chapter to himself in his *History of Western Philosophy* (Allen & Unwin 1961). Covered briefly in Barker (2013) if you want to consult a slimmer volume.

Immediate problems call for instant remedies, for the craft of the apothecary. They do not have to be especially urgent but people do not want to put up with the scratch, cut, bruise, the itch, sore, and insect bite for too long. But you can see that if the practice of a herbalist were to remain focused on remedies, they would have less need for deep knowledge of physiology. After all, if you employ a dispenser, that person needs training in procedure but needs no deep understanding of processes that generated the prescription.

Physic implies a knowledge of (1) human physiology: how, why and where to apply the herb (2) its skilful clinical interpretation: how to make the best of the clinical experience, and only then (3) application: what herbs might you use. Dependent upon an understanding of the medicinal allies and helpers, which in our case are medicinal plants. Even allowing for the naive question asked by the 'consumer' or consumerist practitioner "what herb x is supposed to be good for condition y?" This primer tries to shed light on x and y and to think of their relation to each other and to person z.

Let me summarise:

The trades and the physical crafts make our
domestic lives liveable.
Physicians and other professionals help deal with the
burdens of illness and sustain our wellness.
By extension, a skilled herbalist who is knowledgeable
about plants and people is in a position to provide immense
benefits to others, with very few risks,
to the satisfaction of all.

There are three sides to the therapeutic triangle: person, situation, plant. In three parts, I have tried to show that they sit opposite one another: separated but united.

Part One of this book concerns an energetic approach to the physiology that the herbal physician needs.

Part Two covers the therapeutic approach; and an overview of physiological axes.

Part Three extends the clinical application of plant physic in greater detail.

PART ONE

PHYSIC, PHYSIOLOGY AND PHYSICALITY

Physics of biology

Physiology surveys the processes that permit us to live and flourish. Given the shifting scales of the systems and the unimaginable quantities, the subject is endless.

Medical systems have always tried to extract enough information from these abstract ideas to make them coherent enough for their practices to be workable and as effective as possible. This first Section tries to do just that for the medical herbalist.

Physicality

Physicality makes us who we are.

Endocrine and neurophysiological circuits interpenetrate our locomotor tissue so that we can move (and be moved).

Modern orthodox medicine—in its tendency to separate and specialise—emphasises the mechanical aspect of physicality. It delegates physicality to separate specialities and condescends to leave some of the clinical management of physicality to physiotherapists. Herbalists have many ways to alter the deep control systems that permit healthy musculoskeletal activity.

The human body in time

The physics of physical space and physical beings are equally constrained by time. The time of our lives is cyclical and our histories are constrained by the days, months, seasons and years. The metabolic age of an individual may be higher or lower than their chronological age. Faced with the presenting age of the patient, the herbalist can apply physic towards lowering their metabolic age and help them entrain their lives with the physical circadian world and adapt better to their particular circumstances.

Let's try to define some terms

In nature, parts of the physical world are not really independent: one pole of a magnet "knows" about its opposite. This information is not "thought" but is an inevitable product of a relationship which exists separately from any thinker. Relationships in the physical realm are not random but depend upon one another. Physical laws make no sense unless all of the objects in the world belong to a network of networks as expressed eloquently by Carlo Rovelli as "relative information". When Democritus coined the term 'atom' he meant indivisible, separable but not at all unrelated.

Of course, when humans convert physical information into thoughts and convey them to others by semantic expression, then the information becomes a mental product but did not start that way. A representation of a piece of external information does not make a thought physical any more than a physical object is at all mental.

Bios

Life consists of converting solar or chemical energy into information, using that information to create self-sustaining, self-replicating structures, harnessing energy for that purpose. Information is interconvertible with matter in the same way that matter and energy are interconvertible. For life to emerge, entropy had to be momentarily reversed which required thermodynamically possible structures. Such structures increase or actually become the information for making other structures similar to themselves. It must all happen in a moment, the moment we call our lives here on earth. None of our thoughts, desires, or beliefs can subvert this *bios* or remove it from the core of our lives. The biosphere is the sum of all of Earth's ecosystems. For those organisms, such as humans, that cannot convert solar or chemical energy into information and new forms, feeding on those that can is our only chance of survival. There will always be other organisms—either very large or very small—which will need to feed upon the likes of us.

Food therefore comes before medicine and medicine becomes an intervention in our personal and extended ecosystem. Extensions on and within our person include whole populations that outnumber us, to put it mildly, creating biomes on our skin and mucous membranes. When our boundaries are penetrated or overwhelmed by microbial predators and, from our defensive responses, we develop infectious illness, life changes and medicine take on heightened significance.

Many plants can modify our response to this aggression, making it more effective and so lessening the potential for "friendly fire". Knowledge about them is readily available. This book is not about them but rather with the means whereby we may prepare for any assault and minimise the after-effects of infections as well as increase our capacity to resist them in the first place. This is the place for good dietary and life practices, especially the right amount of exercise and the management of the stages of life.

Duraffourd, Lapraz and Hedayat conceptualise the *terrain* as the constitutional balance of hormones that manages our response to the biosphere both within and without, in the moment and throughout life. Their work is now available in English.[14] In contrast to mainstream anglophone writers, they conceive of the "immune system" as an integral operation of the terrain rather than as an armed force. I like to put a slightly different emphasis on these complex sub-systems of cellular, antibody and cytokine populations and consider them not so much in militaristic terms as in providing providential benefits and assurance of a good life. Think of munity and munificence and municipal dedicated to our sustenance, rather than armies dedicated to our defence. Such an image helps us feel confident and not over-prepared and hyper-vigilant. In this way, medicine begins with culinary herbs, spices and everyday beverages. Medical herbalists only need to be called in when these measures seem inadequate to challenges and circumstantial changes in someone's life or to temporary disruptions at the borders of new territories of ageing and development.

Viruses are thought to be the most numerous of all biological entities. Whether they initiated life or derived from the cross-talk between archaea and bacteria cannot be known but the idea that they can be "defeated" seems to run counter to even the narrowest and crudest conceptions of ecology. The way that bacteria release chemical signal molecules to members of their own group may be analagous to the signalling pathways between our own cells and tissues. Characteristically, they can transpose their genes between individuals as might be anticipated before the evolution of sexual reproduction. In a process known as *quorum sensing*, they can regulate their gene expression in response to fluctuations in the density of a population.

Medicinal plants, of the right kind and appropriate dosage, can enhance the body and the mind as a sensing and signalling entity that needs to look after itself and avoid being swamped by external influences and self-defeating internal circuitry.

Vertical transition of genes from generation to generation as well as the side-shoots of the siblings of parents and wider cousinry provide us with a sphere in which we place ourselves within our social and psychic home. In ancient Greek thought, various terms for life (spirit, soul, animating principle) but Aristotle's bios (though it did not give us

---

[14] Lapraz (201 trans 2020); Hedayat & Lapraz (2013, 2018, 2019, 2020).

the term biology until the nineteenth century) remains the most foundational. Figure 15 *Time Criticality* in Section 2.5b seeks to emphasise this dominance of biology.

Capacity

A person's genome provides the primary source of their range of possibilities, their scope for manoeuvre. The limits may be largely deterministic but not entirely: the terrain can modify gene expression especially if benign and positive conditions of gestation and later experience favour it. The cards we are dealt are never as interesting as the way we play them.

Secondary responses to life and the environment can further expand (or diminish) capacity, because development and experiences modify genomic expression (as can the progress of the microbiome). In a simplistic way, the initial genomic could be visualised as an incline which, for any individual, varies in its steepness. Events that favour the slope becoming gentler will also favour, for instance, methylation of their DNA. This secondary improvement in capacity is reduced by ageing and by chronic, continuous loss of capacitance.

Our capacity for recovery from illness or adverse times indicates resilience, an index of strengthening capacitance and energy restitution.[15] Good attention to the six nurtures will enhance recovery; neglect of them will impede it. (Please see Section 2.1) Medicine can further enhance resilience if applied holistically.

Capacitance

Capacitance refers to the ability of a biological system to recover, restore, and store charge in the face of constant flux. The term is taken from electrical engineering, a reasonable borrowing given that life depends upon electrochemical energy. The control of flow and storage of energy is fundamental to survival.

Put another way: capacitance is the capacity to retain energy yet make available enough of it for the impulse to be discharged and to maintain the same proportion in a reserve store. The *uninterrupted* movement from reserved to available energy is a sign of poise.[16] Reserve is a necessary buffer against changing circumstances and also against an over-optimistic assessment of a task.[17]

Capacitance implies that, even when a person is ill or in a disordered state, a structured response is constantly being requested and provided. This structure, established in the first trimester of our mother's pregnancy, we call the terrain.

---

[15] The application of the concept of resilience applied to adaptive systems like the human person seems intuitively natural, but there are counter-intuitive ideas which may explain some of the effects of herbal medicine. See Taleb (2012) and the discussion on Hormesis in Section 3.3.

[16] To keep the hypothesis in one place, I give a summary in Appendix II.

[17] Reserve is equivalent at the cellular level (from where all biological events proceed) as the bulwark against entropy.

The terrain

The terrain refers to the unique inner physiological landscape of a person. Like all landscapes it responds to environmental pressures and so alters continually at the microscopic level but remains constant—in global configuration—over the years of a human lifetime just as the shape of a terrestrial landscape remains more or less constant in a short geological timespan.

More than a metaphor, it summates the neuroendocrine dynamic that orders and responds from second to second. The terrain refers to all the structures that mobilise the human person, a structure of relationships at every scale: between organelles and the cells that envelope them, between receptors and hormones, between neurohormones and transmitters, and the holoenzyme systems and all of the other matrices that enable life. It is the representative structure from which function arises.

The advantage of the term means that we are not bound to remind ourselves constantly that our division into physiological systems is a useful fictive device: we can talk about phenomena appearing on the skin without constant reference to the cardiovascular system that invests it, nor the ventilatory system that oxygenates the blood, and so on and so on.

Although the terrain subsists at all levels, and throughout the life of an individual it should not be envisaged as a short-term physiological agent but rather the repository of all our physiology, in for the duration. But when a serious accident befalls this whole body or when chronic stress diminishes its reserves, the semi-autonomous regions of the body (see Section 1.2) may assert their independence and overwhelm even the terrain's capacity for self-regulation. Illness of some kind inevitably results.

The terrain emerges from each individual as their basin of attraction, to borrow one of the major ideas of complexity theory.[18] Visualise it as a lake: the waters lapping against its shores slowly but continually refashion the shoreline by tiny amounts, changing it slightly from day to day but conserving the appearance of the whole landscape. It makes no sense to visualise a lake without water or just water without the enclosing landscape. I speak of the individual: this fictional person is a cluster of ecosystems at one centre of a constellation of families and friends, the exits and entrances of each leaving an impression (altering the shoreline) on the person we name the "individual".

The terrain adjusts the metabolic direction as the person moves through life but responds constantly to events as they unfold, like compass and tiller of a boat on water; the terrain and the "person" are no more separated than alloys in a thermocouple. When that direction is getting close to the rocks (back to a watery metaphor) the person gets queasy in some way (illness we call it) and may seek our help. By firmly but gently guiding the terrain to a safer course, by the application of medicinal plants, we allow the terrain itself to relieve the suffering. Deviating from a course is the usual and normal response to challenges, stress and strain and any one of the transition zones we all have to negotiate. This book explores how the practitioner can introduce plants to ease the patient's terrain onto a reset course.

---

[18] Not a single theory but a multidisciplinary approach to complex adaptive systems which are nonlinear and dynamical. This covers the weather, material science and emergent behaviour as seen in human beings.

The post-natal terrain

The neuroendocrine terrain as an imprint—first fashioned in the mother's womb—develops along with the infant. How could it not? The limbic system[19] builds on the already emotional newborn brain, generating spatial learning, memory in its olfactory and tactile world and matures the autonomic systems laid down during gestation. The initial terrain becomes modified because it has to accommodate and integrate the drives of the infant: what it has learnt in the first years of life, and what it has learnt to desire. In infancy and childhood, sensory priming—in which plants can play such an important part—adjusts the terrain to the unfolding world.[20] Of course, the terrain incorporates all childhood and adolescence experience then becomes relatively fixed at age twenty-one,[21] though epigenetic learning has no imprinted end-date.

The terrain is fractal, which is to say that it operates similarly at all physiological scales. As a self-modifying construct it is instrumental in recovering capacitance, as you might expect.

The principal nodes of the terrain: the autonomic nervous system, the hypothalamic-pituitary and pineal axes, and the use of medicinal plants to modify them will be treated in depth in Section 3.6 Therapeutics: Herbal Treatment Strategies by Levels.

The mobile landscape

Just as wind, rain, and chemical weathering forms and alters a terrestrial landscape, so our physiology forms our anatomy. It designs the body to move and so feeds back the messages of the world to the physiology that formulates it.

Surgery is an enterprise that works the other way around: it forces or reverses changes on an anatomy that accidents may have disrupted in a way that physiology could not have anticipated, with ruptures too rapid for it to mend in its slow circadian way. Or, it abruptly changes some of the unfortunate decisions that genetics or behaviour may have obliged physiology to make. Physiology forms anatomy, pathology deforms it.

By analogy, drugs (whether from plants or from synthetic chemistry) transmit forcings onto physiology. The strength of the imposition derives partly from the source and to a great extent the intentions it was supposed to meet.[22] Plants can also provide nurture and nutrient less forcefully in the form of food and culinary modification of digestion. They also afford us opportunities to modify our physiology, nudging it gently but firmly into a more stable position so that our organising capability may be restored. Applied physiology seems the best way to characterise modern herbal medicine because it looks to the horizon of future discovery with rootedness in the past.[23]

---

[19] A term that some neurophysiologists consider due for retirement, but it remains useful common currency.

[20] See Sensory Priming in Section 1.4.

[21] See Barker 2020 *Human Health* p. 207 and references.

[22] How the forcible transmission is received depends on whether the placebo gateway is open. See in Section 2.5a.

[23] The spectrum of plant activity on physiology will be discussed in Therapeutics in Section 3.6. That the Nobel Committee offers a prize for Medicine *or* Physiology shows how concordant they are.

Organising capability

Nature is generous yet economical. Nothing is wasted. When the energy has been fully extracted from material relationships in one ecosphere, it moves up to another where it acts again as substrate of some form, often in the vast system we call the soil (see Figure 1). In this ecological sense, to be soiled is a particularly human concern.[24]

While the terrain persists and maintains our self in the medium and long terms, it cannot in the short term override the organising capacity of the organs, especially the liver and kidney. Both are subject to the capacity of our lungs and circulation to extract and distribute oxygen. Any shortcomings here will rapidly show up as illness and will soon alter settings in other regulatory domains.

Impediments to recovery

As I have borrowed the term capacitance from electrical engineering, another one—impedance—follows on quite logically. Impedance expresses resistance in an electrical circuit to the flow of current. Various devices, like resistors, are inserted in circuits to control dissipative loss or damaging fluctuations in flow. Living beings are open dynamic systems, therefore dissipative, so they have to find some way of controlling energy loss and using, as it were, a complex system of impedances in order to maintain stability and recuperate a former dynamic state.[25]

Recovery is ultimately about replenishing reserves of energy. Sleep and rest remain the primary means of repair, a time for a change in kind of physiological work, at a different pace to activity. Populations of mitochondria have to be increased, particularly in liver and muscle cells; biochemical precursors have to be recruited and metabolic facilitators primed. These operate at the many levels described, for example, in Figures 3–5. All of these systems are absolutely dependent—as is every biochemical reaction—on the matrix of enzymes and cofactors that join every organelle and cell nucleus to the whole enterprise. Time is needed not just to digest and absorb nutrients but to allow for reorganisation and daily repair. Without adequate rest, these processes will complain, will throw up impediments against the stress of overwork. This is the ultimate functional origin of illness, of complaint. They will also intensify structural deficits. Without adequate rest, the municipality of the self becomes susceptible to infectious agents. Infectious disease then brings its own toll with a call on energy but is very often a secondary cause of illness. The immediate cause comes from ignoring or overriding impedance.

Then in its turn, the psyche can resist passive biological impedance: it may actively interrupt recovery of energy by monopolising it out of proportion to actual metabolic demand for glucose. Thereby the psyche may frustrate the soma.

Active impedances at the terrain level may become habituated and certainly generate a great deal of the symptoms commonly seen in clinic. These inhibitors are

---

[24] The theme of *Purity and Danger* the seminal work of the anthropologist Mary Douglas. Eminently sane and readable, it touches on human concerns that pertain to natural medicine.

[25] For further reading, see Maturana, H & Varela, F (1980) whose work may fall short of explaining our biology but provides a useful energetic description.

attempts to restrain continued exertion while the reserves are filling. To borrow a simile from mechanical engineering: lorries fitted with air brakes will not unlock them until the engine has first pumped air into the reserve cylinders; only when the braking gear is replenished will the engine allow you to drive away. With a little mechanical cunning, it is possible to override the system but, from personal experience, I can tell you that, whatever your hurry, this ruse is neither safe nor healthy for driver nor vehicle!

As for the biological driver, a drag will be placed upon flow from energy reserves to prevent demand from active impulses outrunning the speed of response. In the short term we can all choose to ignore the signal offered by fatigue and pain, to resist their inhibition. Just as well: responding effectively to emergencies could be lifesaving. But, rushing prematurely to react to events can set up a pattern of fragile poise so that hyperreactivity becomes an impedance of its own. Rest takes its place among the six nurtures (See Section 2.1).

The call to rest is an intrinsic restraint. If ignored, fatigue and pain tend to follow. If routinely frustrated, the terrain will eventually instal a chronic internal brake upon energy loss so that the overrider will eventually be overridden. The installation of this process may produce the very symptoms which lead to a consultation with the herbalist. The patient will need the six nurtures as much as medication.

The clinical consequences of overriding natural impedances are as varied as they are inevitable as we will discuss next.

Stalling

An aircraft stalls when its angle of climb exceeds available power and it may fall out of the sky. Landing an aircraft is effectively forcing it to stall at just above ground level. Stalling is the most serious consequence of overriding natural impedances. More down to earth, if a child runs up a steep bank and runs out of puff or muscular strength, she might fall backwards or certainly be forced to an abrupt stop.

The incline each person has to approach each day before dawn concerns the rise in cortisol from the adrenal gland, stimulated ultimately by a pulse generated from the hypothalamus. This is the full switch-on to the day that was alerted an hour earlier by the liver's alarm time-piece. If the stimulus is strong but the cardiac response inadequate, or not fully dampened, the resulting stall may be catastrophic. These outcomes are dealt with by emergency medicine and do not come into primary care. Each daily round, then, starts before dawn (whether awake or asleep) with the adrenal gland and liver preparing us for flight. If our terrain is ill-prepared for the terrain because the incline is greater than our resources, we may stall and so become unwell or more susceptible to infectious illness.

Although precipitated abruptly, any mismatch between incline and response was set in motion many years before. In our clinical settings we may have the opportunity to try to persuade—by nurture and herbal treatments—the steepness of the incline to lower and to improve access to reserve energy. Much of that work would be wasted unless we take care to maintain and repair the endothelia of blood vessels and improve organ function, all of which lie well within our scope.

Energy

Matter encloses energy, and life encloses matter to harvest its material, so it is self-making; by harvesting, storing, and releasing that energy, it becomes self-sustaining over time. In this sense, time behaves a little like matter.

Although eukaryote life was a relative late-comer, most of it has depended upon photolysis of water driven by the power obtained from solar radiation, fixing the products in structures, aided by warmth convected in the atmosphere. Plants do not, of course, do this "themselves" but rely on chloroplasts. These organelles were probably free-living ancient archaea or bacteria incorporated into the plant cell as mitochondria are thought to have reached a similar symbiosis in other eukaryote cells.[26]

Chloroplasts are organised into complexes that house the multiple nested series of chlorophyll pigments. The reaction centres can be visualised as vast arenas in relative terms, if you consider that they operate at the scale of the proton. With energy from the sun, protons released from water trigger a hot cascade analagous to the proton flow in mitochondria.

Their reducing power allows for gaseous carbon to be solidified into carbohydrate. This is the material upon which nearly all animal life depends. We can touch and eat the products but are unable to observe all the details as the initial capture endures for some three-trillionths of a second.

All our activities, including writing words like these, depend upon the accumulation and discharge of energy that was first enclosed and then released from chemical bonds. But living creatures cannot wait until the source of energy becomes available. Such a waiting is called death. We depend absolutely upon an ability to store and release energy. This is non-negotiable: our health is a measure of our capacitance, our ability to store and retrieve energy and information. For energy is a signal, a packet released from matter which must

---

[26] For a concise analysis of these processes, see Lane (2016).

be enclosed. Matter encloses energy in atomic structure, life within membranes that are nested in larger and larger conglomerations: organelles, cells, tissue compartments, endo-dermal and epidermal layers and then the thicker carapaces, The signalling devices which intercommunicate between all these structures are vast unseen matrices: webs of enzy-matic filigree, coils of nucleotides and their protein readers and writers.

Although there is a background invariability in the oscillation of atoms, time registers itself in living creatures in variable pulses not as a metrically rigid beat. We take our cues from the sun, moon, and the consequent movement of oceans and atmosphere, setting our timekeepers by them. They are not clocks so much as an internal orchestra-tor and conductor, housed primarily in the hypothalamus but with satellite franchises throughout our bodies, notably the liver but also the kidney. The dark/light cycle can be classed as a rhythm as it features a contrasting strong and weak signal. Although this diurnal rhythm alternates: 1, 2, 1, 2 … the beats are equal in duration only at the two equinoxes. The seasons manifest a different relationship between the stressed and the unstressed signals—the hallmark of rhythm—between the solar light of day and the nocturnal dark.[27] Cloud and fog as well as man-made structures and environments may then obscure and complicate this clear picture. Overlaid on this fundamental binary rhythm flow the movements of oceans and winds: these tides interact with one another producing the complex waves that inform our modes and moods.

Of course, our internal pacemaker not only tracks the time of external events but gen-erates pulses of its own to stimulate and coordinate regularities like heartbeat and match them with the metres of walking, running and dancing.

None of this is controversial, indeed to a musician would be banal, a statement of the obvious, but you can see here a limitation to human discourse made by the scientific method (against which, in physical systems, I wouldn't hear a cross word). The fundamen-tal knowledge of that which can be tested is not at stake but rather the way we interpret that knowledge in ways that are useful to our health and how we conduct our lives.

Physiology of poise

Health, indeed life itself, depends upon energy. How is the flow maintained and controlled? According to the poise hypothesis, health is an outcome of a ratio between available energy and that held in reserve: not a level but a bevelled plane.

According to the Poise Hypothesis, feeling well depends upon an open flow from an adequate reservoir of energy. The flow that feeds us energy from reserve—our ability to store and utilise energy, our capacitance—fluctuates according to age, circumstances, and the stress and strain put upon us.[28]

The physics of health is energetic and cannot be otherwise because life itself manages to reverse the second law of thermodynamics only for as long as it subsists, and then falls prey to it in death. To preserve, conserve and reserve energy is an absolute requirement and depends upon capacitance: the degree to which the organism is capable of storing energy.

---

[27] We say tick-tock not tick-tick nor tock-tock.

[28] Of course, feeling well involves consciousness which makes the simple energetic equation ineffably compli-cated. Consciousness makes itself known to "us" in an obvious way but how it does so is still mysterious but that it depends absolutely on energy can surely not be in doubt.

We use this stored energy to adapt to our circumstances and needs, as do all creatures. When our capacitance is lowered even briefly, we humans experience the stress and strain as a subjective state, which may range from a feeling a little out of sorts to a definite sense of illness. The state might include fatigue, lassitude, aching muscles and a sense of burden with perhaps a transient change in mood, with lightheadedness or even vertigo, or pain may be the dominant sensation.

These experiences send us a clear signal: a call to rest, but we can override this temporary feeling with our will, with a burst of confidence, making us feel sort of well enough again for the time being.[29] But this debt will have to be repaid by rest and sleep; otherwise, it will be repaid by illness.

This temporary loss of capacitance is brought about by an increase in the adaptive load from a wide range of challenges, aggressions, emotional conflict and financial burdens; by loss of agency or a crisis in confidence or a surge of fear.

Disruption to digestion, rest, sleep or enforced inertia will decrease the functional strength of the terrain and will compound the initiating cause of unwellness. This will come from an increase in burden or an abrupt drop in energy to manage it, or both. Usually both.

Restoring capacitance is brought about by:

A: Lowering the adaptive burden:
This is best achieved by change of habit, behaviour, or diet in the broad sense rather than by medical intervention: many "medical" problems are not really medical at all but circumstantial. Applying medication—a "remedy" may be comforting (good) but not a substitute for changes in our way of living.

B: By an increase in the functionality of the terrain:
This can be brought about by changing eating patterns, habits and foods, by rest and better-quality sleep. Dietary and medicinal plants along with culinary herbs and spices provide unique allies in the enterprise of supporting change.

A great drag on capacitance is not so much genetic susceptibility—about which medicine can do so little—but disposition of the terrain, about which herbal medicine can do so much. It is understandable that when someone's circumstances cannot be changed, they reach for medicine, but it comes second best.

Reduced capacitance not only deprives a person of comfort, it also:

i. Increases susceptibility to infection
ii. Increases infectivity to others and reinfection of self
iii. Reduces even further the capacity of the adaptive response
iv. Increases the risk of developing diseases to which the person may be genetically susceptible.

---

[29] Our drives and desires, our will, like energy and its reserves, are dispersed systems and cannot be attributed to any single location. To borrow Edward Said's phrase, "our sense of self is more like a cluster of flowing currents than a solid self". I hope that when the reader is looking for a practical therapeutic approach, the Levels (especially Six and Eight) in section 3.6 bring some help and relief from these inevitably abstract ideas.

Poise describes the point where available energy is sustained by an adequate reservoir with a ratio of approximately ten to sixteen. Self-care reduces any drain on poise. A sense of wellness or of illness—provided ultimately by our physiology—rises to our consciousness and should either give us confidence to continue as we are or tell us that we need to change. Instead of responding to that need for change we may, of course, use medicines to treat our symptoms. This may be a good move if they are a sign of invasion by disease, but it might be a while before you would know. Some modern medicines seek to alter the course of disease but would not be prescribed until the diagnosis is clear, which might take weeks or months.

Whole plant remedies are moderately helpful in reducing symptoms, usually with few if any adverse effects. They cannot, of course, change causal circumstances but by their ability to improve the functionality of the terrain, they may reduce the adaptive burden by ballasting the responsiveness to challenging circumstances; in this way they elevate capacitance. They do so alongside the appropriate nurtures and in this sense and this way of using them, are almost a nurture of their own, an extension of diet. These benefits are more long-lasting than any heroic prescription of plants as pharmaceuticals.[30] The properties of herbs and spices are bestowed upon mucosal surfaces and, if absorbed, on endothelial membranes. In addition, they can enhance organ activity: especially functions of stomach, pancreas, liver and kidney. Over the longer term, they have cumulative nudging effects on the neuro-endocrine settings, imprinted first in the womb that constitutes the initial terrain, and later modified or reinforced by experience.

Aromatic herbs and spices present a subtle but potent influence upon a receptive perception: they have strong flavour and aroma and may strengthen our associative memories with the capacity for neuronal potentiation over the long-term. This cumulative resource contributes to the potential for healthy resilience by this enhancement of sensory priming and what I call stochastic resonance.[31]

As medicine is a practical activity, it is right to have pointed to its application, but we have got ahead of ourselves and need to return to the physical basis of bioenergetics.

Bioenergetics

Chloroplasts in green plants use solar energy to initiate a charge separation in molecules of water to create a source of reductive protons and an energetic flow of electrons to convert radiant into chemical energy. Mitochondria in all eukaryotes take the power of the oxygen formed during photosynthesis to pull electrons through an enzymatic chain

---

[30] When it comes to heroic remedies, perhaps mention should be made of volatile oils—so-called essential—derived from aromatic plants offer us quite a different modality of treatment. Even though the doses used may appear to be low given their dilution in body fluids, their powerful effects in infectious illness and also on mood alteration has been much studied in laboratories across Europe and especially in France since the 1930s where they came to attract clinical attention. By some perverse quirk of consumer culture, these potent remedies are thought to be suitable for use in "aromatherapy" by those who have not studied medicine but would not think themselves competent to use whole plants as medication. For an entertaining history in English, I recommend Levitt 2023.

[31] These two terms have adjacent segments to themselves in Section 1.4. Their connection with the pharmakon follows in Section 3.3. For an enlarged discussion see Barker (2020), Section 20.

simultaneously moving protons across the inner membrane to drive the armature of ATP-synthase. Links in the chain are invariably enzymes and cofactors; chains in the mitochondrion are comparable to those in the chloroplast.

Potential energy is fixed into phosphate bonds by this universal catalytic oxidation of organic compounds from foodstuffs. These are materials anabolised by donor organisms for us to catabolise. The donation is not voluntary but we are part of the huge feeding web that makes up the biosphere.

Feeding, therefore, responds to one of the four continuous essential drives, hydration coming first because biological reactions can only happen in an aqueous environment close to a lipid membrane.[32] The response to the drives can be measured in hours and days but the needs of aerobic respiration have to be addressed within seconds for comfort and within minutes for survival.

Although we may trace our ultimate source of energy reserves to our mitochondria, we have no direct control over them and have to trust in the wonderful sets of integrated structures that magic energy from the organelles to flow up to the consciousness of the (equally magical) individual. Given that health is fundamentally energetic, it might seem sensible to enhance the flow and distribution of energy. But how? As you might expect, muscle cells (skeletal and especially cardiac) and high metabolisers like hepatocytes, contain several thousand mitochondria each. Their numbers and concentrations respond to demand; so, when able, exercise provides the stimulus to optimal development and function with a liver-sparing diet (as discussed in Appendix I) in tandem with an avoidance of toxic environments.

The careless medicinal enhancement of this flow by supplementing diet with precursor compounds such as ubiquinone is of dubious efficacy and may even interfere with energetic differentials within the mitochondrial membranes. Besides, such practices are mechanistic: herbal medicine is best seen as enhancement rather than replacement therapy. Likewise, although free-radical oxygen species are destructive to mitochondrial structure and function, the oversupply of anti-oxidants, whatever the therapeutic intent, can precipitate precisely the opposite action of that intended.[33]

Metabolism is an overarching term for anabolic and catabolic functions. Poise, too, reflects a meta-state of affairs. Even if one could calculate overall mitochondrial function, *poise is a proportion not a measure*. Like energy itself, it is everywhere and nowhere. Poise is precisely not a fixed but a fluctuating ratio that oscillates around a point and eventually converges to *phi*. This is the golden mean: a ratio that resolves to 1:1.61803 (roughly ten to sixteen). Actual amounts are not quantifiable in any practical sense. Besides, the amount of ATP cycling through the system is not the only conduit for energy: structural and enzymatic matrices are necessary for the interconnectedness on which life depends. Quite apart from ATP-synthase itself, the complexity of all the loops and other functional entities almost belies description or enumeration. Thinking to enhance energetic function by supplementing with precursors to the substrate on which the enzyme chain in the

---

[32] To drink, to sleep, to eat, to meet constitute our imperatives; the order is dictated by how long we could survive without responding. As social animals we need to meet to be healthy but also to be fed in due time. To mate as an extension of to meet is a faculty that individuals may dispense with but the species cannot.

[33] Cf. Lane (2016) 268–279.

mitochondria (such as ubiquinone or coenzyme-Q10) might seem to simplify the scale of the task but simplification can only work at the meta-level, not at that of the organelle.

Likewise, using constituents of medicinal plants as if they were replacing endogenous biomolecules misses the point that they operate at the level of the system, and even organism rather than as weak pharmaceuticals targeted to local tissues. However, by contrast, the signals emanating from higher levels *do indeed* influence microstructures, such as mucosae and endothelia. This is where much of the benefit of medicinal plants operates but at the same time they may additionally generate higher-order signals in the limbic system. Thus, low concentrations of complex molecules can generate waves that amplify their strength by feedback loops and generate persistent patterns of responsiveness. That is part of my explanation for the power of plants.

Patients often complain of fatigue and low energy but even if not, the question needs to be asked during the systemic review.

Energy reserves

Energy in physics is an abstract quantity that can move from one system to another. Energy transfer (whether to or from chemical, electrical, thermal or mechanical) implies movement or excitation. Matter itself involves energetic gradients and imply extension in space. So, all is movement: 'still life' (changing scale for a moment) is illusory. While calm may be good for health, immobility is not. The newborn infant matures its brain so that it will be able to walk and so eventually acquire its own food.

Biology emerged from physics. That it emerged at all may not have been inevitable but it could not have been the other way around. We cannot evade our physical world any more than we can our biological one. Nor can we humans escape our psychosocial world and thrive.

Ancient humoral theory amalgamated all of these, uniting the cosmos with physiology and psychology. The inventions of microscope and telescope provided an even more intimate sense of dynamism and scale. It might have aroused a new sense of interrelatedness had not the industrial revolution given us the power to exploit the ecosphere on a colossal scale. Ecology fuses biology with physics in both quantitive and qualitative ways, treating natural systems as processes not objects. The consequences of disregarding such findings are only apparent once you cannot escape the planetary ecosphere. When our hunter-gatherer and pastoralist ancestors degraded their habitats, they just moved on. Australia and Europe were once almost entirely afforested. Now the other continents are catching up at speed.

The abstract method is a powerful and most useful device for solving problems. It consists in making models of reality and applying the results of its analysis to real-world situations. To abstract the individual human from her or his interrelatedness and concentrate on survival may be a useful temporary device in emergency medicine although even here, some context and background is usually required for good clinical judgements. It is not only modern scientific medicine that tends to abstract entities from their background and to demarcate them for treatment. I mentored a herbal student who was doing the same course by correspondence that I had undertaken while studying in America some years earlier. He was required to write a dissertation on *Leonurus cardiaca* but was puzzled by some of the indications and preparations. I suggested he focus on the life cycle of the plant and consider first its habit and habitat. He was surprised at this advice and could not see the sense in it. "I have no idea at all what it looks like. All I need to know is whether it works and what it is good for".

I presume he would not see the point of reading this book but I hope the present reader will see the sense in placing each individual within the entirety of their constellated spheres, like a plant in its natural habitat. Their current state of mind and body, I want to persuade you, cannot be abstracted from the ecological niche into which they were born and the processes they have undergone. The clinical arrangements amalgamate all their spheres into one narrative process for them to witness themselves. Then the herbalist can call into play medicinal and culinary plants more as their allies, friendly and effective, rather than as wilful agents. This may sound rather grandiose but I have found it to be a practical and realistic aspiration. It constitutes my view that the benign and helpful profession of herbal medicine concerns optimisation of a life in the face of inevitable constraints, rather than fighting diseases that are far from inevitable. If you take this approach seriously, you will be taken seriously by extended families and their generations.

Energy and its reserves are non-localisable. They are as wide as our entire system of systems: an organism's need for organisation. The solution to the problem of low energy reserve cannot be found by operating upon a single organelle such as the mitochondrion with some putative supplement. It is true that augmenting the system with a single mineral, such as magnesium, provides great benefit at very little cost to a pregnant woman with pre-eclampsia and *some* benefit to a vagotonic but generally healthy individual. But the problem of low energy reserves have little to do with overall supply and more to do with sub-system weaknesses. Similarly, low vitamin D, has more to do with poor hepato-renal function and bile than with supply. This important subject is discussed in detail in Section 2.5b. Supplementation has been shown to make at best a meagre difference in serum levels in those who have low levels in spite of ingesting adequate amounts in diet and sunshine. The level of activation by kidney enzymes account for the limiting factors.

The web of energy

The number of species in an ecosystem indicates its richness and resilience, serving as an index of the amount of energy extracted from the physical world. The corresponding number of nodes of interaction between these constituent members registers the complexity of the system, though even the simplest organism is itself more complex than the physical system on which it subsists. Multicellular animals and plants raise the level again; sociality increases the size of the interactive web exponentially. Large nervous systems engage and are operated upon by the internal ecosystems they enclose, again as exponents, giving rise to thought.

Ecosystems manage us: we depend for our wellbeing on species colonising our guts, mucosal membranes and skin, but our human minds have created technologies that have enabled us to reduce the biotic complexity of the ecosystems that we call the natural world, the one that provides us with food. That they have been "successful" is difficult to deny, given the rise in the number of individuals of our species and our ability to neutralise competitors and opponents in the search for our food and materials. However, our "goods" come at the cost of a reduction in the biodiversity of our planet.

Discussion of personal immunity, with an exclusive focus on the individual, may tend to disregard the niches we have carved (or even blasted) out of the natural world.

"Our" Ecosphere

All ecospheres nestle within another one and provide a nest to others. That is to say that they are fractal: each one similar in shape though very different in detail to the bigger ones that enfold it and to the smaller ones it encloses. So, when you say "our", it is fair to ask to which one are you referring. Time modifies them all: the disintegrating body enters a different biome just as food scraps on the way to becoming compost do.

Ancient humoral elemental theories remained mainstream until the early modern period. They have survived in cultural consciousness and even in modern immunology where "humoral" refers to antibodies in body fluids in contrast to defences provided by specialised cells. Four element theories remain coherent phenomenological accounts of the world we perceive and through which we move. But our understanding of microscopic interactions has vastly expanded so that we now possess more detailed insights into the dynamics of natural phenomena.

Nor is there anything novel in the observation that time proceeds in cycles. Now we understand in greater detail how circadian rhythms integrate the entangled lives of plants, animals, fungi and all microorganisms within all ecosystems, even if our inventions of agriculture and heavy industry have tended to obscure these relationships.

All is movement in the physical world. Heat is a quantity of movement, not a substance as was once thought. Movement can generate a charge. Charge separation allows chloroplasts and mitochondria to use inorganic sources of power to fix energy and information within them.

Living beings have to detect regular waveforms amidst the hubbub and generate internal pulses to match regular cycles in the environment. In human physiology, perhaps the most obvious example would be the pulsatile release from the hypothalamus of factors that in turn control the hormones of the pituitary gland. Modifying these is one of the several basic approaches open to the phytotherapist.

Our capacity to integrate internal fluctuations with astronomical cycles contributes in very general terms to good health. As walking—our primary movement—is rhythmic so our attention to the sensory streams—auditory, visual and tactile—appears to be rhythmic.[34] If neural networks (as most models postulate) are coupled oscillators, they help us sample stimuli from the world, notice patterns and direct or divert our attention. In social animals, garnering the attention of others confers status while the art of distraction favours all performers from conjurers to hypnotists.

---

[34] See, for example: Zalta, A., Petkoski, S. & Morillon, B. Natural rhythms of periodic temporal attention. *Nat Commun* **11,** 1051 (2020). https://doi.org/10.1038/s41467-020-14888-8

Energy characterises life, with information as mediator.[35] The exclusion of viruses from the living by some biologists rests on the fact that they do not possess a chemical metabolism of their own. Instead, they parasitise a cell, adopt the metabolism of their host, then replicate. Given that they inhabit every ecosystem and the information they encode presents a challenge to each of the lifeforms, this exclusion seems arbitrary and short-sighted. I have sketched the thoughts of this segment into the Figure 1 below:

Astro sphere	Fire	Movement ⇔ Pulses ⇔ Cycles ⇔ Waveforms
Atmo sphere	Air	
Litho sphere	Earth	⇊
Hydro sphere	Water	Charge separation in water molecule
⇩ ⇩		⇊
Bio sphere		*Energy and information fixed in chloroplasts and mitochondria*
⇩ ⇩		*Archaea Bacteria*
Eco Spheres	*Plants*	*Protists Algae*
		Animals

Figure 1: Spheres of activity

Ecosphere, energy and illness

The scale of the figure above is meant as a reminder that although we see an individual—not a system—in the clinic, it is therapeutic to connect the person, if time permits, with all their contingent spheres. When it comes to wellness and lapses into illness, the emphasis may be upon the presenting symptoms. But for clinical practice to mature, it does well to consider the energetic and ecologic basis to presenting complaints, not only in the biologic sense but also the psychosocial situation that has contributed to the current unwell state. In whatever way it was precipitated, some immediate physical state of the blood will always have been moved out of the buffering zone.[36]

Each of the spheres in Figure 1 contain webs of communication. In the biosphere, eukaryotes have made a speciality of finding niches in an ecosphere. An ecosystem manifests the energetic needs of constituent organisms and how each satisfies the others

---

[35] Without the combinatorial power of nitrogenous bases in nucleotides and amino acid sequences in proteins, metabolism would not be possible, nor would mutation. Energy mobilisation depends upon nitrogenous co-enzymes whose precursors are the B-vitamins. See Lehninger (1970) Chapter 14: *Bioenergetic Principles and the ATP cycle*; Bronk (1999) 18, 98.

[36] The concept of buffering in energetic health will be picked up in Section 1.8.

while attempting to attract the energy that flows through the system towards its own niche. Sociality encloses niches in a sphere absent from Figure 1: the socio-sphere. Woody plants are social and prosper in woods and fields bordered with hedgerows. Social animals from ants to elephants and humans are well and prosper or are unwell and struggle to survive according to the energetic and informatic success of their niches.[37]

Our clinical practice operates at many levels at once: we have to integrate horizontal processes (family, friends, the present) with the vertical elements that created this present person and her niche (ancestors, parents, childhood) into a clinical idea and then apply plants, which have their own formative experience, towards a positive consociation.

Proximal physical states that result in illness

Buffering is the capacity of a system to operate within a narrow band of variables such as pH or temperature, to act to restore a fixed point from fluctuations. Whatever the ultimate cause of any illness, whether recent or chronic, blood states as listed below will inevitably create strange sensations, odd discomforts, or pain or some sort of distress:

- Low oxygen extraction
  - With or without low haemoglobin
- High or low pH in one or more fluid compartments
- High or low arterial temperature
- High or low arterial pressure
- High or low blood glucose
- Viscosity of blood—and turbulence in its flow—often affected by:
  - High or low populations of cells or platelets
  - Presence of macromolecules or inflammatory compounds
  - High levels of normal metabolites such as bilirubin or uric acid (ionic disturbance affects the ECF, cells and tissues more than the blood)

Herbal remedies at the appropriate dosage may alter these quickly and offer immediate relief, even if the underlying causes may take months to adjust. Your differential diagnoses will of course consider respiratory tract infection, cardiac causes, and thyroid states as well as the absence of insulin resistance (its presence will be more obvious), keeping the almost constitutional autonomic disturbances such as asthma and migraine always in mind. Whether or not these causes are known or can even be ascertained, blood states such as those listed above will provoke or sustain alarm in the limbic areas where emotional stress may have initiated. In states of psycho-social stress, especially if chronic or even constitutional, a long consultation will be part of the therapy.[38]

The poise hypothesis formulates, if nothing else, the common-sense observation that illness makes us feel weaker and getting better is associated with regaining strength. If you want to visualise it: obtain or imagine a kitchen scale, not electronic nor one with a pointer but a table balance scale.

---

[37] I recommend Odling-Smee, Laland & Feldman (2003) as a very readable introduction to the subject.

[38] See Placebo in Section 2.5a.

Put 100 grams of any material (dried herb, say) on the lefthand pan and 162 grams of material on the righthand pan. The pan on the left will tilt upwards and that on the right will dip down. Now you see a graphic display of poise with the upward available energy depending upon the greater, heavier amount of energy in reserve.

In other words, according to the hypothesis, poise offsets any ten units of available energy by just over sixteen units as *potential* energy in reserve. This ratio is Φ, the golden mean. Here is another way to visualise poise as a distribution of the global flow of energy in constant movement over time:

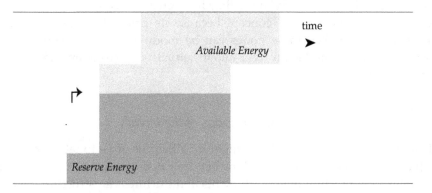

time

Available Energy

Reserve Energy

Figure 2: Graphic depiction of ratio between available and reserve energy

Every cell contains its portion of this reserve in cytoplasm but mostly in mitochondria, especially in skeletal and cardiac muscle. At the larger scale, we exhibit our state of poise in pulmonary and cardiac reserve.

The constancy of the terrain

Movement and change are built upon constancy. You can only move against a resistant force or structure. The terrain constitutes our inner architecture: a foundational virtual structure. Thinking of it as a physiological agent is as illusory as imagining it as some sort of "ghost in the machine". Rather it is a signature tropism imprinted into our body early *in utero* (in late embryonic and early foetal stages) but one that can be modified slightly at every later stage of development both before and after birth.[39]

If you can think of the human body as fundamentally neuroendocrine consisting of a myriad of signalling connective loops, then the terrain is a collective word for the body so constituted.[40] Recent understanding of the pervasive and enormous influence of the microbiome on the terrain might seem to swamp this idea. Yet the microbiome, especially of the colon, is probably part of the adaptive modifications that the terrain is able to make at the key developmental stages. It is the very constancy and stability of

---

[39] Dr Christian Duraffourd taught that the terrain becomes closed and impervious to change at the end of the third heptade. More recent studies in epigenetics suggest that experience can continue to modify the terrain at later stages, even if the fundamental structure remains little altered.

[40] The notion of loops is summarised in the Résumé at the end of Part One.

the terrain that permit changes and so magnifies the effect that can be seen in a person's wellbeing. Once the terrain is more than twenty years old, its capacity to make fundamental changes more or less close. The adult is the inheritor of the child.

Yet small and incremental modifications remain always possible and some powerful infections in childhood and late adolescence will have already done just that. Viral illness' may often attach themselves to weak points in the terrain and amplify the chance of their recurrence but also give some adaptive advantage. Epstein-Barr and Herpes viruses are cases in point. It is not residual viral fragments but the information that the virus left behind and continues to convey. Such infections, current or previous, need to be part of the medical history review as they have great relevance for terrain medicine.

The terrain is such a useful concept because its principle nodes are identifiable and the relations between these nodes can be modulated by the gentle persuasion of medicinal plants. This faculty will allow herbalists to structure their clinical and therapeutic decisions.

The major nodes of the terrain

Details are given elsewhere but here might be a helpful place to tabulate these major nodes (Figure 3). Dysfunctional relations between nodes give rise to many persistent health problems. Adjusting them with plants and nurtures can structure the therapeutics of any clinical practice. The degree to which endogenous pacemakers in any terrain are responsive to and are entrained by external cues and stimuli gives us a fundamental criterion for disposing the person towards or away from health. The primary cues are photic, from the sun and the moon: they involve intensity of illumination and length of daylight. Personal responses to derived secondary cues—climate, weather, and tides—tend to be more idiosyncratic.

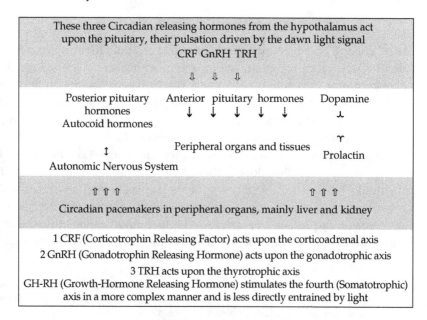

Figure 3: Principle neuroendocrine nodes of the terrain

On the left of Figure 3, the ANS and posterior pituitary hormones operate in the present, from minute to minute. The three hypothalamic-pituitary axes indicated at the foot of the figure operate in several different time scales at the same time but at different intensities. With all these pulses, the interplay between amplitudes and frequencies provides the terrain with its constant buzz.

Dr Christian Duraffourd numbered the H-P axes as in the figure above to reflect his notion of the *sequence* followed horizontally at the pituitary level by day, by season and annually. The fourth axis combines the activities of Growth Hormone with prolactin on most cells and tissues, and on the liver.

The bias in the oscillation between prolactin and dopamine provides a major indicator of temperament, behaviour and mental health. More on that story later.

Of course, the metabolic and digestive organs are the constant obligatory organisers and custodians of these nodes. They provide us with additional therapeutic opportunities. You could put it more strongly: the organs oblige us to pay attention to them when we attempt to modify the terrain and its pacemakers, taking stock of their diurnal, menstrual, seasonal, annual and septennial characteristics.[41]

Semi-autonomous systems or regions of the body

Our terrain embodies our medium and long-term potential because it is both stable yet modifiable to a certain extent both by experience and therapeutic intervention. As well as being a slow tropism acting in the background, the terrain registers the amount and kind of leeway available to us. This dynamic responds well to therapeutic nudging. Indeed, the most effective long-term use of herbs is indirect in that they allow the terrain to manage an illness rather than doing so directly.

But they can do both and, anyway, in a life-threatening emergency, an immediate response is needed, with a speed the terrain cannot match. In such extremes, the body does not await control signals from adaptive circuits of the blood but responds rapidly by reflex alerts from loss of fluid, hypoxia, and the attendant threats of blood loss. So much is obvious to first aid if not to common observation.

Also, not entirely distinct from the terrain, there are other quasi-independent domains which operate within hours or days. Their semi-autonomous reactivity may act against long-term interests, as may their under-performance. Leaving aside ionic and respiratory control of extracellular fluid pH and immediate responses to tissue injury, primary examples of these domains would include:

The haemopoetic system in bone marrow and in circulation	↔	Microbiomes of skin, colon, and other mucosal surfaces
↕		↕
The adaptive immune system	↔	Mast cells and other regulatory domains

Figure 4: Quasi-independent domains

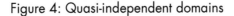

[41] The significance of septennial will be addressed in Section 1.6: Lifespan: Counting out and down the years.

These domains respond quite quickly but may misinterpret signals so that they under-produce (as in anaemia or low platelet count) or over-produce (as in polycythaemia), under-react as in immunodeficiency syndromes or overshoot as in auto-immunity. The pluripotent stem cells—analogous to meristematic tissue in flowering plants—retain some native pre-gastrulation capabilities. Platelets are messengers with several portfolios and are implicated in many chronic disorders, notably migraine. From the clinical perspective, these systems are modifiable by signals from the terrain which is not surprising as they and the terrain belonged together in the embryonic and foetal periods. Multiple sources generate these signals, chiefly as the microbiomes and limbic system responds to the world and to diet and other nurtures.

The genome of the new individual is unique and distinct. Its terrain—an emergent pattern of hormonal relationships imprinted at a very early stage—can be thought of as the "reader" of this new genome.

This terrain—this inner landscape—is itself, like any landscape, modified by patterns in the local environment. The developing individual in the late embryonic and early foetal stages has to negotiate uterine life, which must include the current experiences of the maternal terrain which is also responding to *her* environment. Not forgetting the influence of the grandmother who fashioned this egg that has been fertilised so very recently. This process constitutes a neuroendocrine imprinting and is estimated to take place between the sixth and thirteenth week of pregnancy. As our fingerprints are formed during the tenth week, it is a fair assumption that individuation occurs in this phase. Survival from the twelfth day until the sixth week and beyond depends upon the placenta.

The human placenta is unique in mammals and even in primates.[42] It could be interpreted as the organ that initiates and instals the innate immune system and does so by a delicate negotiation between maternal and foetal interests so that the foetus is able to receive adequate nutrient supply from the mother's blood and the mother does not interpret foetal signals as alien. The diplomacy between the two municipalities is far from trivial because the embryo and foetus contain both self and non-self genes.

So, we have an energetic system that communicates and, as with all animals, we have to move: towards nutrient and thermal comfort and away from predation and toxic threat. It is impossible to separate movement from perception so let us deal first with movement and take up perception again in Section 1.4.

---

[42] Cf. Ashley Moffett, professor of reproductive immunology at Cambridge University, Centre for Trophoblast Research whose work within The International Society for Stem Cell Research (ISSCR) has released new guidance in response to emerging areas of stem cell and embryo research. For a brief overview see her piece in *London Review of Books* 43:22, p. 20.

Movement

Without a physical body we could not think, indeed 'we' would not exist. Yet, with our physical brains we can think things that do not otherwise exist. There begins our great strength and also our vulnerability to mental overload and all the suffering that entails. We can elaborate worlds in a world that is already overwhelmingly elaborate. When we suffer we contrast the world as it is with the way it might be. As social animals, all our problems are connected with other people, with physical proximity or distant threat, unwanted absence or intrusive presence.

Moving and being moved

If arithmetic, algebra and calculus express the energetic relations of the material and informatic world, then physiology, geometry and mechanics define the movement of our bodies through space.

Physical movement is inherently less prone to ambiguity than is the cycling through psychosocial space.

Tensegrity, a term coined by Buckminster Fuller[43] to mean "tensional integrity" was originally applied to physical structures.[44] Some two decades before he did so, I stood as a child beneath the Skylon at the 1951 Festival of Britain. This iconic, metal structure seemed to float on its plinth on a site on the South Bank of the Thames still bearing the

---

[43] A brilliant engineering thinker, he did not unfortunately take the advice given to Nobel Prize-winning chemist Frances Arnold "don't talk about things you know nothing about". I stood with him in a small group after a performance of WB Yeats's Dance Plays at an Oxford college in 1971 where he was expected to pontificate and reluctantly obliged. He did not know what he was talking about.

[44] Often called 'floating compression' by those—such as sculptors, architects and bridge engineers—who use pre-stressed materials.

ravages of war. While marvelling at it, I somehow "got it" that this is exactly how a standing child looking up is *able* to stand and look up. This was two years before the 3D structure of DNA had been discovered in detail. This oscillating material demonstrated that molecular structures have to conform to space and time just as large objects must.

The term *bio-tensegrity*[45] is usually applied to palpable structures such as the human spine, which works something like a cantilever bridge with bone as the pre-stressed material. Bones get stronger when subjected to stress and tension. If this makes it sound more the territory of osteopaths and physiotherapists than that of herbalists, I would ask you to think again. Remind yourself of the cytoskeleton. In each of our cells (and in those of all creatures, including bacteria) this structure—composed as it is of protein filaments—conforms to the same principles of tension and compression as seen in the boughs of a forest tree. Enclosing the cell, other mixed polymers such as glycolipids maintain the integrity of the outer membrane, which is itself composed of phospholipids that are amphiphilic, that is: composed of both polar heads and non-polar tails. This arrangement allows them to self-form a phospholipid bilayer. Large compounds from plants can penetrate to bone as well as any other tissue; they likewise are held in solution as geometrical structures.

I have treated many cases of supposed "mechanical" strain in men with very physical jobs for whom physical treatments offer no relief.[46] When I started in herbal practice I thought it right and sensible to understand the limits of my chosen field, but I was wrong about musculoskeletal complaints (we do not treat individual joints but the whole system) as I was wrong about neurological complaints.[47]

At a very small scale, polymers may be read off as sequential series (of hexoses, lipids and amino-acids, for example) but the folding and unfolding of proteins happens not just in a sequence but in full three dimensions, directed by the forces of bio-tensegrity. Our cells and our organs have to maintain their shape and resist deformation if they are to function. What is muscular contraction by which we breathe and move, but a change in the cytoskeleton? We speak of structure and function as if they are separable but this is as artificial as separating matter and information: all the signalling proteins have a structure. Cytoplasmic streaming, so much more visible in plant cells, enables the migration of material through tissues and the removal of waste.

All of our days are enabled by folded enzymes and most disease is expressed or even created by a failure of proteins or nucleotides to fold properly.[48] Bio-tensegrity announces

---

[45] Coined by the surgeon Dr Stephen Levin but see also the work of Graham Scarr, an osteopath, chartered biologist and fellow of the Linnean Society (Scarr 2018). See Swanson RL (2013).

[46] I particularly remember the words of the wife of a furniture lorry driver when picking up his medicine for chronic back pain "it is the only thing that has ever done him any good".

[47] In this I was rightly remonstrated by the Austrian neurologist Dr Robert Egg when he came to England to study phytotherapy.

[48] Glycosylation of proteins into glycoproteins like the immunoglobulins has less to do with folding but more with affinity with antigens or to cell surface receptors in the case of the pituitary hormones follicle stimulating hormone (FSH), luteinising hormone (LH) and thyroid stimulating hormone (TSH). Yet affinity is a three-dimensional event. Mucins, yet another class of glycoproteins, contribute to many of the symptoms of tissue congestion that confront us in the clinic.

our arrival: the waving of the cilia of the ovum and the flagellae of the spermatozoon initiate life. Then the zygote could not divide without centrioles and microtubules. After nuclear division, a contractile ring cleaves the cytoplasm into the two daughter cells. Then the sphere of pluripotential cells known as the morula,[49] under mechanical tension, prepares for implantation and eventual gastrulation generating a wave of differentiation by sheets of dividing cells.[50]

I hope that I have said enough to dissuade the herbal apprentice from separating the body into physical and mental elements, from being too ready to separate structure from function, and from being too literal and territorial about the limits of phytotherapy. It is perfectly possible to do all this without falling into the opposite trap of self-aggrandisement.

Motion

Galen held that all sickness was a form of motion sickness or at least that stillness was wellness. Physics, on the other hand, would maintain the opposite: that when the universe lacks movement it arrives at a state of total entropy, or statelessness. These contrasting ideas are not really contradictory: any chemical reaction stops when it reaches equilibrium so we die when all our biochemistry finally reaches its end state. But we live in a steady state whereby we break down nutrients and evacuate our waste. Our whole-body experience, however, equates to more than chemistry on a reactive plane: it constitutes a summation of sensory and mental events. So, a sense of resolution, a balance between tension and compression gives us a pleasurable experience of stillness, so intense that pleasure is hardly the word.

Motion therefore is our motive force, our emotive drive. The universe of objects out there may not be conscious or capable of caring about us but if we cease to feel emotion we almost cease to be. That is our motor, with our cognitive skills at the helm. We can only steer a vessel that has motion: motility and emotion, to rather labour the point.

Balance and proprioception

Tensegrity applied to physical structures shows that though they appear to be at rest, their strength comes from their potential for movement—through tension and compression—against loading and in the face of external forces. Bio-tensegrity can be thought of as an extension of this principle to complex living systems. It is common for clinicians to focus on the internal organs contained within the cavities of the axial skeleton with scarce attention to the feet. I think this is an oversight and recommend herbalists evaluate them in every case because ankles provide the stabilising stance that is fundamental to posture

---

[49] Named from a resemblance to the fruit of mulberry, *Morus nigra*.

[50] Later on during embryogenesis microtubules develop within neurones. The Nobel-laureate mathematician Roger Penrose has proposed that their vibration functions at the root of human consciousness; see Penrose, Roger *The Emperor's New Mind—concerning computers, minds, and the laws of physics* Oxford 1989. I touch on the hypothesis in greater detail in *Human Health*.

and good movement. The answer may be recommend appropriate supportive foot-ware rather than medicine.[51]

As I have emphasised in the last segment, our strength comes from our capacity for movement at all scales but in order to move our whole body we have to know the starting position and that initial posture has to be stabilised for the impetus to move to result in an efficient (energy-saving) series of movements. Our power to move depends upon enough energy (*and* information) being available; this immediate energy depends upon an unimpeded flow from reserves.

Movements themselves depend also, of course, on a set of clear signals. But these do not of themselves originate the impulse to move. The real originator is the perception of the physical body in space, from our proprioceptive mind. Proprioception provides us with a sense of where all parts of us are situated in space. This is both central and peripheral all at the same time and space. If this mind is coherent and energised, balance will be stable, not displaced. Movement and posture result, then, from a coupling of central and peripheral states of being. They are integrated at various levels in the brain without having to consult the left cerebral hemisphere to analyse the position in space.

In common with all vertebrates, humans depend upon proprioception. In us certainly, proprioception links seamlessly to interoception—the sense of wellness in our viscera. Interoception centres itself on the enteric nervous system and gives us a holistic overview of our current state. Interoception (signalling by tissue hormones and neurotransmitters of the gut), sends us the primary signal of wellness or the contrasting alert to illness.[52] Linked to balance, this alert registers vague nausea and disquiet or the more definite motion sickness.

So, poise in the energetic sense results in physical poise. Stumbling may come from contradictory or ambiguous signals, or our stabilisers fail to receive enough energy in time. A clear signal needs adequate power just as smooth movements requires an uninterrupted flow of ions and energy into the neuromuscular endplates. The result is sensory-motor coupling.

The proprioceptive mind has something of the character of music: the rhythmicity and cadence necessary for walking. Like music, movement is necessary for balance.[53] This is the mind in all animals that lets them know where they are in space. It is physical thinking that does not need thinking about. It knows that rubbing a back against a tree will satisfy an itch. All creatures have knowledge of where and how and what they are. It comes from this deep relationship between the body and the world. This knowledge of position, extension and movement through space gives us our bearings, in common with all creatures. Analytical knowledge—information that is communicable—is abstracted from the sensorium; it comes to us as a secondary competence.

Balance is most sensitive to proprioceptive sensors in the ankles. Signals from these long tracts can easily be disrupted by injury, made worse by enforced rest. Delayed proprioceptive signals account for much of the uncertain movement of old age.

---

[51] See Mapping the body in Section 2.5a.

[52] For a very accessible account of Interoception see Damasio (2021).

[53] As Albert Einstein quipped "Life is like riding a bicycle. To keep your balance, you must keep moving."

Keeping eyes down on trip hazards actually make this worse so I recommend patients keep an eye also on the horizon: this helps with visual reassurance, rather as one does at sea. As falls become more common in old age and may lead to hospitalisation and therefore further deterioration and a greater risk of death, this is far from a trivial matter. Elders need the space and time not to be flustered so that their delayed energy–plus-information has time to stabilise their balance and movement. Speed becomes a trip hazard. The herbs they need are those that slow the fluster, stabilise the mental tremor, and will be those that strengthen peripheral circulation and reduce alpha-sympathetic autonomic drive while sustaining their beta-sympathetic response. Beta-blockers are nearly always contra-indicated in old age.[54]

Balance depends upon poise: energy, strength and flow. Energy comes from charge separation, the prototype of which may be seen in the photolysis of water within chloroplasts prior to photosynthesis and the fixation of carbon from air to bios.

Posture, position and personality

Human beings may have abstracted information from the world to create the Anthropocene Age but physicality remains the deepest kind of knowledge, inherent in life. It allows us to act before learning and is how the lioness knows how far she can safely tighten her jaw when picking up her cub by the scruff of its neck with her teeth.

There are different ways of being well and most of them require feeling comfortable in the skin. Comfort here consists of a state of adequate sensation without sharp peaks of intensity, without point loads, irritation or itch. Attuned, no doubt, with peaceful brain-waves, feeling well depends also on the sensation that the self fully occupies the physical body, with the sense of power in reserve to animate it, moving from a bed of repose and quiet breath to action. As the self fills the physical body, perception fills the external space with no sense of barrier. This needs more than barely adequate reserves of energy, this needs poise.

Theories about human personality tend to categorise traits that are behavioural and thus are assigned to the mental and psychosocial spheres as much as to physicality. This is understandable given that they aim in principle to be predictive about behaviour, but our personality is also an outcome. The flavour of a personality, like perfume, results from a composite of many different notes and strands, often contrasting. If our personality is mainly a result of following determinants: biological, hereditary, social (where we are brought up in and our role in family and community), our values and beliefs, our behaviour, emotions and inner thought patterns, then it may be more productive to *characterise* rather than *categorise* a person just as we speak of characters in fiction. In myth and literature, characterisation brings revelation, not chastisement.[55]

The full clinical experience is the perfect arena to enable this characterisation to be formulated for the first time for both patient and practitioner as will be discussed in Section 2.1.

---

[54] This is a simplification, of course, especially with congestive cardiac failure, but best to find ways to sustain rather than incapacitate further.

[55] Disposition as it may show up in our practice is enlarged in Section 1.9.

Clinical note

Assess patients' style from gaze, gait, posture, and degree of physical repose.
Assess their autonomic disposition from history and systemic review.
Assess their temperament from your analysis of their neuroendocrine terrain.

Comfort is a necessary concomitant of health. I describe comfort as an absence of point loads and is felt first in the skin and will be attuned with a sense of peace and calm. Life counts on quiet breathing: animation (in the usual sense) requires a discharge of energy from repose and reserve. To animate is to give life. To move our patients towards animated comfort is a precise and sufficient aim. When patients ask if the medicine will have any side-effects, I tell them it may make them calmer and more comfortable. And usually that is what they report.

Praxis

As the natural world is three-dimensional, it seems intuitive that threes must be structural (and complex life is impossible without the trio of air, water, earth). Although the number three is odd and the first prime, it is necessary to syntax and narrative sequence: beginning, middle, end. Physical and mental tasks necessarily involve doing one particular thing before another.

Clinical medicine can become more coherent when we think of the body in relational terms, when we review the physiological basis of our patient's problems from the interaction between the three germ layers.[56]

Tensegrity of geodesic domes rely for strength upon the rigidity of triangles. Molecular bio-tensegrity has been used to explain the formation of cytoskeletons and the helical structure of DNA, and to the spontaneous self-assembly of proteins, and even organs. The free and efficient movement between gel and sol states in the cell depends upon a degree of rigidity in the enclosing structure. This rigidity is energy-saving as it permits control and effective movement in the whole body. This is why hyper-laxity in ligaments presents so many diverse challenges to the patient and practitioner. Always examine the arches in your patients' feet and the range of movement within wrists and ankles. The tensile state of ligaments connects intimately with the motor cortex. If the signal is one of laxity, energy must be diverted to compensatory mechanisms which will show up in the disposition of the terrain. I hope that Figures 4, 5, 6 and 13 will help with the clinical orientation.

Praxis is the default and obligatory state that we have in common with all vertebrates: we know where we are and where things are and how to navigate amongst them. Human abstract thinking is an add-on that is minute in computational size compared with running a physical body. Physical capacity enables mental ease because the

---

[56] Clinical assessment may be helped by revising gastrulation in embryology!

proprioceptive mind cannot escape its rational knowledge. The critical factor is mobility. To quote Hans Moravec:

> Encoded in the large, highly evolved sensory and motor portions of the human brain is a billion years of experience about the nature of the world and how to survive in it.[57]

At least praxis is visible. Unlike cardiovascular disease or cancer, it is not silent at any stage—nor is running out of breath.

Dyspraxia

Comfort can take place only when flow from the well of reserve energy is unimpeded. Control of the physical self requires the same poise. Clumsiness (which patients often cite as a symptom of premenstrual dysphoric disorder) or other instances of dyspraxia indicate an inability to mobilise energy towards the task in hand. Such a state makes a person prone to accidents and even misfortunes in the sense of being unable to remove themselves from the wrong place at the wrong time. Dyspraxia in this wider sense undermines the ability to make good choices, to see and seize opportunities. Accident-proneness, especially in youth and childhood, is a sign of an attention diverted away from the proprioceptive mind. During your case history, if these elements predominate, it is your cue to find a way to sustain that patient's poise.

Walking and other modes of rhythmic movement, with a fuller expression in dance, are fundamental modes of improving kinaesthetic intelligence and self-healing: a kind of medicine that relies on the self.[58] Kinaesthetic resonance is the relational feel of our being. Whenever our situation changes, even minutely, there is some change in the felt quality of movement and a change in the overall muscular tone of the body. Although these ideas might seem to belong to the realm of physical body therapists, they can play a great part in our work in therapy and nurture to be discussed in Sections 2.1 and 2.2.

Look before you leap

Just as musicians understand that music cannot happen without silence, so dancers know best that movement cannot happen without stillness. In both, sound and movement are types of thinking. Analytic thinking is typified by thinking long and *hard* when faced with multiple choices. Tactical empathic thinking, by contrast, happens during a good clinical consultation: thinking long and *soft*.

Medicine attends to the practical needs of the people it serves, so the utilitarian rightly takes precedence over the philosophical. Yet a way of looking precedes a way of acting.

---

[57] *Mind Children*, 1988 Harvard University Press. The theme of Praxis is more fully developed in *Configuration of the Terrain within the Human Body* Barker (2020) 101–103. See also Minsky (1986).

[58] The great American dance teacher Margaret H'Doubler (1889–1982) pioneered movement and kinaesthetic awareness for health as did her student Anna Halprin (1920–2021) (who worked with terminally ill patients) and my own teacher who extended dance into the Alexander Technique: Winearls (1990).

In the Western tradition, the pre-Socratic philosophers were not analytic in the way that came to dominate the thought systems that succeeded them. Both slow day-dreaming and lightning swiftness can be adaptive ways of arriving at conclusions. By contrast, impatience when making important decisions, may lead to dyspraxia and loss of poise.[59] Decisions about the deep, important directions in life come best from soft thinking, whether fast or slow. Then comes the moment of surrender that makes for good out-comes: you do look and yet you do leap.

Impulsivity and its opposite—the tendency to be cautious, analytic, considered—are poles between which human life and physiology oscillate. These polarities are mediated by the very hormones that medicinal plants have the power to moderate in us and so are crucial to our understanding of their therapeutic potential. As we saw in the segment on motion earlier in this section, tension and compression are pre-requisites for the resolution that results in pleasure. In the reproductive sphere (on which evolution ultimately depends), orgasm and ovulation are the leaps which an age of dreaming do not reverse. They involve fast-acting neurohormones from the posterior pituitary like oxytocin that switch from negative to posi-tive feedback.[60] We will take another look at the constitutional domains of these polarities in Section 1.9 and consider the therapeutic possibilities in parts two and three.

Movement in plants

As movement is to animals, chemistry is to plants. You can be a herbalist without know-ing the finer details but knowing nothing would be like visiting a foreign country and not knowing their words for "thank you". Plant bodies may not change their original loca-tion but they do extend their territory gradually and also periodically by dispersion of their propagules. Movement within vascular tissues is unceasing as it is within their cells. The plant body lifts itself up in the air from seedling to mature height by elongating the internodes within its stems and even more so within its roots. By their movements and com-munications, plants unite the atmosphere, hydrosphere and their inherent medium, the soil.

The other movements that plants make are molecular: in a constant storm of synthesis and rearrangement, they metabolise chemicals just as we synthesise and rearrange neurotransmitters, hormones and proteins. They cannot do this on their own and need all the other domains of life to accomplish their growth, just as we do.

Plants, then, however they might seem on the surface to be 'other', are dependent upon us as we are on them. If the human infant does not grow and evolve with them, poor health is the likely outcome. The point I wish to emphasise is that the influence of culinary plants in the diet primes our senses of taste and smell. In this sense the divide between culinary and medicinal is false. The earlier this priming is introduced to the infant terrain, the better they will be set up: more for the great preventative potential of plants, their mitigation of infectious illness when it inevitably occurs. Good herbal inputs in the early years will set the stage for their medicinal activity when required later in life.[61]

---

[59] I am not attempting to reinterpret the distinction made by Daniel Kahneman in *Thinking Fast and Slow* (2011) but to draw attention to endocrine dispositions that have clinical importance.

[60] Cf. Section 3.6 Level Six.

[61] I developed these ideas in greater detail in *The Multi-Modal Hypothesis for the Actions of Medicinal Plants: Sensory Priming and Stochastic Resonance*: Barker (2020) Section 20.

Signalling and perception

The biology of perception is complex almost beyond description yet percepts form the basis of human interests. Percepts foster sociality so that if indeed we all hallucinate, we share in the hallucination. I will argue in this Section that qualities of percepts must involve quantities as much as modes of perception. Ambiguity in a visual field may come from low light levels in the field or a lack of focus in the eye, but ambiguity in other modalities can be a quality of affect, as in how one might respond to an aroma. Vision defines space, seeks fixity, but the other senses are conducted more in relation to time than space, like music. Ambiguity in the olfactory sense may contribute to the allure of a perfume or the memorious effect of a familiar smell, a familiarity which cannot be pinned down or it may seize one with the full accuracy and plenitude of its gestalt. Medicinal plants introduce qualities into the perceptual field. We would be impoverished without them. I shall pick up the subject again in Quantity and Quality at the end of Section 2.2.

From cell to person to culture via tiers of organisation

The following integrated arrangements form the biological relationships from which our being arises and generate the psycho-social constellation from which our individuality emerges:

1	Congregation of cells ➤	tissues
2	Congregation of specialised tissues ➤	organs
3	Congregation of organs ➤	organising systems
4	Congregation of organising systems ➤	individual bodily unit
5	Congregation of bodies ➤	family or societal unit
6	Congregation of societal units ➤	culture

Figure 5: From physiology to ecology to human culture

This stacking hierarchical table makes little sense unless it is appreciated that each stage is mediated by microbiomes and other ecosystems as in any landscape. Each of the nodes in each congregation sends out a material signal which is reciprocated by the return message, closing the loop. These organised loops tell us who we are and where we find ourselves. In humans, the questions of "what if we were other, where else might we be" lead to the philosophical question four-year olds ask, the pinnacle of perceptions: Why?

Qualia

Consciousness is said to be the "hard problem" by philosophers and some scientists.[62] Qualia—the ineffable quality of experience—holds out against demonstration by the scientific or any other method unless you count poetry as a method.[63] Biologists might counter that the question "what is it like to be" displays an exclusionary anthropomorphism in that only humans so far as we know ask that question.

An alternative response could postulate that as all communication requires redundancy of information, all complex systems generate a surplus or they could not communicate and if they could not communicate they could not be complex.[64] The argument is as circular as an informatic loop itself. Bacteria communicate by quorum sensing and lateral gene transfer but such direct communication would be too slow, unwieldy, and error-prone in multicellular organisms with their partitioned cell nuclei. Proteins stand in for signals that can transfer larger amounts of information more precisely. The larger the system the more nodes will it contain, the more nodes the greater the opportunities for signals to interact and form a perceptual complex. A perceptual complex with a surplus cannot help but recognise itself and its perceptual borders, or it could not operate, so resulting in a kind of condominium.

---

[62] Others, like Marvin Minsky and perhaps Steven Pinker, claim it is a question of computational competence and cellular diversity. For further discussion and references see *Moravec's Paradox* in Barker (2020) 102–3.

[63] The question is notably explored by Thomas Nagel in *"What is it like to be a bat?"* (The Philosophical Review 1974).

[64] See Shannon in next segment.

This surplus, so the argument goes, generates an emergent or higher order property that cannot operate unless it becomes aware, the awareness generating a quality commensurate with the *quantity* of interactions.[65] If this explanation is acceptable, *Qualia* becomes an index of connectedness dependent upon numbers. Only a bat could answer its own question if it could pose it in the first place but why would it bother to answer a question posed by humans?

The question of how our perceptual sphere reacts with the world is of great practical concern:

Energy as information

Energy and matter are interconverted in the ratio that Einstein famously demonstrated.[66] The physicist Giovanni Vignale perhaps goes further in maintaining that the universe is composed of information not matter or rather that all matter itself *is* information.[67] As I am not a physicist, I am in no position even to agree with him but there is a remarkable symmetry between the following paired theorems:

| The second law of thermodynamics | Entropy is inevitable in physical systems |
| Shannon's Theory of Information | Redundancy is inevitable in informational systems |

This goes to the heart of physic because although we treat tissues and systems, not individual cells, energy distribution is bottom-up and all signalling is cellular: tissues and systems may collect and organise signals but they do not initiate them. I hope to show in part three that the way we use medicinal plants as adaptogens influences signalling. Over a course of treatment with repeated prescriptions (and the use of culinary herbs over a lifetime), these signalling pathways can be enhanced and incorporated.

Matter in biological systems organises itself into informational circuits. These are the *micro-events of life*, referred to as S–O–R circuits in the Résumé at the end of Part One. They are subject to many of the constraints faced by any thermodynamic system. The interconversions between energy, matter and information stand behind all iterative operations. We see them in clinic when they become turbulent and manifest as illness. Metabolic systems work effectively only when there is inbuilt redundancy.[68]

Perhaps Giovanni Vignale will permit me to modify his assertion and suggest that living beings constitute information that interacts with matter. They do this by always pairing information into a template and catalyst. So, for example, signalling molecules interact with protein signal receptors that sit on repetitive membranes. Strands of nucleic

---

[65] See Quantity and Quality at the end of Section 2.2.

[66] For a succinct, comprehensive, highly readable account of the relationship between information, energy and matter see von Baeyer (2003).

[67] Vignale, Giovanni *The Beautiful Invisible—creativity, imagination and theoretical physics* Oxford UP 2011.

[68] As we observe from our computers: the size of a file has to be larger than its data because extra capacity is needed to store it and to interact with the storage device and external media.

acids such as RNA and DNA act as templates for signal receptors or for their complementary strands. All made from precursors from the environment: carbon dioxide, nitrogen, water. All mediated by phosphorus, sulphur, monoatomic ions (especially sodium and potassium—the gatekeepers to communication), and a few trace elements.[69]

Interpretation: complex molecules as informatic systems

If in the psychosocial realm "there are no facts, only interpretations", as Nietzsche would have it, in our biological lives, misinterpretation can be fatal. Hermeneutics is the philosophy of interpretation and proceeds as if humans with their language are the only beings who think that what they think matters. It matters in medicine, of course, where it is difficult to imagine medical practice without some kind of divination and, as interpretive beings, we should treat information as our currency. The deepest level, far below language, must be the movement of enzymes and substrate with their emission and reception of signals. At this level, the complex molecules synthesised by plants, enter our systems and organise signals, with those of taste and smell closest to our desires.

The visual field, more than any other sense, deserves to be seen as a shared hallucination even though it is the sense (as in seeing sense) most associated with objectivity. Yet it is highly sensitive to local conditions, quickly altered by changes in blood sugar, pH, and temperature, how well we slept and current mood. Vision gives us data about depth of field and from which we can abstract the relational. As such, it holds strong biological importance (and also cultural sway in visually dominant literate cultures). The other senses can be experienced (even enhanced) in the dark and contribute to what Marshall McLuhan called Acoustic Space, the integrating function of the right hemisphere. This is where complex substances from plants may provoke a complex response.

Interpretation happens at different speeds in different people. Processing speed relates in part to available energy but also the dominant qualitative dominance of the senses says much about the perceptual style of a person: visual predominance compared with the acoustic and tactile. As practitioners, we do best to attune our interpretive style with the sensorium of the patient.[70] "I see what you mean. I hear what you say. I don't like the smell of that. It leaves a bad taste." Give William Blake, who combined etching and drawing with poetry and what today would pass as communication theory, the last word: "If Perceptive Organs vary, Objects of Perceptions seem to vary:/If Perceptive Organs close, their Objects seem to close also."[71]

Percepts as information rely upon our internal electronics and complex biochemistry but these are inherited from the realms of life that preceded us, notably plants and fungi. The informatic codes that constitute our structure and function are sequential (as in

---

[69] Buffering of tissue pH depends upon bicarbonate, chloride, hydroxyl and other ions.

[70] Marshal McLuhan defined this field of cybernetics for a generation. Criticised for conflating messages with channels, nonetheless, he predicted the connectivity of electronic media some thirty years before the internet came to dominate our lives. He, along with scholars like Northrop Frye, Peter Fisher and Harold Bloom, detected cybernetic understanding in Blake ahead of his era. See also McGilchrist (2019).

[71] *Jerusalem* Plate 34 lines 55–56 1804 from *The Complete Writings of William Blake* Nonesuch Press Ed Keynes 1957, p. 661.

DNA, RNA and proteins). Yet, as percepts, our minds appear to convert such digital information into a summative analogue configuration. Digital is precise and repeatable but has to be read, word after word. Analogue is capable of more ambiguity and variance, but can be seen holistically, not sequentially, all in one go.

The calculus of poise

The informatic output of a system is obliged to be larger than the system itself. Shannon's Theory of Information[72] tells us that the inbuilt redundancy of a system cannot exceed certain limits which is another way of saying that if we interconverted information and energy, reserve beyond a certain level is a hindrance and below it, the system ceases to operate effectively, if at all. The ratio between the system and its reserve is not a fixed amount but will return after excursions, converging to a characteristic ratio and so can vary within the expression of its means. To take a well-known example that occurs widely in plant forms, the output of the fractions expressed by numbers in the Fibonacci series starts widely enough, at 0.5 but never larger, and converges rapidly to the Golden Mean. Actually, random numbers will also converge, but less rapidly. This extra speed conserves our precious energy.

This energetic ratio, necessarily conserved for life to continue, is founded upon an immense architecture of interdependent compounds and structures that permit the extraction of energy in the first place. Nutrient supply depends upon an array of compounds that are essential over time. Of them all, the one that behaves analogously to poise in that it needs always to be available and requires a larger reserve is the calcium ion.

Reality, rules, tact, and subtlety

Perception combines physics with biology and then generates the inner and outer psychosocial worlds. As babies we experiment and learn that all objects obey the invariant law of gravity. We notice also that this invariance does not apply to other interactions, notably those between people. People react when baby falls over but the stack of bricks seem mute in the face of being thwacked by the experimenter's tiny hand.

The bricks have primary qualities of shape, colour and texture but do not seem to have agency beyond responding to forces whereas the faces of those who feed us in infancy do, and so do we in gaining their attention. The baby as scientist observes invariances in the world—gravity, friction, mechanical behaviour of objects—but can only learn from observation when provided with emotional security and warmth.

Touch, smell, taste, the texture of material in the mouth starts with feeding and the sense of feeling comfort in a place. After milk, plants will inevitably be primary materials to be introduced into this realm and the child's response will become a secondary

---

[72] Shannon's Theory of Communication was first published as a paper in 1949; soon republished in book form, it has since been much reprinted. See bibliography. One of the most important developments in Information Theory, it is congruent with the cyclical loops of endocrine systems. Berlo's Model of Communication (1960) stripped this down for use in behavioural topdown business management but is of doubtful use in medicine as it downplays biofeedback and fails to distinguish variance in human personality and belief.

quality: one that is registered and processed inside its own limbic system. I would argue from first principles that the greater the richness and complexity of such plant materials, the wider the individual's acceptance and tolerance base (or munity) will become. Plants form a primary experience, the sooner integrated in life the better. Of course, smell, taste and texture cannot be separated from the emotional warmth of the environment in which early nurture takes place. Sensory richness runs in parallel with a good enough home without overt or covert danger signals to foster the cognitive, physical, social, and emotional well-being of children.

Touch communicates its meaning, almost like a primary quality but acquiring language introduces the child into a realm of ambiguity. What did he *really* mean?

Language and sociality introduce us to rules and to interpretation. We move from the world of primary percepts—invariant gravity and material physicality—where the rules are never contradicted, where proprioception rules universally, into our own self-constructing world of secondary characteristics that form our personal mind view. Yet the process of learning leads us forever to compare and contrast interpretations, seeking the just solution, often with a conflictual sense. Such is social life. We may choose strict adherence to some rules in some situations and rather looser interpretation when it suits us. There is no ambiguity in a command: "Though shalt not kill" but rules are there to be interpreted holistically, taking into account the detailed context. What does a white lie entail? Surely it is a question of tact, sparing someone an uncomfortable truth.

Languages universally embody the important existential and intimate facts of life. Latin scholars had to learn the four principal parts of irregular verbs. Two are critical to interpretation, to give and to touch: *do, dare, dedi, datum; tango, tangere, tegi, tactum.* Datum: what is donated, given; tactum: the touched. To define tact would be tactless in the extreme. Touch is not ambiguous because, though rules may surround it, it can only be its complete self.

Medical diagnosis claims to deal only in primary percepts and concepts, often at variance with our world view or at least refusing to incorporate it in the medical encounter. Personalised medicine does not condescend to ideas that the practitioner considers unhelpful nor patronise the patient as if an infant but seeks to find common purpose for the benefit of the patient, not the sense of being right, assured of the correct diagnosis. Touch is an important component of medical interactions which aim to reach the truth with kindness, tact and subtlety.

Subtlety allows the echo of words to resonate with meanings in their range of synonymy, just as a musical note vibrates with its enharmonic. The upper and lower aromatic notes of basil, for example, are perceived qualities, not definitions. We are primed for subtlety and perceiving relations.

Sensory priming

Perceptual signals rely upon channel strength and in turn depends upon a *quantity* of energy and information from which emerges a *quality* of perception. Compare standing in a desert or up a rocky mountain with standing in a moist forest beside a running stream. Both have qualities, but one is quantitatively (and therefore qualitatively) denuded, which may possess its own beauty.

So far in this Section I have compressed ideas from several sources, notably Gestalt Psychology (not to be confused with Gestalt Psychotherapy), which itself has been criticised as *merely* descriptive, not explanatory.[73] Successful life depends upon pattern recognition: the continuum of processes that permit humans to perceive the world and communicate with one another unifies cognitive and emotional indexes of health.[74]

But I cannot attribute to anyone else the following ideas of sensory priming, which I hope the aspiring and the seasoned herbalist will consider worthy of attention.

Newborns explore the world with all their senses, the tongue exploring in tandem with the receptive sampling of the olfactory bulb, visual recognition playing a confirmatory and discriminatory role. Olfactory and gustatory sampling of our environment establishes qualitative distinctions. The primary search operated by taste and smell is for feeding and hydration and connectedness. They formulate an archive that constitutes our successful belonging, the basis of emotional health.[75]

At weaning, when maternal resources are to be supplemented, the taste buds are further engaged, favouring sweetness and smooth texture to enable growth. The sweetness usually come from plants, perhaps augmented occasionally by honey. Bit by bit, the introduction of other plant material will recruit the other taste buds, so beginning the lifelong pilgrimage into the life governed by sensory priming. The terrain—imprinted in the womb—will incorporate this exploratory investigation of the plant world, to be archived in the structures and neural connections of the limbic system. Plant foods have been selected and modified by cultivation over centuries and millennia. Originally more bitter and sour than we now are used to, plants create our culture.

By experimentation in the natural environment, some plants would have such profound physiological effects by ingestion of even small quantities. These effects, known to everyone, would derive from molecules entering the blood stream in quantities that are now measurable. These form the basis of drug plants and are integral both to medicine as analgesics and also to human culture (via the autonomic nervous system) as mood modifiers. The resultant changes in mood and energy provide the basis for shared experience that tends to become socially endorsed (or reviled) and ritualised. Opium and coffee, marijuana and tea, to say nothing of fermented beverages. Many of these social pleasures are associated with the recognition of taste and aroma as a shared experience. This sensory priming is uncontroversial to the extent that the plant is culturally accredited.

Industrialised societies have segregated plants that were formerly used as medicines from the drug plants (much modified) that have been retained and the rest discarded.

Herbalists reclaim the value of these plants as medicines. I will discuss in Part Three that they may act pharmacologically along a spectrum as drug plants, simples and as adaptogens. Their effect upon our health will, I maintain, be more profound and

---

[73] 'Merely' is rich. As if scientific explanation (with its inherently provisional nature) is the only approach to discussing phenomena. I have found Mitchell Ash's *Gestalt Psychology in German Culture, 1890–1967 Holism and the Quest for Objectivity* Cambridge UP (1999) to be the most reasonable and interesting account of the subject.

[74] Valuable insights are offered in Gibson (1979 & 1986).

[75] Readers wanting less sketchy information might like to reach for Varela, Thompson, & Rosch (2017).

long-lasting if they come via the path of sensory priming. Depending upon the plant and the dosage taken, they may then amplify and extend the effect by stochastic resonance (See Impurities in Part Three).

Stochastic resonance

Pharmaceutical science is an example of a field that searches resolutely for perfect signals in the form of perfect molecules, uncontaminated by the stochastic effects of organic molecules and the oligo-complexes typically found in medicinal plants. A multitude of organic molecules from industry and agriculture are toxic in concentration but when extremely diluted are found to be potent endocrine disruptors.[76] As good a reason as any to advise patients never to wrap food in clingfilm and always to rinse detergent thoroughly after washing dishes.

The approach taken by herbal medicine, in contradistinction to the purification process demanded by the pharmaceutical trend, seeks to adopt the "noisy" signature from whole plant extracts or plant material to strengthen what is actually quite a weak signal from a dilute complex mixture, from a single plant even before it is mixed with others. The dilution is made by the water in the plant and that which is added in the preparation, and then further diluted by the several litres of body fluids when ingested. Our medicines are strengthened in their relative weakness by their very noisiness. These are already high levels of dilution but we may even be able to appreciate these noisy signals diluted by an order of parts per 10^{-6} or even 10^{-8}. Going any higher than these dilutions would seem to overextend the theory and stretch credulity.

Resonance is the transmission of a force or oscillation from one system to another. Simplest to appreciate in music, it can also be demonstrated in a mechanical system when an object is struck and makes a noise. Vibration is movement within a material. The orbital motions of the earth, sun and moon (and to some extent other bodies in the solar system) create resonance. Randomness of events is stabilised for living creatures by the periodic punctuations in time provided by the movements of these three bodies. But, of course, the routine of our days is variously interrupted by unexpected events, the weather and a host of unpredicted tasks. The contribution made by our entrainment of circadian and other periods to health will be discussed in the section that follows.

The discovery of random motion in suspended materials was discovered by the botanist Robert Brown as he worked upon pollen. The word *stochastic* originally meant to make estimates towards a target,[77] a kind of guessing through a sea of random variables, and first found use in mid-seventeenth century mathematics. Life flows stochastically from moment to moment but every movement is strictly dependent upon only the previous movement, with a finite number of possibilities for the next, although predispositions may narrow the scope of probabilities.

---

[76] Dr Jean–Claude Lapraz devotes a Section to the phenomenon in La Medicine Personalisée 2012. Translated into English 2020. See also, for example: *The occurrence of pharmaceuticals, personal care products, endocrine disruptors and illicit drugs in surface water in South Wales, UK* Kasprzyk-Hordernab et al. 2008 Water Research Elsevier 42, 13.

[77] στόχος = 'target' in Greek.

In modern times, the term stochastic resonance resurfaced in climate studies in the early 1980s, but the mathematical work was applied in electronic engineering, especially in acoustics. The goal of sound recording had been to find and preserve the perfect signal and to exclude the disruptive influence of noise. But "high fidelity" turned out to be a misconception: there are no perfect signals in nature and in many circumstances, the addition of a certain amount of noise actually strengthened the signal. The effect is known as the noise-to-signal ratio, a measure that may be critical to complex dynamic systems. In the 1990s, stochastic resonance was applied to other fields, all of which depended upon the modern formalisation of probability theory, made by Alexei Kolmogorov in the 1930s. Computational Biology in common with other dynamical systems requires these mathematical analyses; contemporary genomic analysis depends upon algorithms generated by them.

The idea can be expressed relatively simply: life is a sequence of events: where you are now is more or less likely depending upon what happened to you immediately before. The range of possibilities is huge but not infinite: it depends upon some probability found within a certain range.[78] The set of probabilities that relates to you is constant within bounds: outcomes for each individual depends probabilistically upon previous outcomes. In other words, the apparent randomness is constrained. Entropy in the physical world is hidden in living beings, but only during a lifetime. Yet entropy operates silently throughout our lives and generates the dynamic search for energy that constitutes our survival and, with enough of it, our health.

---

[78] I think this is what 'ballpark estimate' is meant to convey.

Rhythms: tuning in—adjusting our inside to the world

One day/night span provides living beings with a basic beat, the unit of our time on earth. Such notes in succession orchestrate feeding, growth and reproduction. They make riffs and patterns in the human mind, turning these cumulative quantities into qualities. Time, at least in this sense, is not linear but tracks an elliptical order of months and years, mirroring the orbits of sun and moon. Each annual ellipse stacks upon its predecessor, drawing the stack up and along into a spiral. Between the day and the year, the months will wax and wane. Transition from one season to another will alter thresholds of response, creating turbulence, confusing signalling, creating uncertainties.

Every person that comes to your clinic is constructed thus. They will present an animated physical structure but also one set in time. Disjunction in their rhythms will have contributed to some lack in their sense of wellness. Assessment of their interior adjustments will lead you to founding a treatment that takes account of the particular stresses and strains. Just as their years will be composed of months and days, so the treatment will need to assess their patterned responses at different scales of time. The following table suggests how you might match signs and symptoms with different physical sub-systems.[79] Although inevitably over-schematic, it has the practical value that medicinal plants will influence these areas of human response in ways that are generally predictable. Theoretically, this schema could be more finely grained, more inclusive, more detailed, but it would lose sight of the primary aim of focussing on prescribing and dispensing medicinal plants. All schemas lead to further questions—they can be no more than a provisional beginning. The student will want to follow up leads to the fascinating

---

[79] I make a distinction between autocoid hormones (such as histamine), that are generated by the posterior hypothalamus and extend throughout the brain and have important responders in peripheral tissues, and the many diverse autacoids that are produced and metabolised locally with paracrine activity. These terms continue to develop in medical physiology and nomenclature is far from settled.

details in more comprehensive textbooks of endocrine physiology and develop more interesting ideas than these.

Rhythm	Evaluate
Daily	Autonomic tendencies
Entrainment [discussed in The Major Nodes of the Terrain in Section 1.2, and in Figure 3]	Autocoids: biogenic hormones and amines
Menstrual	Anterior pituitary hormones
Tidal	The precession of hormones within the anterior pituitary
Seasonal	Alterations of relations between the four pituitary axes, between catabolic and anabolic drives
Annual	Stage in life
Septennial [heptades are discussed fully in following section 1.5b]	Transitions in life

Life, of course, is never so straightforward: although we are patterned our survival depends upon us disrupting our own responses to take account of circumstances as they face us. Besides, none of these sub-systems are really autonomous: it is the relations between them that manifest in our responses and behaviours. So, in the table below, although they may be separated for the purposes of discussion (and formulating a prescription), we cannot influence one drive without exerting some change in another.

These are preliminary remarks about complex interactions which will be expanded in Part Two and, with therapeutics in mind, in Section 3.6. But it is worth mentioning here that anti-diuretic hormone (ADH) from the posterior pituitary stimulates rhythmic secretions of CRF from the hypothalamus, as well as its more obvious connection with renal function. This makes sense if you consider that restraining diuresis would facilitate undisturbed sleep until the circadian pacemaker signals the start of a new endocrine day at 4 am.

Arrhythmic adaptive response	
Responsiveness	Hypothalamic drives
Impulsivity	Biogenic amines
Reactivity	Post-pituitary hormones
Capacity for rapid adaptation	Adrenal medulla\Vascular Autocoids

These responses tend to amplify tensions in underlying patterns. The cumulative effect of our capacity to adapt by matching our actions and internal patterns to the outside world will show up in our ailments.

Biological structures and functions are materials that generate cyclical waves in response to astronomical cycles and the physical cycles they generate on earth.

These depend primarily upon the rotation of our planet, its tilt towards the plane and its orbit, producing circadian, seasonal, and circannual cycles. The moon perturbs these with its own cycles and produces circatidal resonance on earth. As discussed in Section 1.4, physiology derives from these interactions between physics and living organisms.

This means that every biochemical reaction will resonate to some cycle.[80] Most of these are incalculable in detail but we can at least make some overall assessments from symptoms. Fatigue if you accept the poise hypothesis, but headache, vestibular disorders, insomnia, digestive upset (see Fragmentation in Section 2.5c) and general malaise will call for nurtures (Section 2.2) before herbal treatment.

We cycle and recycle many thousands of compounds many of which (for example folate and adenosine) coordinate immunity, nutrition and sleep with external cycles. Cycling conserves energy and reduces randomness. Metabolism is an integrated assemblage of cycles, the fundamental ones being catabolising nutrient to compounds that store then release energy to do our work, our life which in turn is cyclical. These constitute the "state cycle" of our days. Whatever consciousness may be (see Qualia in Section 1.4), it is the dominant cycle of our waking lives and even infiltrates our sleep in dreaming.

We behave cyclically in response to internal and external signals, some of which are vital and some we consider volitional.[81] All behaviours depend ultimately upon the cycle of cell division for which folic acid and adenosine are necessary, if not entirely sufficient.

Some of the more important meta-cycles tabulated below are those we can modulate or even modify with medicinal plants. Separated by type and time magnitude, they are:

- Respiratory cycle of inspiration and expiration, cardiac cycles and cardiac variance.
- Cyclical movements within the peripheral autonomic nervous system, and its central generators.
- Circadian cycles of blood temperature and glucose, often driving energy and mood. They provide useful guides to timing of medication; only in acute illness should one disregard them and resort to as banal an instruction as "take three times a day"; in most chronic conditions go for a bipolar approach—morning and evening—with two different but complementary prescriptions as detailed in Section 3.8.
- The five phases of the sleep cycle, alternating between NREM and REM into a roughly ninety-minute episode, which must be repeated more or less unbroken three times a night at the very least but preferably double that for sustained good health. REM is shorthand for the type of sleep characterised by rapid eye movements, N for non-REM.
- Metabolic cycles of catabolism and anabolism are primarily circadian but echo with the seasons
- Feed\fast cycles; digestive cycles, especially bile which circulates from liver and back again in the enterohepatic circulation, matching the tides, detailed towards the end of Section 2.5b

---

[80] Inevitably, then, the symptoms of your patient will follow a cyclical path. One function of herbal medicine that they will notice is that the peaks and troughs of their symptom-provoking cycles will be smoother and less extreme.

[81] Whether or not these are truly "free", they will be subject to some constraints. Without constraints we would dissipate energy.

- Endocrine cycles: self-organising signalling systems of the form signalling-organisation or optimisation-response (S-O-R)
- Lunar and lunisolar cycles which feature strongly in our reproductive lives but also the metabolism that generates them

In common with other species, transitions between phases and cycles are associated with physiological risk and stress. As the alpha-sympathetic is a transition between para and beta sympathetic, too long in this zone will reduce capacitance.

Early developmental cycles generate new structures and functions as they progress. Later cycles consolidate. Progression can be a phase of learning and change or one of entrenching the past. A bit of both may be inevitable.

Cyclothymia, in spite of the name, is a condition of mood change where entrainment by external cycles is weak and so the psyche tends to float free on the winds of chance rather than cycling with fixed cues like dawn light. Because they lack heavy ballast, their thoughts may float free but results in poor buffering as we will discuss in Section 1.8. Cyclothymic persons are buffeted by contingent events and respond physiologically to changes in the weather. As this painful sensitivity may correlate with a creative sensibility it might be unfair to ask patients who are visual artists whether they would swap their condition for a symptom-free life, but it may help to gently point out that seeing more is feeling more, and that may hurt.

A moral sense is as prone to symptom as an aesthetic one.[82] All mental and emotional life generates its own cycles. Because doubt is inherent in faith, in terms of cycling, psychopathy is an extreme opposite to cyclothymia where the ballast of self-belief is heavy and if they cycle ideas at all, doubt is a way-station rarely visited.

Cycles, whether stable or variable in amplitude, are usually measured by their frequency. In human life we mark and name frequencies as days, months and years. We remember (and, most importantly, count) these durations as episodic events while the cycles continue to repeat. Our physiology is most aware of the daily resetting but the tides flow beneath them. Seasonal resets that occur at least twice each year can come as a jolt and especially disturb the H-P axes and set off autocoid hormones. These step-changes are linked primarily to regional day length rather than local weather. Daily rhythms are the focus of Section 1.5c while annual and septennial periods of lifespan, with their clinical importance, are considered in Section 1.6. How past and future devolve onto the present feature in Section 1.9.

All creatures are subject to circadian cycles and all mammals are entrained by at least one of the other astronomical rhythms: tidal, lunar, seasonal, circannual. In humans, both the pulse generator for sleep and the impulse to drink and feed are generated in the hypothalamus.[83]

---

[82] Wittgenstein claimed that: "Aesthetics and Ethics are one and the same." Ruskin and William Morris would have probably concurred.

[83] Poets may make much of it, but there is great variability in human response to the lunar cycle. I would guess from reading and (unscientific) observation that maritime cultures are more tidal, landlocked ones more lunar. In these, there would be only two fortnights per lunar month that would drift slowly through the solar year, as was the case with the hunting calendar of the Oglala Sioux, an icon of which stands on one side of the shield of the National Institute of Medical Herbalists in Britain.

But as our bodies can contain as much as 67% water and the oceans exceed earth's landmass, and the thermal density of water is high, a short digression into the how the mass flow of water may cycle within our bodies may be in order, especially for its implications for our present physicality and our ancestral past.

Tidal flow: vertical and horizontal

Light is the signal that drives the nycthemeral (day/night) rhythm and may also play a part in the lunar cycle on account of the sunlight reflected by the moon.[84] All manner of nocturnal interruptions are possible (and modern electric life is full of them), but they are not usually patterned. While the luminosity of both daylight and moonlight depends upon variable weather, the rate of change of daylength is slow compared to that in the lunar cycle. This might seem obvious given that we are comparing cycles of 29.7 with 365.2 days, but the physiological effects are not always noticeable at the time.[85] Also there is a ten minute difference between the solar day and the lunar day which flows on, drifting through the days and nights instead of being periodically reset.

Tides are driven by the pull on water from the three bodies of sun, moon and earth. The strength of a tide reflects the height and vertical motion of a body of water drawn up then released by gravitational forces. Tides interact with the horizontal movement of streams and currents.

As tides rise and fall in response to moon and sun throughout this twenty-three hour fifty minute cycle, so bile (the confluence of water and oil in the gallbladder) circulates six times a day and may resonate between high, slack and low water in earth's tidal rhythms.[86] The cephalic phase of the digestive cycle (in the hypothalamus) has the *potential* for being optimised by the circadian reset but can be pulled off-course by all manner of contingent factors, from grief and penury to constraints on resources, from internal deficiencies to the demands and needs of others. With our erect bipedal posture, feeding is usually vertical; while digestive organs feed in horizontally from left and right. The tube itself can accommodate to either posture.

There are two deeper vertical and horizontal features of time and tide that organise our biological and social lives. The hypothalamic pulses drive our organs vertically through the agency of the pituitary gland, which has half a dozen messengers to regulate circadian timing with the periphery. As they do so, these hormones generate a tide within the gland. This horizontal ripple circulates along the day and night thereby regulating themselves and integrating their vertical drives along with return in formation about how the world is behaving and how the body is coping. Figure 3 presented an

---

[84] The range of variation in luminosity is between 0.1 lux at full moon & 0.001 lux at new moon. Daylight, by contrast typically provides >10,000 lux.

[85] Women with premenstrual dysphoria say of themselves that it is not until their menstrual flow that they appreciate the phase that preceded it.

[86] Fishing and boating are organised between two high and two low tides. These four periods of 6.2 hours are further divided into modules of 3.1 hours that centre on the slack tide. Sleep and the entero-hepatic circulation are similarly modularised as discussed in Bile, Gut motility, Mood and Sleep in Section 2.5b.

overview of these vertical and horizontal tides (where the abbreviations are expanded); greater detail to this scheme is given in Figure 6 below:

Hypothalamic pulse	CRF	GnRH		TRH	GH-RH	Dopamine
Pituitary response	MSH ACTH	FSH	LH	TSH	Growth Hormone	Prolactin
Primary organ responders	Adrenal glands	Gonads		T4/T3	Long bones	Most tissues, especially skin and breast
Peripheral products & responses	Steroids as at ▼ below	Oestrogens	Progestogens	All tissues	Most tissues	Central and peripheral effects

Figure 6: Hypothalamic vertical pulses and pituitary horizontal tides
(after Duraffourd & Lapraz)

▼ 1 Glucocorticoids 2 mineralocorticoids 3 DHEA & other sex hormones
This vertical and horizontal orchestration was Dr Christian Duraffourd's key insight into the neuroendocrine management of human life, along with his understanding of how medicinal plants can and do influence it along with autonomic regulation as we shall survey in Section 3.6.[87]

* * *

Harmony is vertical because the component pitches register at different heights at the same moment. Rhythm is horizontal in that it marks repeated moments. Mostly we perceive time as a flow, even if we retrospectively revolve this horizontal stream in our minds into cycles of months and years. Our own lives may seem sequential but separate generations stack up vertically above us as we grow. Their influence upon us does not fade as they move gradually into the past. Brought about by the differentiation of somatic tissue from germ cells (mitosis then meiosis, as in flowering plants), parents and parental figures anchor us in the human family and the older generations root us vertically in deep time. Siblings and cousins figure in our horizontal web, which collects, if we are lucky, teachers and friends.

These vertical and horizontal relationships—with all their gifts and challenges—orbit around the spindle of our lives. They are the outward projection of the terrain and need to be surveyed and experienced by patient and practitioner as outlined in Section 2.4a.

That the vertical human is also bilateral may be obvious but is not trivial. Patients very often remark how all their problems are on the left or the right. Whether or not they notice, we must. Doctor Duraffourd considered manifestations on the right to be

---

[87] By contrast, orthodox medicine concerns itself with a binary view of solely the vertical so that, e.g., adrenal, ovarian and thyroid disease or diabetes or pituitary adenomas are either diagnosed or excluded. Diseases are treated as singular states without reference to transverse relations.

constitutional and those on the left to reflect our adaptive response. This followed from his conception that FSH is the great initiator of metabolism in the foetus while LH completes the cycle. Breast tissue shows this most clearly with receptors for FSH (and ACTH) more expressed in the right and LH (and TSH) more on the left. Prolactin up-regulates all receptors including its own. It builds the areola in conjunction with oestrogen, FSH and oxytocin.

Laterality affects the unpaired organs more obviously but probably also the paired because the symmetry is approximate and the lungs are not even that.[88] The left-sided adaptive effect can usually be seen in legs and feet. If strong palpation below the knees medially elicits pain, the side is diagnostic as in Figure 7.

	Right		Left	
	Cerebral hemisphere	Brain	Cerebral hemisphere	See McGilchrist (2019, 2021)
		Thymus		
	Lung	Heart	Lung	
FSH & ACTH receptors predominate	Breast		Breast	LH & TSH receptors predominate
	Splanchnic circulation crucial for marginating platelets, spleen for storing them			
	Liver	Pancreas	Spleen	
	Colon		Colon	
Basal	Testicle & ovary		Testicle & ovary	Reactive
Pain signals biliary congestion	Knee		Knee	Pain signals pelvic congestion
	Ankle and foot structure		Ankle and foot structure	Usually more everted, nails more fungal

The work of the neurophysiologist and psychiatrist McGilchrist (Bibliography) refers to laterality of the hemispheres

Figure 7: Anatomical bi-lateral associated with asymmetric physiology

---

[88] See Kidney in Section 2.5c.

Flexible adherence to natural cycles is good both for sleep and digestion. A very long or very short circadian cycle (range 19–28 hours) makes a strong case for encouraging entrainment by front loading the day's intake of food ("breakfast like a king, dine like a pauper") with protein, fat, and complex carbohydrate thereby taking advantage of the morning's high thyroid yield.[89]

Timing is said to be the secret of comedy and so it is with herbal medicine and all the plant humanities.

At the larger scale of months, the seasonal trimester can be viewed as an important indicator of how best to strategise the use of medicinal plants. If you prescribe according to the phase within the season as well as within the day you will provide the most appropriate treatments, as discussed later.[90] Always, then, locate your patient's request in the following scheme where metabolic change is initiated, expressed and culminates, leading to the next transition:

Initiating	February	May	August	November
Expressing	March	June	September	December
Culminating	April	July	October	January

Figure 8: The tripos of seasonal metabolic progression

This works for north and south hemispheres but would need rethinking in the tropics where three seasons predominate.

---

[89] See nurtures in 2.2 and gut motility in 2.5b.

[90] In Section 3.6 Therapeutics: Herbal Treatment Strategies by Levels

Cycles, rhythms and seasons

Health from a biological point of view may be defined as the fitness of an individual to match challenges from the environment. Some of these challenges will be random, or appear to be so, and therefore unpredictable. Our fitness to manage random fluctuations in our environments seems to be enhanced if we are able to conserve stable strategies for meeting fluctuations that *are* predictable. The tricky manoeuvre is to make our adaptive behaviour flexible enough to deal with alteration yet regular enough to resist responding to every mild perturbation. In other words, our health requires that we are adequately sensitive to external events while at the same time capable of ignoring some signals. For survival, we need both reasonable concern and healthy indifference; the trick is to learn when to invoke one and not the other. Health requires us to develop a buffer zone that is robust without rigidity.

An important attribute of the healthy response, then, is the ability to discriminate between isolated chance events and predictable change. One cannot judge whether an event is part of a pattern unless one has an internal pattern book against which it can be matched. Only then can the secondary assessment be made about whether the event is a risk or an opportunity.

Fluctuations in the physical world outside challenge the stability of our internal environment, putting pressure on homeostasis. These environmental fluctuations are predictable insofar as they are rhythmic. The most important observable and predictable rhythms in nature derive from the movements of the three bodies: earth, sun and moon:

1. Earth's spin produces a single dian period divided into the binary cycle of night and day
2. Emergence from one phase of the cycle into its opposite, produces transition zones: the narrow crepuscular phases of dusk and dawn
3. Earth's tilt produces the binary cycling of winter and summer, especially marked in high latitudes

4. Emergence from each phase of this longer cycle also produces transition zones: the seasons of autumn and spring
5. The movement of tides influence most creatures, especially those who feed in the transition zones between land and sea. Generated by the moon, their influence on humans seems ambiguous and has yet to be fully explored.
6. The annual cycle derived from earth's orbit is a cumulative measure of ageing and success in feeding and reproduction.

These fluctuations would give us clues about the availability of food during the pre-technological ages in which we evolved. They determine the behaviour of most creatures, humans not excepted. Aperiodicity is potentially dangerous because it is unknown; periodicity can be accommodated because known. Such knowledge may lead hunter to prey and alert hunted to the presence of predators. These ancient patterns still live within us.

To take account of such rhythms after the event serves no adaptive purpose. For organisms to use the information, they must be able reliably to predict it and to be alert before its onset. For such an operational device, there must exist some internal analogue of external periodic events. While the existence of such a timing mechanism was postulated in ancient times, it was not located until late in the twentieth century and its functions validated experimentally. This central timer consists of paired structures in the forebrain, each containing about 8000 nerve cells, known as the supra-chiasmatic nuclei (SCN). These clumps of nuclei lie close to other well-known regulatory centres, which are known to determine rhythmic vital functions such as respiration, heartbeat and temperature control, as well as the less determinate periodic needs of feeding and excretion. The SCN is not the only body-clock: rather it seems an indispensable regulator of all the other pacemakers and oscillators that are distributed throughout the body, with the liver taking primacy. Internal processes have to regulate themselves while responding to external variance. The diurnal light-dark cycle regulates the activities of organs.[91]

To be adaptive, all oscillators need to perceive and respond to rhythmicity in the external world, and to learn from the outcomes. To respond effectively, the clock itself must be able to adjust its rhythm to changes in the environment. These changes must be periodic: it would be of no value responding to yesterday's weather (especially in the British Isles). The six cycles listed above do not vary a great deal within a human lifetime while many other cycles are too variable to measure. Even temperature is secondary to light and daylength as useful predictor. It needs to be read in conjunction with the primary external cues, night and day: the regular alternation between light and dark, known as the photophase and scotophase.

Variability

Variability is a signal characteristic of living organisms, and variance—the range of characters which any individual may exhibit and the bounds within which any individual may inhabit—provides an important measure for biologists. In this respect, living beings resemble the weather, which is forever changing but within certain bounds: winds of 400mph have never been recorded on this planet, though they are a constant manifestation on the surface of Jupiter. Weather derives in turn from climate which shows a much slower

---

[91] Summa KC, Turek FW (2015) The clocks within us *Sci Am* **312**: 50–55.

variability, thus climatic change is generally more predictable than the weather. Climatic change is likely to alter the bounds of variance of weather in a particular place over a timescale usually measured in decades and often longer than a human lifespan. Climate derives in the main from the obliquity of the earth's axis about its orbital path around the sun, but is also profoundly influenced by latitude and other geographical effects, especially proximity to thermal reservoirs. Earth's spin and orbital velocity have changed and will continue to do so but with predictable and astronomically slow periods. There are cycles on the surface of the sun which seem to affect weather but other solar cycles and those within the earth's magnetic core probably influence climate, but these have long periods which we are not yet able to predict. Other changes in the crust and mantle produce both slow and fast effects like tectonic drift, which cannot affect human lifetimes, and earthquakes and volcanism, which do very often in all our lifetimes. Solar irradiance decreases with latitude simply because of the spherical curve of the earth but while high latitudes receive less irradiance, their seasonal climates derive more from the tilt of the earth's axis. While this angle of obliquity varies a little, the period of this variation is 41,000 years. Together with the equinoxes which precess every 22,000 years, these variations, whatever their effects on climate, must place negligible strains upon human adaptability, to say nothing of the fluctuation in the eccentricity of earth's orbit, which clocks in at 96,000 years. None of these fluctuations could be detectable by direct human perception.[92]

Weather and climate provide us with expected bounds of variance against which we may plan our lives. The measure of predictability is itself variable, depending upon where we live. By accommodating variability we reduce the adaptive strain upon ourselves, that is: if we adapt we remain healthy, if not, we become ill. Accommodation involves both anticipatory behaviour and internal mechanisms which constantly sample the outside world and calibrate responses, and our responsiveness. Most of our adaptive mechanisms reduce our responsiveness to predicted change and increase our responsiveness to unexpected change. In Britain, cyclonic low pressure weather tends to dominate over more stable anti-cyclonic systems. It has been shown that some individuals are very susceptible to the alternation between these two periods of weather, and that it is the relative speed and the amplitude of the oscillation at the boundaries of the two phases that causes their transient illness, manifesting as headache, nausea, visual and balance disturbances, irritability and other disorders of mood.

Health as a state of a stable median in the face of variability is a biological and ecological idea to which herbal medicine has much to offer.

Life as information

We do not know what the day will bring but we know that it will be a day. This is the primary unit of adaptive life about which all change must be calibrated. Night and day orchestrate our movement through life but—with this two-step rhythm at our backs—the search for food and mates has also to sample environments: to differentiate between helpful directions and those full of uncertainty, even opposition. This tasting the air is performed at different scales by all creatures.

---

[92] Temperature fluctuations can flip in decades as we are all now too aware but global warming can only emphasise these other trends.

The life of tiny single-celled animals such as amoebae, which are capable of movement, is dominated by the chemical environment in which they find themselves. They move away from impoverished, toxic or hostile places and move towards those that are rich in nutrients. This ability to move along chemical gradients provides the necessary precursor to multicellular life. I have hypothesised that this bias—to which I give the term 'mindedness' persists in all living beings and is a fundamental driver and integrator of the rhythms of human life.[93]

Not only in animals: inside the apparently static plant body, all is movement and flux using chemistry and physics just as amoebae do, even seeming in extreme environments to defy physics. While most bacteria are *relatively* passive to the environments they exploit, they share with all strains of life the ability, by means of chemical codes, to learn and replicate, and so evolve. As for green plants and fungi, the bodies do not themselves move but colonise environments by growth and dispersal in and above the soil.

Periodic

Biological systems are sequential, phasic and periodic and therefore numerical. Unless it were so, embryological development and all the later staging would not be possible. The chromosomes and DNA strands themselves oscillate under the impulse of ultraviolet light—one of the most important external signals—so that sequences, phases, and periods register time in our lives. Time is an oscillation and an approximation at that—life has pacemakers and, unlike clocks, does not work on exactitude, more like music. Even percepts like smell oscillate so that an inherent ambiguity characterises our limbic identity.

Menstruation gives its colloquial name to periods but of course all life is periodic. The defining period for all life is the light/dark cycle of approximately twenty-four hours. Unlike most things in life, this is entirely predictable.

As for the week, in spite of concerted effort, no convincing evidence for a natural seven-day natural cycle has emerged, its only contender being roughly the length of one of the moon's phases, but this is more of a visual presentation. It also divides the average menstrual cycle into quarters but that rather implies greater equivalence between its phases than is really the case. However, the circa-tidal rhythm of about half a circa-lunar day of 12.4 hours (itself derived largely from the Circa-lunar cycle, ranging between 27.2 and 29.5 days) means that high and low tides precess around the 24 hours getting earlier or later each day. If we were solely tidal, breakfast would get later each day! Tidal creatures like crabs respond primarily to low tide when they feed but even this rhythm may be influenced by the photoperiod.

Unlike these rhythms, we can (and do) reset the daily (circadian) period like a timer.[94] The circadian pacemaker entrains everybody to do this at 4 a.m. (after housekeeping by the liver at 3 a.m.) so that, before dawn, the day gets off on as firm a footing as possible.[95]

---

[93] I developed this and four other interlocking ideas in Barker (2020) pp. 22–42.

[94] The body "clock" is more like a stopwatch.

[95] It is the invariance of the rhythm not only in people but in all forms of life. A comprehensive textbook for the subject is Refinetti, Roberto *Circadian Physiology* Boca Raton CRC Press 2006.

This reset sets off hypothalamic pulses to the adrenal axis which has been dormant since 10 pm the previous evening. Once initiated, the adrenal hormones permit the activity of the other axes and generates cycles of endocrine peaks and troughs, metabolic highs and lows resulting in fluctuations of body temperature, blood sugar and other measurable phenomena. All organs—not just the obvious example of the heart—oscillate in tune with internal signalling circuits and resonate in complex harmonics.

This resetting of endogenous rhythms to external cues is known in circadian physiology as *entrainment*. More of a departure point than a homeostatic fixed point, it calls upon all players to initiate the day.

> *The clinical relevance of all this for us as diurnal creatures is critical: the daily excursions through the phases of the autonomic nervous system largely define our behaviour and response to the world.*
>
> Crepuscular creatures who live in transition zones of dusk and dawn are hyper-vigilant because there is just enough light for predators to find them; they are particularly anxious because their feeding time is the shortest of all.
>
> This degree of excitation is found in people who are caught in the alpha-sympathetic, the transition zone between para-sympathetic and beta-sympathetic.
>
> The H-P axes and the pineal gland direct the alternation between catabolism and anabolism.
>
> These metabolic periods cycle within the circadian period mediating between activity, rest, feeding and sleep.
>
> *The influence of medicinal plants on all these cycles is at the core of our practice.*

At the larger scale of a lifetime, seasons, years and larger periods pattern our memories and personal experience. Though some of us are more "calendric" than others, these patterns are crucial to horticulture and infuse literature and the arts. As a science, chronobiology and circadian physiology did not emerge fully into mainstream consciousness until the millennium and even now is more of a speciality than is warranted.[96]

Circadian physiology played no part in my training so, when I started out in clinical practice, I had no preconception of its importance. In my first three years, however, clear patterns emerged: people whose problems seemed resolved in April, would return in the same month the following year with a "different" presentation but, beneath the surface, one could detect a manifestation of the same complaint. Beyond hay-fever and Seasonal Affective Disorder, I found seasonal and annual patterns in most cases. The longer I practised, the more I discerned periodicities within a patient's lifespan and was able to see the correlations with plant life. This led me to the midpoint hypothesis,[97] which happily correlates with the observations of Drs Duraffourd and Lapraz.[98] In the simplest terms, it points out that in early February, the internal central heating goes *off* when we may be experiencing snow and ice, while in early August it goes back *on* during weather that may be the hottest in the year, a paradox to which we now turn attention.

---

[96] For a historical treatment see Refinetti (2006) 3–19.

[97] Barker (2011).

[98] Duraffourd & Lapraz (2002) pp. 710–719.

The photic year

Meteorologists determine the start of each season by the average local weather rather than other climatic considerations. So, in a conventional calendar, the first day of March is heralded, at least in Britain, as the first day of spring even though the vernal equinox is only three weeks away; likewise, June the first is taken to be the beginning of summer even though it too is only three weeks before the solstice that marks the actual *middle* of summer from the point of view of the sun's height. In making August part of summer rather than autumn, meteorologists are more in tune with our usual weather and culture, but they make no sense from an astronomical, solar, point of view.

By contrast, a calendar built upon day-lengths exhibits the solar structure of the year. These photic cues (rather than temperature alone) trigger the seasonal hormonal shifts that affect all living creatures and on which human health depends. Critical changes in day-length go some way to explaining why February and August have always shown peaks in hospital admissions for certain conditions. The ganglion cells in our retinae are photovoltaic cells and reset thermostats in our metabolism on a seasonal basis.

The solstices and the equinoxes represent the sun's apparent movement: being over-head at each of the two tropics at 23.5 degrees of latitude in June and December, then turning back, crossing the zero degree of the equator in March and September when days and nights are equal. These four—solar limits and crossing points—identify the true *middle* of each of the four seasons. We should calculate their *starting point* midway between them. True: the weather will always lag behind, because it takes time for the atmosphere to heat up and oceans to cool down.

If we take the four seasons to be roughly equivalent in length, it follows that the start of each season is not that of the weather-forecaster but is to be found at the midpoint intervals that lie equidistant between these four solar events. These four transitional midpoints—on the sixth of each of February, May, August, November—show the true start of each of the four seasons and are highlighted in the calendar in Figure 9. Start days might be hot or cold and more like the season that immediately preceded it, but plants and migrating birds have to look ahead and plan for breeding and feeding. They use increasing or decreasing day-length to do so.[99] Homologies exist between their hormonal systems and ours, so, even if we reach for overcoats, scarves and gloves or sun-hats, swimsuits and sunscreen before we venture out into the local season, our metabolism is not so persuaded by today's weather alone.[100]

Throughout the year, the actual lengths of complete day/night cycles are not equal because of the eccentricity of earth's orbit. Calendars try to squeeze these unequal day-lengths into equal-sized boxes. We create these human devices for our own purposes: to accommodate the fact that measurements of the tropical and sidereal year do not match exactly and nei-ther one constitutes a whole number of days. They are our best approximations and why we have leap years to prevent our numbered years drifting apart from astronomical reality,

---

[99] See Foster & Kreitzman (2009).

[100] I have elaborated these physiological ideas in a paper written for the Order of Bards, Ovates & Druids and delivered as their 12th Mount Haemus Lecture in 2012.

as happened historically between the Old Roman, the Julian and the Gregorian calendars, forcing the British Parliament to shave off eleven calendar days in 1752.

With all necessary caution in any search for temporal exactitude, I present my calendric ideas as an approximate guide to our physiological seasons as the sun ascends from Capricorn across the equator to Cancer and back down again. The calendar best fits people in latitudes of between 34 and 60 degrees. The seasons of course are reversed in the southern hemisphere.

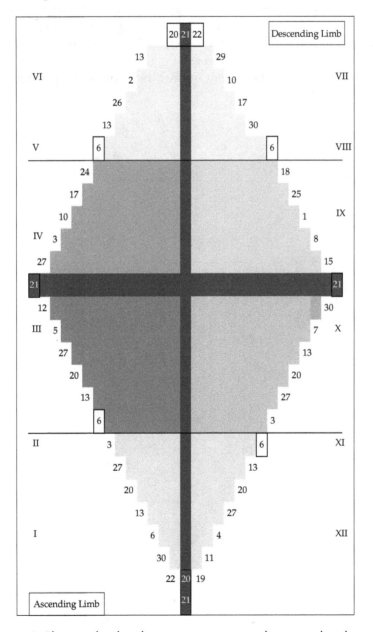

Figure 9: Photic calendar showing equinoxes, solstices and midpoints
Days are shown in Arabic numerals, months in roman.

A year is not made up of a whole number of days so cannot fit neatly into any plan. As the seven pitch intervals do not fit exactly into an octave, keyboard musicians have to use the fudge of equal temperament. Figure 9 represents my attempt to fit the circannual cycle into a plan that is circular but not circa!

Much clinical physiology relates to time more in the universal sense of birth, reproduction and death than to the calendar. One of the great privileges of practising for more than forty years has been to help three generations with herbal medicine. A middle-aged woman with arthritis decides to bring her daughter, first with a difficult menarche before helping her overcome difficulty with conceiving, then treating *her* young daughter (without forgetting the ailing grandmother) and now helping with hot flushes, having seen her from menarche to menopause.

Plotting the biography of the patient against the periods of their biological lifespan comes in the next Section.

Lifespan: counting out and down the years

M usic is said to be our way of counting without knowing that we are counting. Most information is sequential, encoding the time interval. In biology, nucleotides and proteins depend upon sequence, as does the cell cycle when replicating these informatics for passing them on to the progeny. In an important sense, then, systems count out their lives without perhaps being "conscious" that they are counting.

Cell division is a self-counting system, the period of which may be generated from within or without and varies between tissues.[101] The collection of ideas in this section are meant to contribute towards a rough and simple heuristic about human development to help concentrate attention on the patient's life in a clinical setting.[102] I propose that metabolic markers in the lifespan can be grouped conveniently in periods of seven years.

When clerking a new patient, we note their age and date of birth but biology suggests that this information is more than a convenient index: age contains a cumulative metabolic total. The metabolic age of an individual may be greater or lesser than the chronological number of days. The length of the cell cycle and its stages, rates of division and DNA methylation, of apoptosis and cellular damage all proceed with the push of genes and the pull of environmental stressors. The timing is not exact but similar within a range as you invariably find in complex systems. The range is not so variable that we cannot discern the evolution of an individual and put a name on each stage and expect it to occur according to a plan of sequences within a certain duration. That is the basis of developmental biology, which takes over from embryology once the baby is born.

---

[101] See Yamagishi, MEB & Shimabukuro, AI Nucleotide Frequencies in Human Genome and Fibonacci Numbers Bulletin of Mathematical Biology **70**, 3: 2007; Perez, Jean Claude Codon populations in single-stranded whole human genome DNA are fractal and fine-tuned by the Golden Ratio 1.618 Interdisciplinary Sciences: Computational Life Sciences **2**, 3: 2010.

[102] I have developed these ideas in greater detail in Barker (2020) Section 13: Patterns of Life.

Critical stages are essential to human development and there are thresholds of time and space that have to be passed for good outcomes: normality is nothing more than a statistical range. It does mean that some outliers must be anticipated. Studies in human development are fundamental to embryology and neonatal development. Early cognitive and social development preoccupies paediatrics, and necessarily informs educational theory. Once development is complete, scientific interest switches to reproduction and ageing. Medicine is left with the job of finding empirical solutions to the problems of adult patients. These derive in large part, as saints and psychologists have argued, from their earlier development.

As circadian physiology tells us, perception of the oscillation in luminosity exerts control over all metabolic and endocrine systems. Melatonin crosses the placenta and enters the foetal circulation thereby allowing the maternal melatonin rhythm to inform the foetus about day length and circadian rhythm and so synchronise its physiology. With this template, the newborn will come to note a pattern of variation in ambient light at some point. Depending surely upon season and latitude and hemisphere of birth and the home environment, my guess (from limited observation) is that entrainment can begin as little as six weeks after birth though such evidence that there is suggests that the process is not fully installed until at least a full year has passed.[103] Growing perception of this rhythmic alternation between day and night will permit the vast cellular proliferation in the developing brain and body eventually to become entrained so that it makes sense to speak of developmental days, weeks and months. While the names we give to timespans may be arbitrary, the periods themselves are biological events.

Eventually, the infant—passing many "milestones"—graduates to being identified by its years, at the age of four being capable of distinguishing portions of a year.[104] By the age of seven (eighty-four months) the year as a measure has become consolidated, both socially and biologically. During the following seven years, the endocrine software for puberty is being run and materialises at highly variable times either during this heptade or delayed until the next. At age twenty-one, epiphyseal plates are closed to growth hormone in most people, marking the culmination of somatic growth. Further metabolic development is mostly marked by neuroendocrine change: for instance, the decline in progesterone at age forty-two and of oestrogen at forty-nine years.[105] This would suggest that staging persists long after our primary development as infants.

You will notice the number seven and its multiples making their appearance so that it seems more realistic to measure lifespan in heptades rather than the culturally usual decades, as in: thirty-somethings, three score-and-ten, itself a factor of seven, and so on. Jaques' speech in *As You Like It* on the seven ages of Man makes mention of qualitative

[103] *Programming of the fetal suprachiasmic nucleus and subsequent adult rhythmicity* Trends in Endocrinology and Metabolism Kennaway D University of Adelaide 2002 DOI: 10.1016 S1043-2760(02)00692-6.

[104] My next door neighbour announces herself not as four but four and three-quarters, putting me in mind of my baby sister introducing herself to the world with identical delight, seventy-five years ago!

[105] Gynaecologists recognise that women lose progesterone quite abruptly as they embark on their sixth heptade and it is not controversial to expect the abrupt loss of oestrogen at their seventh.

not quantitative stages.[106] Well, dividing larger numbers into bite-sized chunks is normal in both biography and biology. Cultural and political life is mostly marked by some term or another: whether annual, biennial, presidential, parliamentary. These periods are probably not as arbitrary as they might appear.

In childhood, a portion of a year seems an interminable wait. Even in late adolescence, prospects of two or three years may seem to all intents and purposes eternal. From a clinical perspective, marking the phases of metabolic and endocrine life in heptades correlates better than decades with life events. There is statistical evidence from epidemiology that *about* every seven years (circa again) the alacrity of our immune response reduces by about 11% per annum.[107]

Lifespans in comparative developmental biology are staged in numbers so by focussing on heptades I am only seeking to correlate qualitative clinical phases with age.

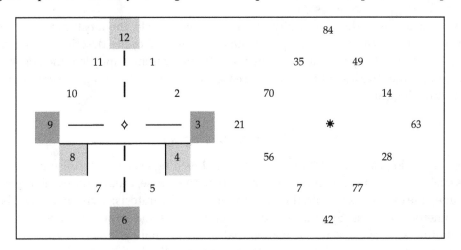

Figure 10: Multiples of seven fill the clock face once only without gaps

Ancient cartographers and astronomers employed a sexagesimal rather than a decimal system because of its greater number of factors.[108] On the left of the figure of a standard clock-face in the figure above, if you count around the clock from the top position, the numbers two, three, four (all multiples of twelve) cannot fill all twelve positions on the clock face: they leave gaps. Five can, but takes you only to 60, and would anyone measure a life in half-decades? Eleven also can cycle and fill but that would take you to the improbable old age of 132 and is anyway longer than a decade. It is the cells and tissues that count and unlikely for them to be decimal, having neither fingers nor toes! Counting out the years by the numbers on the clock, one by one, multiples of seven fill the clock face once only without gaps, like leaves filling a stem. (It works for the first

---

[106] Act 2, scene 7 in Complete Works, Clarendon Press, Oxford 1988, p. 638.

[107] Reported by the Biostatistician Professor David Spiegelhalter during the Covid–19 pandemic on 23 April 2020 Radio 4 at 21:00.

[108] Factors express what you can do and how you can do it. Primes have none but themselves.

seven years measured in months.)[109] If cells are self-counting, they must do so in the most economical manner, energetically, geometrically and arithmetically.

By analogy with angiosperm anatomy, leaf insertion on the stem (phyllotaxy) is not arbitrary; in the commonest arrangement, the angle between successive buds divides the axis of the stem according to the golden mean as the stem interval (plastochrone or internode) elevates the leaves towards the sun.[110] A logarithmic spiral between leaf apices fulfils optimal space-packing around the initiating tissue, known as the meristem. This placing of leaves creates vertical columns arrayed to reduce shading and optimises solar energy. So do we proceed in our lives from one plastochrone (metabolic interval) to another. As in space, so in time.

As a simile this does not work at all: we are mobile and do not photosynthesise. But as a deep analogy it does combine the universal obligatory relations between structure, time and energy in living systems.

When it comes to the plausibility of the seven-year cycle, the most important prefix to bear in mind is *circa*: roughly, approximately. Biological cycles describe an oscillation about a mean.[111] The cycles—initiated by intrauterine priming—may lengthen or shorten according to the stresses of life, and by disease, giving rise to tissue age shorter or longer than chronological age.

Prime number ages

There are biological examples of animals using breeding cycles that utilise prime numbers such as 13 and 17 to avoid predation.[112] In our own case, though tissues may contain innumerable quantities of cells, they were all initiated by mitosis; division into two being a symmetrical process. Symmetry reduces randomness and so reduces energetic load. In counting systems (given that we internalise the annual cycle and beyond a certain age count our summers, winters or birthdays) we can divide our ordinals to see how far we have come but prime numbers break this symmetry, having no antecedents. Symmetrical information is compressible (and computable) and so saves energy. Numerical ages that are prime present us therefore with challenges and opportunities for change, so my prime number age hypothesis goes. Each such age finds us losing and seeking a handhold and so we are more likely to get ill if we fail to find new ones. After the age of

---

[109] No surprise, really as even a round clock fits into a square matrix of 7x7 columns.

[110] As an instructive exercise, try drawing the spiral from leaf tips of *Plantago major*; I trust your lawn has some. For a detailed and beautiful account of the beauty of phyllotactic variety, I recommend *Strasburger's Text-book of Botany* (English translation Coombe & Bell 1976) 123–128 or the smaller *Plant Form* by Adrian Bell (OUP 1991) which "can be treated as an illustrated dictionary." Slicing through the middle of a spear of red chicory shows you space filling with beautiful clarity.

[111] Aside from being one less than the octave, another internal property of seven that may correlate cycles with energy conservation is that its reciprocal generates a cyclic number, with a repeating period of one less than the seven digits (viz., 142857...). Multiplication by all digits up to seven cycle the same sequence. The harmonics of these make it as good a candidate as any other for human developmental periods to converge.

[112] For a more detailed discussion, see *the primes of life* in Barker (2020) Section 13.

seven, we summate the steps of our genetic spiral in years. Prime numbers are just cracks in our pavement over which we have to pause and step.

Clinical audit in my own practice finds a good correlation and tends to support this idea. I wish I could succeed in persuading educators in herbal medicine to extend an audit to other practitioners on this and many other actualities. At critical phases such as the forties (slipping into decade mode), there are three primes, so this phase should show up more patients seeking appointments.

For all this arithmetic, the important clinical need will always be to relate the patient's stage in life at first visit to their previous biological and psychosocial stages, with particular emphasis on their prenatal development as inferred from parental and grandparental influences. The overview of the lifespan in the following segment highlights critical elements of each septennial phase.

The septennial lifespan

In the womb, the limbs including the toes are defined by day fifty-six of the foetal period, and fingerprints are present by week ten. The registration and initialising of our identity, and therefore our unique terrain (invisible to ultrasound) establishes itself between the sixth and thirteenth week.

As an important note to the following table, I would emphasise that the greatest disturbance of the terrain occurs at or close to the transition between heptades as well as the prime number ages within them.

Heptade	The nodes about which the tides of life swirl	Primes
First 0–7	As the three domains (Figure 12) develop in concert the opportunity for sensory priming (Section 1.4) is at its greatest. The four H-P axes are in a constant complex relationship with each other to build the CNS and musculoskeletal system. From age four, thyroid axis dominates to provide the energy to finish the formation of the child.	5,7
Second 7–14	At age seven in girls (nine in boys) the phase moves to adrenal dominance to run the software for puberty and to prepare the ground for steroid receptors in the respective organs. The coordination between them and growing limbs requires a full staging of the H-P axis, both horizontally—within the pituitary gland itself—and in the vertical axes between the pituitary and peripheral glands, namely: adrenal, gonads, thyroid, and the cells and tissues of the soma. From age eleven, medicinal plants particularly help with prolactin-dopamine axis, especially in males. At age thirteen, scope for irresolution high so a good call for plants.	11,13

(Continued)

(Continued)

Heptade	The nodes about which the tides of life swirl	Primes
Third 14–21	Both before and after adrenarche and menarche in both sexes, the two anabolic arms of metabolism—the gonadotrophic and somatotrophic axes—compete in the growing individual, the former providing the architecture in the form of bone and muscle, the latter the size of cells and tissue. If a female reaches her adult height at puberty and does grow taller after this transition, gonadic congestion will not be offset by lengthening of bones and so tend to characterise the follicular phase of menstruation as congestive (and may make for a difficult menopause when it arrives). By contrast, if there is a pronounced post-pubertal growth spurt, it will tend to influence the luteal phase of menstruation, but not necessarily adversely. In both sexes, psychosocial transitions may be especially difficult. In males, transition from late puberty is helped by growth of long bones unless it exceeds an adequate dietary intake. In both sexes, tension between drives, desires and responsibilities (sought or imposed) will manifest as autonomic dispositions or display contrasts in differential expression of dopamine and prolactin: sources of many syndromes and symptoms, migraine being a notable example. As central circuits become formed and receptors recruited, experimentation with alcohol, amphetamines, and cannabinoids especially harmful in long term. If psychotic episodes seem threatened or are precipitated, clinical opportunities should be taken to prevent them from spilling into the following few years. Strong drive at nineteen provides an opportunity for resolution, sometimes missed.	17,19
Fourth 21–28	Unless channelled, conflictual conditions are likely, especially in the prime year period of irresolution; calls for strong and compassionate mentoring as much as medication. If drives remain unresolved or unchannelled, alternating conditions of mood or bowel habit likely.	23
Fifth 28–35	Drives likely to mature as physical peaks are approached. Problems likely to be situated in thyroid and gonadic axes. In this and the following heptade, couples experiencing difficulty with conceiving are likely to seek the assistance of a medical herbalist.	29,31

(Continued)

(Continued)

Heptade	The nodes about which the tides of life swirl	Primes
Sixth 35–42	Problems continue to be situated in thyroid and gonadic axes. From 38–42, according to Dr Lapraz, some women experience a "dress rehearsal" of the menopause, a mini-phase, which may last as long as eighteen months.	37,41
Seventh 42–49	Loss of progesterone makes this phase potentially critical to wellbeing *throughout* this heptade and into the next: luteopause and andropause. As forty-eight is the median age for stroke, be alert to asymptomatic atrial fibrillation.	43,47
Eighth 49–56	Menopause and Andropause in both sexes. Be alert from at least this phase but preferably the previous one, of asymptomatic atrial fibrillation. If this and the previous phase has been managed well with herbal medicine, a phase of strong recovery and good decisions can be expected.	53
Ninth 56–63	Vitamin D storage deteriorates during this phase; don't supplement without a concurrent good supply of vitamin A obtained from the diet. Remain vigilant to silent atrial fibrillation and its entrenchment. Be alert to possibility of local tumour growth in head on legs as much as breast and womb.	59,61
Tenth 63–70	If it is not already fully in train, anabolic resistance leads to more rapid loss of muscle bulk with corresponding pain, especially in hands and small joints. The end of this phase marks double the putative physical peak and perhaps the median of life expectancy. Whether humankind will regress to the mean after the recent extension in longevity remains for some of us to see.	67
Eleventh 70–77	Collaboration with others in the care of your patient in this phase may be particularly important.	71,73
Twelfth heptade 77–84	Doubling of the sixth heptade: critical for the reproductive axis, that is the maintenance of tissues. At age 86, life expectancy actually increases slightly.	79,83

Though linked with the past, the current ideation of self is also isolated and not entirely commensurable with its past self-images. One of the burdens of consciousness.

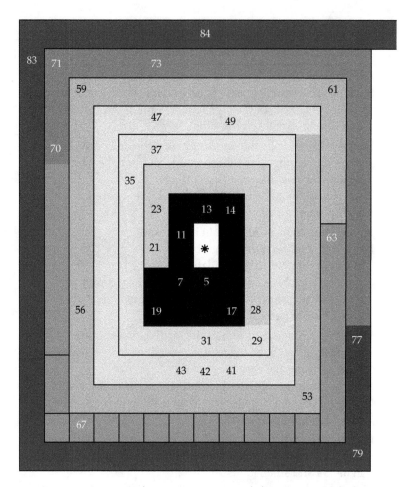

Figure 11: Heptades as genetic spiral: key to stages below

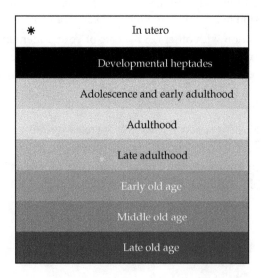

Another way of viewing the heptades as life phases:

1st, 2nd, and 3rd heptades—Developmental Phases

1	2	3	4	5	6	7
8	9	10	11	12	13	14
15	16	17	18	19	20	21

4th, 5th, and 6th—Activation Phases

22	23	24	25	26	27	28
29	30	31	32	33	34	35
36	37	38	39	40	41	42

7th, 8th, and 9th—Consolidation Phases

43	44	45	46	47	48	49
50	51	52	53	54	55	56
57	58	59	60	61	62	63

10th, 11th, and 12th Phases: Reconciling Possibilities with Acceptance

64	65	66	67	68	69	70
71	72	73	74	75	76	77
78	79	80	81	82	83	84

13th and 14th Phases: Acceptance

85	86	87	88	89	90	91
92	93	94	95	96	97	98

Key:	Prime number age	Transition

Beneath the arithmetic, one could divide the lifespan into eight post-natal clinical stages without assigning ages:

- Infancy and toddlerhood
- Early childhood
- Middle childhood
- Late childhood and adolescence
- Early adulthood

- Middle adulthood
- Late adulthood
- Dying and death

The ninth stage—prenatal development—is really the first and depends upon what influences came to bear upon the parents, which might have included herbal medicine. Ageing is inevitable (arriving more or less in heptades) but staging is not always fully realised.

When attending the dying, denial of the outcome will be devastating for them and, apart from making them lonely and desolate, you will have missed a privileged opportunity for reviewing the life span, for appreciating that a sense of humour is rooted in our mortality.

Elements of cyclic management that tend to loss of poise

The autonomic nervous system (ANS) manifests the cycling between day and night itself and from moment to moment within waking hours. Cycling between the resting and acting arms of para- and ortho-sympathetic systems characterise our lives like night and day. The ANS provides herbalists with the primary arena for strategic intervention. If you do nothing else in your therapy, you will have accomplished a good deal, assuming that you also include plants that have direct effects on surface tissues, maintained mostly by plants in the diet, aided by sensory priming.

Bacterial and viral infections dislocate both central and peripheral clocks but the SCN reasserts itself when the bout is resolved. Acute illness can remove us from circadian entrainment so we become free-running for a time. Convalescence is recovering entrainment. Most syndromes of chronic fatigue will invariably involve involuntary dislocation of circadian management, whether or not an infection was the initiator. Most of the dysautonomias likewise are linked to the range of capabilities of managing the cyclicity of life.

Uncoupling liver clocks from the SCN can be occasioned by midnight feasts and other interruptions to circadian rhythm, whether planned or spontaneous. But, to maintain a healthy regularity, such delights can happen only in the short term for a short while though for them sadly never to happen might be injurious to health.

Control

Poise—maintaining the flow, the ratio—depends upon control: sustaining the flow of energy but restraining it from uncontrolled surge, from turbulence. Speaking only of motor control, herbal dispensers are familiar with controlling the flow as they pour medicine from a measure into a bottle. Docking a boat negotiates between solid and fluid movement. Steady as she goes!

The metaphor of steering a ship, responding to tides and winds was foundational in cybernetics which has seen applications in all control systems.[113] Circular, recursive, self-correcting causal events inform physiological, informatic, and social circuits. Energy flow depends upon a self-replenishing system, whatever the scale of focus. Control is lost when energy flow is disrupted. Its availability relies on the trail of ions, enzymes and cofactors from a reservoir that well exceeds current demand. Control of output states depends upon energy reserve. States of low control therefore can be regarded as deficiency states and corrected accordingly by increasing capacitance and reducing stress as we will discuss further in the next Section, How to Remedy Loss of Poise.

Involuntary signs such as tremor denote some interruption in signal flow or loss at source. Fidgeting or racing ahead of oneself or other restless states suggest impulses that cannot be contained before discharge. This disorganisation may attest to an irresolution at higher levels. When a balance between excitatory and inhibitory drives cannot be contained, the conflict is usually central not peripheral. Even so, restless states are energy consuming and may also indicate reduced reserves. Sometimes using beta-sympatholytic herbs actually releases the energy that is not being effectively channelled but would not, of course, be appropriate usually in states of chronic fatigue. Even in such cases, reducing the available energy in the short term for the patient to achieve long stretches of natural sleep, may be just what is needed, so that reserves can be replenished. In short, we need to control the flow of signals and nutrient in order to conserve and distribute energy, to generate and release charge.

Self-control appears as a character trait when it is invariant. If the highly controlled individual happens to suffer from fatigue, a nutrient-dense diet and very long bouts of rest and sleep are remedial but if the person is anhedonic, this remedy may be resisted. Self-control usually protects other people, but if never relaxed will exhaust the person. If carers are unable to control their flow of energy, they will have little left to give. Some are faced with choices beyond medical control but for which sustaining plants can offer some solace.

Filtration

All animals are tasked with feeding and are most receptive to cues that facilitate it, distractible mostly by cues that interfere with that end or pose some threat. Social animals have to be alert to a wider range of subtler, often ambiguous, ranked cues. Our minds use filters to sort out information that is extraneous to the task in hand. Less task–orientated individuals who ponder and speculate a great deal are less inclined to filtration and want to amass all the material information before coming, if ever they do, to a conclusion. The paring down may come later, if at all. Receptivity to the environment and our filtering activity (when not contingent upon the pressure of a task at hand) may be strong indicators of personality and therefore the default disposition of our ANS. This disposition tends to choose our pattern of life even as it might feel thrust upon us.

An extreme inability to filter is seen in bipolar mental disorders where the highly rapid inner mental voice is externalised into speech and behaviour. Filtration operates

---

[113] The term cybernetics—coined by Norbert Weiner and colleagues in the 1940s—was taken from the Greek for steersman, helmsman: κυβερνήτης.

differently in schizophrenia where the normal inner voice is interpreted as belonging to an external source, often dictatorial or mocking.

Thoughtful people will always be prone to eczema, which does not mean that those who are free of it are thoughtless but you cannot process that much that slowly without accumulation. Whether your patient is atopic or not, their sensitivities will in some measure reflect their ability to filter out and select from a barrage of signals what matters to them, and what might be disagreeable. This data sampling is how we negotiate the world: how much we let in or preselect with our dispositional filters. Creative artists and scientists cannot do original work if they reduce their receptivity. Others see what has to be done and want to filter out extraneous distractions. As a crude distinction, some overthink to the point of discomforting their lives while others are impatient to get on to the action. Sleep eventually provides the great filtration bed, and dreams a response to the archiving.

Stabilising the influx of information depends upon control as do the output states. The capacity for oscillating swiftly between para- and ortho-sympathetic is a sign of good adaptation. If such people become your patients, their complaints are likely to be deep-seated and constitutional because of the energetic cost of this speedy adaptation.

High energy complaints like anxiety and low or inhibited flows of energy like the psychomotor retardation of depression cannot, of course, be assigned a simplistic energetic explanation but, using a somatopsychic approach with herbal medicine is a large part of our efficacy.

As the amount of information we let in depends upon filtration, how we organise and deal with influx characterises our autonomic style and relates to our processing speed.

Processing speed

Tortoise and hare are both effective in their own ways. People who appear to be slow learners may appear slow because they filter out fewer signals from the influx of stimuli open to a greater range to by. More accurately, they eject options only after scrutiny, which takes time and energetic capacity. They then have to spend time picking over the material towards arriving at some synthesis. This is completed by dreaming, especially in vagotonic individuals with capacious memories. Like horses they learn slowly but do not forget, (except for short-term details as in King Alfred and the cakes)!

Hares cut to the chase as if time is chasing them. They streamline their responses to stimuli and whittle them down in an instant, freeing up energy to move fast. Actors, comedians and compère hosts are true hybrids, thinking on their feet while in view and, tortoising when not. Whether nimble politicians are hares or hybrids probably depends upon their wider disposition, the subject of Section 1.9.

The psyche of a tortoise in our modern world of proliferating obsolescent *stuff* may wish to externalise thoughts and memories and be unable or unwilling to extricate him or herself from the objects that may declutter the mind but fill the house. The modern malady of hoarding may lurk behind your patient's inability to manage their thought processes.[114]

How physic can influence processing speed is part of the therapeutic discussion in Section 3.6 but next we need to outline how poise can be recovered physiologically.

---

[114] Recommended and very sympathetic reading on the subject (and an antidote to anti-clutter instructionistas) is *Possessed: A Cultural History of Hoarding* Rebecca Falkoff (Cornell, 2021).

How to remedy loss of poise

When patients ask me how I can help them, I tell them that it is quite simple to explain: I will prescribe and dispense herbs to lighten their burden and to increase their carrying capacity. The reader might be posing the very same question. Even if we reframe the response in terms of reducing the expression of unhelpful genes and facilitating helpful epigenetic expression, we might well ask—to step down from the general to the particular—how that might be achieved.

Well, first of all it is not brought about by medicinal plants alone as the first Sections in Part Two are dedicated to explore. We have to situate the patient in the therapeutic environment with the practitioner as conduit for the healing process.

Poise points to the energetic basis of biology and so we have to remedy its loss in the medium that conjoins cells, tissues and the whole organism—the medium of water. It sustains life so we cannot modify the terrain unless its aqueous foundation finds itself in optimal homeostatic state.

As discussed in Section 1.3, motion can only arise from an unmoving base. Homeostasis refers to the nexus of fixed points about which our drive towards nutrient and away from danger and the final stasis of chemical equilibrium (death). Homeostasis maintains and buffers internal environments close to steady points by means of negative feedback loops. These maintain each variable—notably core temperature and pH, also blood glucose and electrolytes—within narrow bounds. By stabilising inner variation, by resisting change, homeostasis permits the organism to deal with unpredictable local variations. It is a blind system that allows us to see. By automatising our response to events, it frees up the energy it has conserved and allows us to act.

The circadian system generates a pattern of *predictable* variation that acts like a template to recognise the sequentiality of life. By riding on a bedrock of homeostasis our forward drive can interact with the world in an energetically efficacious way. A fluid system with a fixed range of pH needs to be buffered to avoid unstable fluctuation.

Buffer

All biochemical reactions in the body are enzyme dependent and these can only operate within a narrow temperature range and need a pH between 7.35–7.45. The bicarbonate/carbonic acid buffer system regulates the pH of body fluids so that life is even possible. As for energy supply, the liver is the largest of the body's buffers. Stable blood sugar depends upon effective relationships between liver, endocrine pancreas and glucocorticoids from the adrenal cortex, all of which can be modified by medicinal plants. Adequate function of each assure the buffers to our adaptive response.

The sense of resisting change to keep within a normal range leads effortlessly to the metaphorical notion of a cushion or barrier zone that makes life more comfortable and safe. Buffering and ballast go together. Almost any load on a person that lacks them will lead to their illness.

Ballast

Physical ballast in physical transport systems such as ships prevent rocking or yawing motions. They provide the necessary stability against perturbations as buoyancy compensators do in balloons or in gliders when thermals are strong. The metaphorical notion of ballast has the same general point of resisting flux and anchoring response.

The hull of a sailing boat could serve as a metaphor, almost as a model, for ourselves travelling through life. It needs ballast in the form of a keel but also sails to capture fortuitous winds. Although the keel produces drag it provides essential stability to a hull exposed to lateral forces and contributes to the righting of an overturning boat. This models an example of a reciprocal oscillatory system like ourselves who self-correct deviations from course by way of feedback.[115] Knowledge from experience is an input into our system and so modifies how feedback operates: this feed-forward impulse sets the course. Otherwise, becalmed by homeostasis, and stasis gives the clue, we would not move forward, never innovate.

Heavy craft respond slowly to changing circumstances but are not easily capsized. A fast, nimble light craft is versatile in good weather but can easily be destabilised by a sudden squall. Just so, a sensitive soul can be flustered by a chance remark and capsized by an abrupt encounter.

Cyclothymic persons (whom we encountered first in Section 1.5a) are both nimble and steadfast, with a terrain heavily anchored in one of the two catabolic H-P axes with a forceful but untethered oscillation between dopamine and prolactin. They are hyperresponsive with their spirits thrown on and off course with a very irregular short period.[116] Their reactive tendency in the posterior pituitary hormones makes them blow hot and cold in affect and intimate responsiveness. They tend not to regress to the mean in cyclical terms though in fundamental belief and direction they are paradoxically strongly anchored. This self-belief, like stoicism, makes them slow to seek help but can be helped very much by medicinal plants.

---

[115] As discussed in the segment on Control in the previous section.

[116] In great contrast in period and severity to those with bipolar disorder.

Depleted ballast is restored primarily by rest, buffers by repletion of ions and other cat-alytic elements, primarily from diet and good intestinal absorption. So are replenished. Occasionally, mineral supplementation along with plant-based proteolytic enzymes may be advised. Herbal medicine will help with absorption and the quality of the patient's rest, replenishing ballast. Prescribed plants will recalibrate neuroendocrine systems that have deviated from course. They do this by providing buffers between stimulant hor-mones and their receptors so that the circuits (S-O-Rs) are smoothed and dampened by feedback as we will examine in Section 3.6.

Just to put all this in some clinical context and remind ourselves that medicine is physic, not physics, let us say, paraphrasing the first paragraph of this section: illness will always result from a loss of reserve energy. Restoring capacitance is brought about by:

- Lowering the adaptive burden
- Increasing adaptive capacity

Achieved by:

- Restoring cyclicity (Section 1.5a)
- Smoothing the functionality of the terrain (Section 3.6)

How do we do this? Complexity Theory follows the interactions between physics and biology and describes living beings as coupled oscillators. Nurtures and medicines need, then, to integrate our cycles (Section 1.5a)

Oscillation between binary reciprocating poles along a spectrum

The closest we come to fixture is our attempt to match the alternation between day-light and night. There are other rhythms derived from this alternation as discussed in previous sections. Nothing in biology is fixed because everything is constantly moving against the *relative* stability of physics. Physical and mental events travel in channels but even these are liable to flip from one path to another, seeking the path of least resistance, the pathway energetically the most fluid.

The yin-yang taijitu expresses the fundamental polarities involved in our own bodies and how these are mirrored in life outside us and within our bodies.

Poles are places not objects and certainly not impenetrable opposites. They mark the extent of a flow at the edge of a moving field or of the swing of a pendulum. Day flows into night. The dynamics of a system determines its poles which flow and change place as in a dance. In human affairs, power is a bordered field while love is unbounded. I raise the question again in Quantity and Quality in Section 2.2.

Movement between poles create phenomena. Even if we do not go so far as Galen when he said that stillness was wellness,[117] one could say that all symptoms are the prod-uct of turbulent movement. The clinician observes and records during the consultation and examination how movement between polarities express themselves in the patient.

---

[117] See Motion in Section 1.3.

The crucial point is that oscillation is the healthy norm but some people (and they may become your patients) are fixated at one pole and do not budge. This is an extreme but it is clinically significant the extent to which a patient hovers over one pole and does not gravitate to the other.

When they move too readily, and react as if opposite poles are walls that oppose rather than absorb the high wave they have created, symptoms often generate as a cascade. The clinical response is to calm the waves. Maybe Galen had a point when there is too much movement.

Symmetry and complementarity

The Danish physicist and philosopher Niels Bohr made foundational contributions to quantum theory and atomic structure. He had the yin-yang taijitu on his coat of arms above the motto *contraria sunt complementa*: opposites are complementary.[118] Perhaps in our physiology we should have as broad a mind when we are trying to help reduce the asymmetries in the oscillating fields of our patients.

Let us cite some of these major polarities which manifest in the physical, physiological and psychosocial worlds. I hope the reader will spot where the particulars emerge in various sections throughout all three parts of the text.

DARK	LIGHT
COLD	HOT
CENTRAL	PERIPHERAL
MOIST	DRY
ORDER	DISORDER
CONTROL	ABANDON
SEDATION	STIMULATION
ANIMATION	AGITATION
RETENTION	DISCHARGE
HEARING	LISTENING
ROBUST	FRAGILE
PROCESS	OBJECT
RELATIONAL	REDUCTIVE
ENHANCEMENT	REPLACEMENT
SYMMETRY	ASYMMETRY
EXUBERANCE	RESTRAINT

Our tissues are required—as homeostatic organisms—to set fixed points (especially pH, temperature). This enables each system to revolve around a viable centre. If the centres were also mobile, there would be no point about which we could oscillate.

---

[118] From the website Escutcheons of Science.

In any one body, there will be islands of the opposite and contrasts of form and texture, as so profoundly intimated by the dots of opposite colour in each swirl of the yin-yang taijitu.

Categories are differentiated and ordered qualities. Symmetry can conserve information and therefore energy, and so becomes a sought quality in many categories. Where asymmetry becomes marked, complementary qualities may be sought to return the composite whole to a higher order symmetry.

A number of second order symmetries match the alternation between accumulation of a charge and its subsequent discharge. At the level of organelles, this is electronic. At the tissue level, the alternation is between contraction and release, operated by the ANS. A large separation between the two results in explosive release, for instance in orgasm, ovulation, ejaculation and uterine contractions.

We assimilate energy as we rest, feed and sleep, permitted by the nicotinic and muscarinic receptors for acetylcholine.[119] These operate to lower smooth muscle tone in vessels and the digestive tract, with dampening of cardiac activity.

Whether this resting state is perturbed or calm depends upon the concurrent balance and relative strengths of the biogenic amines, especially serotonin and histamine. Freedom from illness depends upon smooth gradients between these contrasting complementary states. They flow ultimately from alternations in the physical world: between darkness and sunlight. Symmetry between impulse and resolution—broken briefly, restored promptly—moves us towards an adaptive state.

Patterns of oscillation from charge separation to discharge in motor activity characterise our energetic lives. Spending too long in the transit zone is fraught with problems. Extended transition time between these contrasting states generates more symptoms and functional syndromes than almost anything else.

These are the people herbalists can most help.

To care is to pursue precision in an approximate world. To care is adaptive, providing the tolerances are varied according to circumstances, so that we do not become fixated on caring too much or too little. Between enormity and minuteness we can settle well into a harmonic median if we have the right help.

Discharge

An overall characteristic of the human organism that shows up in movement and behaviour relates to the accumulation and discharge of energy. Discharge of energy and information is positively discharged in all circumstances where the parasympathetic gives way cordially to the beta-sympathetic without alpha-sympathetic interference as in:

- Dancing, athletic exercise, love
- Laughter
- The certainty of creative flow from the ludic impulse

---

[119] Named after the plant and fungal alkaloids that mimic parasympathetic activity.

- Well-honed repertoires of physical practice (e.g. operators in busy street markets, bars, skilled building trades; actors on stage)
- Command postures, notably when stance is holistic and ethical

By contrast, movement and discharge across the autonomic system can be disorganised and disjointed when some of the following circumstances prevail in an individual:

1	Subject to high filtration		Discussed in… Section 1.7
2	Low or absent filtration	Unfiltered stimuli overwhelm so that output cannot self-organise; manifest in restless fingers, fidgeting, tremor, procrastination (if not in madness)	Here!
3	Subject to strong inhibition	Where para or alpha sympathetic dominance inhibits release of beta	3.7
		Inhibition of desire by low oxytocic discharge	3.7
4	Subject to counter-currents	Turning over alternatives in rumination	2.2 in nurtures 3 & 5
		Turning over alternatives by Memorialists	1.9
5	Subject to restless impatience	so that any outcome is better than no outcome: fear of inaction or indecision; gambling	1.9
6	Fear of mutiny	Dictatorial personalities with higher levels of adrenal androgens relative to gonadic	3.7

Fear of conflict coupled with fear of being contradicted, intolerance of frustration, all lead to poor autonomic synchrony. A seemingly unrelated symptom correlates with such disordered synchrony and is worth asking patients about: whether they are prone to bouts of *pruritus ani*, presumably from poor timing of *chole*, which we will discuss fully in Section 2.5b.

Temperament: temporal attitude and physics of personality

> For the gods perceive future events, men what is happening now, but wise men approaching things
>
> —Philostrates Life of Appollonius of Tyana viii, 7.[120]

Temperament in the traditional sense meant the quality of admixture of the four humours—choler, blood, black bile, and yellow bile, relating to the four elements—and so flowed with the constant movement of life, tending downwards as sluggish sediment or upwards into mobile air and warmth. Temperament, in the sense of movement inevitably involves time and timing. Comedians and humorists tell us that a sense of timing define a sense of humour. Good timing satisfies us as if randomness in the world had been defeated for the moment.

Personality, as an assemblage of characteristic traits, reflects our trend away from the cosmos towards individualism. As a unit that can be insured with tastes that can buy stuff, classifying personality suits behavioural psychology, advertising agencies and contemporary politics. There is nothing new in the human tendency to characterise (even caricature) people with whom we interact and recent years have seen a trend in an opposite direction: towards viewing traits as situated upon a spectrum rather than inside a labelled box. Just as temperature is measured in degrees along a range, so a person's disposition for such and such is true only within the extent of their gamut and depends upon context, and even the state of the weather. As clinicians, we try to assess the *range* of behavioural response and move a person back towards the midpoint of their own scale. Rather than typify them, we seek to move their own physiology to a place where the symptoms evaporate.

---

[120] Quoted in *The Complete Poems of C.P. Cafavy* translated by Rae Dalven London Hogarth 1961, p. 53.

If temperament means dynamic admixture, tempo (like temperature) refers to a rate of movement and, as life is locked in step with time, a person's temporal attitude is a key to their autonomic disposition.

Though we can alter course and change direction, our ability to fundamentally change our temporal outlook is more limited than other aspects of personality. A person's approach to the three tenses of time and how they organise all three is significant and—because related to the ANS and the neuroendocrine terrain—has potential for modulation by medicinal plants.

Our species holds a unique capacity for visualising time and imagining a large set of future possibilities including a discursive imaging apparatus for how one might respond to each of them. We are the great anticipators who try to separate risk from opportunity. The physics of personality lies within this capacity for formulating options, for turning them over in one's mind and choosing which path to take. Although we make mental images of impending events (and of the past once we have slept on current events), these images are virtual. Time seems sequential to us: "Time and tide wait for no-one". Although images dominate, giving us our "view", sound is the most sequential and temporal of the senses, so language (and music) reflect movement in time. Time sense is central to human experience and personality because behaviour and attitude are inherent to it.[121]

Every moment of time involves some choice, even the choice to do next to nothing. All choice is made under conditions of some uncertainty and the choice made is irrevocable. Routine and habit compress our sense of time and so save energy. Circadian entrainment reinforces habitual patterns and so can be adaptive but to rely entirely upon previous experience would stultify novel ideas and insight.

The work of the Nobel laureate economist Daniel Kahneman found that most people are (a) more afraid of loss than motivated by gain, (b) more anxious about *changes* in their situation and (c) think about the future from a position anchored in their beliefs.[122] These insights have relevance for our response to the patient's narrative during the clinical assessment and Kahneman's latest work focusses on medicine and law.[123]

Decision-making, therefore, relates the current situation to the future. Leaving aside humdrum and quotidian choices we make all the time, styles of making important decisions are (according to the psychiatrist Raj Persaud) a good guide to personality and one I find useful in practice. Those who try to maximise their outcomes or optimise them can be called futurists. Maximising contrasts with being good enough or *satisficing* (a merger between satisfy and suffice).[124]

The physiological problem facing futurists is that maximising maintains high levels of tone in the system which cannot be discharged. Whatever result is obtained will always be less than perfect to the envisioned perfection, making them liable to continual disappointment and regret.

---

[121] According to the physicist Carlo Rovelli, (Bibliography) time is always a percept.

[122] For this seminal work in contemporary psychology of human behaviour, see Kahneman (2011).

[123] Kahneman & Sibony (2021).

[124] Coined by HA Simon in *Administrative Behavior* Macmillan New York 1947.

Regret in the nostalgic sense afflicts those we might call pastists. By deferring, reducing, or even eliminating choice they drown in the recollection of all that might have happened or did take place in all its bittersweet ambivalence.

Futurists will no doubt have made excellent pension arrangements but no forward plan can eliminate unforeseen circumstances.[125] Having deposited so much energy into the future, they may find themselves stranded if their choices—dictated by naive rationalism—turn out to be less than providential. The rich life of the heart can never be reduced to a variable in an equation. My futurist patients are surrounded by everything they could have wished for but are disabled by a perfection that has failed to materialise. For maintaining such high tone over such a long time, they are prone to deep deficiencies and will therefore need remedies to sustain their depleted ballast. But, trusting only in certainties (the opposite of a gambler) they may discontinue treatment if they cannot discern benefits among the variables.

> There is an entirely different kind of anticipator and these patients may account for the majority of clinical presentations of non-communicable disorders. They are the hyper-vigilant, always on the outlook for a threat, held in a state that should be a stepping stone to action. Often resulting from early experience, this anticipatory anxiety comes to characterise the terrain. The passage from impulse via preparation to action becomes vitiated by the computations not so much of gaining benefit but of avoiding harm. Noradrenaline, this great initiator, outstays its time. We'll discuss how we might help this alpha-sympathetic dominance in the Section on the ANS in Section 3.6.

Pastists or memorialists may often be creative or inventive personalities on account of the material they amass and patterns they discern. They do so by maintaining high parasympathetic tone. But because they are very slow to discharge and eliminate residues they inevitably become very congested, with all the consequences for respiratory and digestive systems. At least there is no ambiguity about how to prescribe for them! Pastists, if liable to dither in the present, will have slow reflexes (unless they have also high alpha-sympathetic tone). In the longer term, they may be prone more to regret but less to disappointment: more a gentle melancholy and less a toxic depression. Rumination can be productive, educative, establishing meaning from the past and a potential future. Melancholy can open the door for long-term learning.

How long does the present moment last? It seems that the duration from unseen and unknowable intention (a deep human deception thinks we are somehow in charge!) to the execution of an event lasts about six seconds.[126] Performing a practised routine can reduce this considerably and also depends upon the profession: actors and comedians are used to responding on their feet. Even greater reductions of the "present" duration is seen in lifelong martial artists and zen buddhist monks. If time is physical, the present is shorter than any biological function. If it is a percept (Rovelli again) the current moments will depend upon brainwave states and (when alert) will congregate into an episode.

---

[125] Appointment diaries make relative futurists of all professionals.

[126] I have reviewed the literature in *Human Health* (2020). For an enjoyable account of relative biological time periods, I recommend Money (2023).

To "live in the present", as is commonly exhorted, can take opposite forms: to escape into hedonism or enjoy the sensuality of the moment, knowing that it will never return. Both recognise mortality. There is a long cultural tradition of savouring the present moment—*carpe diem*—usually translated as "seize the day".[127] Or from the English poet Robert Herrick: 'gather ye rosebuds while ye may' to Edward FitzGerald's *Rubáiyat of Omár Khayyám* and the rich Sufi tradition that inspired it. All this poetic and philosophic meditation on the brevity of life is quite distant from the presentist temperament.

Presentists are impatient empiricists who get easily bored. They want to get on with things. Often hedonic, they discharge easily and impulsively so are toned only briefly. They may be choleric but the most pertinent feature is their ready expression of dopamine which can usefully be dampened. Gamblers and chancers are presentists who—viewed in a positive light—are those who spot opportunities not seen by most. They perhaps understand that as we can do nothing about random events and may misunderstand the nature of risk (as Nassim Nicholas Taleb would have us accept), we may as well surrender and so gain.[128] Presentist patients will visit you from time to time on a whim but do not repeat treatments as they want things 'sorted' in a trice. Schizophrenics who show extreme levels of dopaminergic discharge are locked in the present. Far from savouring it, they are cruelly cut off from the rest of time and life.

Childhood is a presentist state until they become burdened with history and once they have to face independent decisions. Presentists perhaps refuse to take the burden of the past too seriously.

The distance in time and space between desire and locating its object can range from a few steps in the direction of the cupboard to crossing continents in a frenzy. Desire in the life-changing sense doesn't arrive too often (there just isn't time) but even satisfying the daily wants can be delayed or seized in an instant. The literature on delayed or deferred gratification is extensive and interesting but I want to draw attention to the relation between adult temporal style with the capacity to discharge, tabulated in the previous, discussed in fifth nurture (Section 2.2) and its follow on in therapeutic levels in Section 3.6. It connects with another temporal function—telling stories. My take on narratology (Section 2.4b) may not sound as cosy perhaps as might currently be popular.

Humans are anticipators, so we all survey, feel our way through and calculate the options. All of us live tripartite lives distributed across the three tenses. How we do so and how we deal with outcomes offer clues to personality. Locked into one at the expense of the other two ignores the opportunities of the present.

Although our temperaments are embedded in the terrain, they come up for re-election, as it were, at transitions between heptades. So, vagotonic pastists storing memories, maximising futurists who retain money but shop around obsessively in the present to secure the future, and impulsive presentists who run out of time can, if they are fortunate, respond to life events and nurtures to modify their temporal natures. Otherwise, we'd be out of a job.

---

[127] Horace, Odes 1.11; better might be: 'pick the fruit of the day now it is ripe'. He continues: 'trust tomorrow as little as you can'.

[128] His work (see Bibliography) asserts the fragility of seemingly robust systems of human thought and our tendency to retrospectively rationalise our mistakes.

Inflexibility is only adaptive in tyrants and other disorders of the will, where the will is not tempered by the thoughts of others (unless in delusional 'others' as in schizophrenia). Psychotic states cannot manage or afford empathy unlike psychopaths who know how to employ it to manipulate others so they have a perfectly good, indeed devastating theory of mind.

On a much lower scale, fixation is a major key to the operation of personality: how stuck in one mode compares with the facility to oscillate between opposite modes. Anchoring behaviour in a value system is socially adaptive with great biological benefit but fixation as a permanent disposition rarely so. Obsessive compulsives are fixated on routines that hinder them from progressing to more pleasant or more purposeful tasks. Very difficult to approach let alone treat, I have seen some modest improvements with diversionary tactics, distracting them from their fixation along with herbs that soothe and encourage, notably *Sambucus*, *Tilia*, and *Lamium*, aided by a diet rich in pumpkins, aubergines, potatoes, and lady's fingers.

In both fixated and impulsive patients, relative dominances between dopamine, prolactin, and oxytocin are most amenable to therapeutic balancing. Temperament is embedded in these as well as the autocoid hormones. These are at the core of herbal therapeutics and will be discussed fully in Section 3.6, Level Seven.

The three tenses correlate with temporal faculties everyone displays in different measure: planning and remembering in order to act and reenact. Perhaps a more realistic version of Persaud's hypothesis would identify those who manage the current episode with an accurate eye to its immediate future within the day and a good memory for the past are the greatest exponents of poise.

When the current episode with its immediate future is not besieged with options, this state may be considered contentment or drudgery, depending upon the individual and circumstances. But usually, choices present themselves or are even forced upon our attention. The unknown is fraught with risk and opportunity. Those who predict risk quite accurately contrast strongly with those who minimise in the hope of maximising reward. They stand polarised in temperament as pessimist and optimist respectively.

Optimist and pessimist

What may look like risk aversion can be realism and an openness to evidence that the optimist disregards. Pessimists may show, against stereotype, a greater ability to change their minds. Optimists tend to be resistant to evidence and see only narrow chances. Unrealistic people do often win through and over-cautious ones miss opportunities but they are outliers. Is the distinction as humoral as "hothead" versus "cool head"—fiery versus airy? Pessimists seem more discerning about context so may be less fixated about evaluating the worst case than optimists are about accepting everything at face value. Against that, a great deal of energy can be spent on avoiding danger. Whether consciousness overestimates reserves or is pessimistic about them is an important index of personality. Life must conserve but not hoard energy and needs to both look and then leap as discussed in Section 1.3.

Optimists tend to strong beta-sympathetic drive while pessimists are likely vagotonic. Medicinal plants operate against this crude distinction in that a little *Rosmarinus* mixed with vagolytic plants like *Thymus* and *Achillea* can sharpen the mettle of a pessimist and beta-lytic plants like *Tilia* can relax the spring of an optimist. In temperament, *always* and *never* are more polarised extremes than optimist and pessimist. Herbal medicine can be a useful lubricant for stiff habits.

Perfectionists—subject to the tyranny of the ideal—are intolerant of uncertainty and ambiguity: they cannot accept and shrug off mistakes. But because they are fastidious, being treated impeccably (and surely that is the ambition of a therapist) the patient practitioner will reap rich rewards. Personality traits that need extra care are found in phobic, obsessive and squeamish people and those anhedonic souls who fear ecstasy. Herbs that raise courage, soften borders and increase gusto such as *Borago, Verbena, Trigonella, Foeniculum, Melissa, Menyanthes* and *Turnera* and others will need to make an appearance. Resistance to change as a hurdle may be softened by the kind of relaxed recommendation implied by "I used to do that, and now no longer do".

An optimist is happy with the day. The pessimist hopes tomorrow will be better. The ironic interpenetration of supposed opposites as in the complementary dots in the yin/yang taijitu. In autonomic terms, the optimist perhaps discharges more forcefully and cannot tolerate dithering while the pessimist thinks through all the options (perhaps until it is too late to act on them, at least immediately). Each could learn from the other.

Hot and cold

Caricatures are easy to read and tempting to make. They create the tools which music-hall used and now stand-up comedians employ to make people laugh. Our appetite for them—from seaside postcards to ladybird books—never wanes. Caricatures accommodate well to a theory of types. For this very reason, the social sciences and prudent political comment warn us off them. Are they too conveniently true or false by misrepresentation? They provide fodder for prejudice.

One day, a large lady in a pink blazer (here we go) launched into my consulting room. She had on bright red lipstick which set off her complexion (contrasting ruddy and pale) topped by enormous blonde hair. With a badge on her lapel, she had all the command and posture of a colonel in the WRAF and was built for the task. "Phew it's hot in here!" she exclaimed on this mild spring morning with the door open to the garden. She wanted to know what the hell I could do about her blazing psoriasis.

You didn't need to invoke ancient humoral or even modern endobiogenic medicine to know that her metabolic turnover and her thermostat were set too high. Caricatures are not fictional but not as common as caricaturists would have us believe. This lady is the only entirely hot person I have treated in all the years; neither have I been presented with too many entirely cold people. The better question to ask of heat may be to find out whether it is central or in the periphery (see Section 2.5a) because vagal tone conserves and sympathetic tone dissipates. Either way it will show up in the skin (Section 2.5b). Life is all mixture: caricaturists are over-eager diagnosticians; their exemplars may be true to type but not to life.[129]

---

[129] Hippocrates is scathing about uncritical ideas of hot and dry. See Lloyd (Ed) (1983) *Tradition in Medicine* in *Hippocratic Writings* p. 79. Details in Bibliography.

Some physiological generalisation is justified, however: an over enthusiastic thyroid output will aways produce heat. Inflammation will invoke the sense of heat rising and dispersing (the sense of being hot, bothered and restless). Beta-adrenergic output may be high but not translate into muscular activity. A person with parasympathetic strong enough to inhibit or delay beta-adrenergic output will feel cold, as will most spasmophiles when they constrict. Spasmophilia is a term current in French herbal medicine[130] that denotes the tendency for certain individuals whose health is generally very good to respond to stressful challenge by a generalised vasoconstriction in smooth muscle. I have adapted the concept to the poise hypothesis as a temporary impedance and will take it up again in the segment on diagnosis in Section 2.3.

Moist and dry

Still, hot and cold metaphors serve us very well for movements in a person whose blood may be up, or the opposite—run cold. Dilation does of course result in perfusion while constriction will dry out tissues. These movements do have clinical relevance but to codify them as qualities is to oversimplify, and to project human qualities onto plants is sentimental. One of the four humours—choler—really does sit at a core of metabolism and needs a segment to itself (in Section 2.5b). The autocoid hormones—acting in concert—are involved in thermoregulation and vascular tone, mood and sleep and (behaving like humours) certainly contribute to the quality of personhood.[131]

But hydration belongs to the skin, lungs, heart and kidney. If someone is really moist, are their sweat glands compensating for failing kidneys? Sjögren's and other types of severe dryness (known as sicca syndromes) are serious and common enough. Rather than typify, it makes more sense to understand what is going on in the municipality. Naming is the prelude to understanding, not knowledge in itself. Reverence for the four humours seem to be a condescending falsehood: who does it help to pretend we do not know what we do? It seems like an ingratitude to some of the benefits of the modern world. We endure the downsides enough without looking to the ancients for a way out of our troubles.

Phlegm is a defensive process of normal physiology and reflects the importance of sol/gel alteration that is so important to cell functioning and tissue health. It is a process not a category. If its flow is excessive, our job should be to find what is being protected and where in the municipality perceived threats are producing defensive mucus. Then we diminish the sense of threat by central means and reduce reactivity in the peripheral locations of the two other domains (See Figure 12).

Character trait theories

Modern theories of character trait or disposition are based on a history of factor and lexical analysis from questionnaires which (like the development of IQ) has been charged with a range of cultural biasses. A brief summary will suffice: Carl Jung (1875–1961), the

---

[130] Discussed in some detail (but not in English) in the *Traité* of Duraffourd & Lapraz (2002) p. 494.

[131] For therapeutics, see Section 3.6.

Swiss psychiatrist who founded analytic psychoanalysis introduced the notion of personality and behaviour emerging from two cardinal traits—introversion and extroversion.[132] Gordon Allport (1897–1967), an American psychologist who taught at Harvard for most of his career, was the major contributor to what became known as Five Trait Theory (openness, conscientiousness, extroversion, agreeableness, neuroticism). This remains dominant theory to this day along with that developed by the German born British psychologist Hans Eysenck which reduced traits to three (neuroticism, extroversion, and psychoticism)[133] Hexaco, as well as telling us it is a six-trait model, is an acronym. It adds "Honesty-Humility" to Five Trait Theory.[134] Sixteen-trait theory was developed Raymond Cattell using multivariate factor analysis.[135]

All of them use questionnaires that serve the hypothesis and not the subject. They fail to enumerate varieties of context, they fail to express the oscillation between opposite traits common in ourselves and our patients. They do not permit you to express sub-categories that contradict the category. In that (and *permit* is ominous), they serve a futurist mentality well: academic and professional psychologists have slipped unobtrusively into consumerist culture. We can find more realistic, more contextualised depictions of character in drama, literature and myth (and in the oral traditions of non-literate cultures) than we can in the attempt at a scientific taxonomy of personality.

They may only be trying to do what we all do: derive general patterns from the particularities of social life. However, their findings, it seems to me, are generated from inauthentic, unrealistic studies which cannot mimic the varying and evolving contexts that people face in their lives. These results can indeed be replicated but in the same narrowly defined cohorts in conditions equally untrue to life. Of course, they show trends, distributions and even some truth about dispositions, but all this scoring does not help us help people.

In botany, a taxon refers to a species not to an individual plant. It is difficult to conceive a taxonomy of personality authentic to life and one that incorporates differing norms between cultures—nor between generations within them. Trait theories do not adequately factor in the maturation effect (nor that of birth order): matching a patient's current heptade with their past experience gives us a timeline to their character.

It may, however, to be helpful to match Five-Trait Theory with elements of temperament. For example, introverts may be absent-minded because they are distracted from what is going on outside from what they thoughts absorb them at that moment and so may forget whether or not they switched off the heating. This forgetfulness may impel obsessive or conscientious introverts to keep checking the switch and generate an additional layer of anxiety to the one that inhabits their personality. Their working memory is

---

[132] In his address to the Fourth International Psychoanalytical Congress in September 1913 in Munich that marked his final break with Sigmund Freud.

[133] Eysenck (1916–1997) was always a controversial figure (as I remember from my student days) and accused of unsafe practice, data not replicable (even concocted) and scientific racism.

[134] This sixth trait emerged as a finding in the early years of our current century when previous research was applied to a wider range of languages and cultures.

[135] Cattell (1905–1998) was controversial and like Eysenck was accused of scientific racism, probably unfairly in his case.

not so much absent as less present in the physical world than in their minds. Extroverts are all for doing and thinking later, if at all. This shows up early enough for no-one to suspect cognitive impairment. On the contrary.

The distribution of temperament into the three tenses are no more than nodes at which character traits converge. They are not categorical but heuristic and they do represent traits that we can modify to some extent in herbal clinics. Personality is a psycho-social construct while temperament more expresses underlying biology which botanical agents can modulate.

> If temperament points to a tropism rather than a category it rather reflects the way we conceptualise the properties of medicinal plants. To project human tropisms onto medicinal plants—an idea much espoused by the old herbals and still has some adherents today—is an unrealistic anthropomorphism. The Tropisms of herbal remedies reflect our shared evolutionary and ecological pathways but it seems just as wrong to categorise them as it would be to place human personality into boxes. Our world is awash with labels: full of scores, vacant in value.

Physiological regulatory networks

Returning to physiology from the psychosocial sphere, lest we get lost in human labelling, the architecture of the human multi-dimensional experience is built upon biology, a view I defend in *Time Criticality* in Figure 15. These elements rely on homeostasis to keep us alive long enough to respond to events and challenges. Body temperature and blood pH are regulated from moment to moment by chemoreceptors and sensors in the hypothalamus in tandem with effectors in the brainstem that control and maintain respiration, renal filtration and output. Ultimately these depend upon endocrine, sensory and motor systems as well as circadian regulation.

Beneath all of them reside gene regulatory networks that permit the multiple components of gene expression in the formation of proteins and the management of DNA and RNA replication.

None of these networks can operate without the informatic circuitry discussed in Section 1.4. I have made the point in many of the nine sections so far that information can be described as such only if it operates in a loop whereby a receptor responds to a signal. In most circumstances (ones that are not emergency reflexes), a sub-routine interpolates this circuit with some organisational modulation as I repeat in the résumé that follows.

Résumé of ideas in Part One

- Life is energetic by definition.
- This energy fuels the formation of membranes to give some separation of life from the material world. Life within the barriers contains more information than without and is chemically more reduced.
- Life-forms interact with other life-forms to generate ecosystems.
- Ecosystems are interpenetrative so that all eukaryotes are obliged to share, to be mutual in the face of multiple levels of competition.
- These mutualisms depend in turn upon myriad microbiomes, components of which will be mainly protists and procaryotes.
- The biology of the human individual is an array of interpenetrative ecosystems and microbiomes. Physiology responds to regular events, the most predictable being the dark/light alteration signalled by blue light at dawn (opportunity) and yellow light at dusk (potential risk). This anchoring by regular astronomical events (known as *entrainment*) frees us to respond to random irregularities in the environment so that we can extract energy from it. This stability is disturbed and reset by seasonal change, with great potential for illness.
- Life is polycyclic, phasic, patterned, and sequential. Cellular life is pulsatile and lives on a sea of waves: solar, lunar, lunisolar, tidal, lunitidal.
- Many immediate and basic responses to external stimuli are reflex events (stimulus—response, SR) but life is mediated by more than just a response to a sequence of accidents, a point that Behaviourists refused to take. In complex organisms—and necessarily those with *organs*—an interpolation of an organising feature between S and R dominates so that animals who move for food are characterised

88

by architectures of: stimulus-organisation-response (S-O-R).[136] The dominant organising centres are found in the brain, liver and other digestive organs; these organs regulate the homespace with respect to the microbiomes. Others maintain the inner environment and respond to change. They include the kidney, bone marrow and musculoskeletal matrix.[137]

- Neural circuits constitute special forms of an S-O-R that stack in reverberatory assemblages. Their output in human consciousness and behaviour creates complexity almost beyond reckoning.
- A more definable characteristic of the human organism relates to the accumulation and discharge of energy.
- The physics and biology of human life depend upon an array of ecosystems and so are irreducible and not negotiable (at least not over a lifetime).
- The human infant develops and builds emotional, mental and linguistic structures upon these physical ones. Clinical psychologists often speak as if these events trump the biological ones.
- All of these integrated systems grow and develop by learning and in so doing embody our psychosocial world to make us part of a group, usually familial in some sense. Collectively these virtual structures create culture. Our introduction into one or more of these begins each person's biography. Our entry into social life and the extent and quality of our participation as we negotiate tribal and subcultural allegiances creates the collectivity we call the self and which different personalities demarcate in different ways and perform socially in different modes. Sociologists often speak as if these events trump the biological ones.
- Our investment in sociality repays inevitably with emotionality. Anthropologists and ecologists (and herbalists too, I hope) tend away from hierarchies and favour the importance of the web of interactions. Even so, to emphasise the fundament of biology, ceasing to breathe for more than four minutes leads to harm beyond therapy to repair.
- Qualities of health depend upon qualities of perception and quantities of energy and information. Health depends upon reliability of channels so that ambiguity in the sense of a threat that is difficult to assess does not get confused with the inherent and desirable uncertainty of social niceties. Tact consist in the avoidance of literal truth when negotiating sensitive and difficult matters without being evasive. It seeks to enhance comfort and avoid distress. This discriminatory function enhances social understanding and is a large part of a good bedside manner.
- All creatures are subject to circadian cycles and all mammals are entrained by at least one of the other astronomical rhythms: tidal, lunar, seasonal, circannual. In humans, both the pulse generator for sleep and the impulse to drink and feed are generated in the hypothalamus.

---

[136] An overview of the manifestation of circuits in physical structures feature in the work of RL Swanson on Biotensegrity in the Journal of the American Osteopathic Association, January 2013.

[137] Clinical note: Cascades discharge energy in a way that abruptly disintegrates SORs, coagulation of blood being a notable example.

- In times of danger, basal tendencies may be binary: approach/avoid, attach/detach but during human development we learn to qualify situations, to interpret according to context so that trait theories of personality consider opposite poles not as separate but tendencies along a continuous scale. If we allow the two basal tropisms: introvert and extrovert, we can at least generalise that there are those like quiet contemplation and those who enjoy noise and distraction. I have suggested that this binary, whatever its merits, revolves around a disposition towards the sense and tense of time.
- What is more certain is that everyone responds in a particular way to the events of the moment but is entirely general in that the autonomic nervous system is implicated, along with its modifying autocoid hormones. The majority of medicinal plants modify the branches of the ANS and many also the autocoids. These effects are fundamental to our process and the basis of our materia medica, to be discussed in Part 3.

PART TWO

PATIENTS AND THEIR NEEDS OF PHYSIC
PHYSICIANS AND THEIR PRACTICE

Where to begin?

Medicine is both lofty (in that it deals with human suffering in an almost altruistic way) and down to earth, because it concerns human bodies in their pain and vulnerability. Medicine is not ideally conducted in the market place but rather in a space set aside. As in the theatre (and surgery is conducted in a theatre), performances of medicine may look similar but they are all different. They cannot be repeated exactly or packaged: just as though similarities converge in people, each person is unique.

The pandemic of 2019 has extended (so far) to 2022. The enforced separation has given rise to the fond illusion that medicine can be conducted virtually at a distance. This suits a managerial, detached style of medicine that operates on people rather than with them and tends to place the process in the market place, where it does not belong. This tendency may be the signal pathology of our age.

Other ages have had their problems and people have had to deal with them, with or without help from medicine. The great insight of Hippocrates and his colleagues who practised on the Greek island of Cos between 430 and 330 BC was to tell his students and patients that life was about process, not about things, not solely utilitarian. He placed the emphasis for healing within regimen and the therapeutic encounter and repudiated the search for a panacea to all ills. In his day and for most of human history nearly all panaceas were plant remedies.

Life proceeds from the senses: touch, taste and aroma before sight. The wish for haptic harmony is congenital but our socialisation inevitably attenuates or submerges it. Harmony—a state rather than an impulse—reminds us that we are innately sewn into the fabric of the natural world. As much as plants and all things under the sun.

In the hope that the herbal apprentice will seek to maintain that innate sense, I trust that the therapeutic process will win out over hopes of a panacea. Hippocrates was not at all against herbal remedies, he just taught they did not act alone. In the sections that follow, I give detail about the process of medicine in which plant-based medication comes an important third in a sequence of priorities. To repeat the sequence, I suggested at the end of the Introduction: "first the witness, then the nurture, only then the herb".

The therapeutic space

The therapeutic space gives the patient the opportunity to not be themselves. Not themselves as others see them or denote them: Maria's mother, Gwendoline's aunt, Bill's wife, Sacha's partner. They can tell their history as they and not others see it. When you see a husband and wife together with only one as the patient or even when they take it in turns, one often corrects the other which might launch a gentle debate about what really happened and what it might have meant. If you happen to do a home visit, or bump into the patient in the street or at a social event, or if you come to know them a bit in some wider context, you will begin to appreciate if it wasn't already obvious to you that the way we present is always a construction and that in the therapeutic space, our presentation is always a performance not because we are inauthentic but because that is the way social humans are.[138] In the course of the consultation, we may come across our mythic selves or begin to edit the necessary fiction we have created in our attempt to come to a truth or present ourselves as deserving of therapy.

The herbalist as therapist provides the very important physical space that does not double as domestic place. With a dispensary close by but not obtruding, the patient knows the encounter comes, at least in Britain, with a medicinal intention. No surprise there, or presumably they wouldn't have come. Apart from a welcome, an invitation to be open and not constrained by preconceptions will help the consultation come to fruition. This is stronger, as always, if it is sensed rather than spoken. Explicit comes later, at the end. As for implicit, the most auspicious and relaxing start will be to somehow impart the sense, if you can find how to do it, of having all the time in the world. It is the opposite of calling time, as some traditions do, rather sternly. There are practical difficulties here and maybe the patient has later appointments and it will not work with people who have developed advanced logorrhoea. My own early experiences of running a busy (and costly) multi-disciplinary clinic made me at times so tense that I was not able to conduct things the way I would have liked. Later on, having my own space, I was able to make time and first consultations could take more than two or even three hours and the patient was surprised at the time that had passed. In this later phase of my practice, follow-up appointments were less needed or sometimes even dispensable, to make a small pun.

Space for special purposes needs rubrics and rituals: surgical operations take place in a theatre, religious observances in a temple. The temple has always provided a refuge from the market place to which it stood in contrast.[139] Modern secular life may seem to avoid formality, oppressed as it is by the market place, yet this avoidance can feed

---

[138] Further Reading: Goffman (1959).

[139] Cf. John's Gospel in the Christian Bible Chapter 2, verse15.

a yearning for the uncrowded space. Natural environments are at a premium and the great outdoors relieves us of our particularity but we also need to examine our particular state in parallel but separated from our social selves, a need provided by therapy. Herbal medicine introduces a truly natural medium in a contemporary setting. It is ageless, too: no need to invoke the past or make a piety of tradition: plants co-evolve with us.

First the witness

"Attention is the rarest and purest form of generosity"

—Simone Weil

Illness invites us to change. The primary agent for change is oneself: in our interaction with the world and with others. We have been too long acquainted with ourselves to know who we are entirely and we may be better able to predict the behaviour of others than our own. We cannot see ourselves as others see us. The mirror can only reflect our own perception. To be witnessed in a therapeutic situation where the therapist has the primary intention for the client to be heard in full—without interruption— provides an opportunity for them to know themselves. Human hurt calls for recognition as much as sympathy. Therapy is not so much a technical skill as one of compassion, empathy and affect.

But it is also one of restraint, a special kind of tact: the practitioner must suspend all prejudice and whatever *preconceptions* have arisen from first impressions. To have had no first impressions would be not only improbable, but clinically negligent. They must, however, be put to one side for the moment. This holding two modes of thought apart for a while without dividing the self is the skill to be acquired. A difference may exist, even a gulf, between the age and world-view of the two parties but this must be bridged.

Medicine must be a composite practice if it is to reflect the three modes of behaviour that characterise human life:

1. Natural biological actions
2. Technical activity
3. Expressive actions

All three are involved in how we manage to stay alive and operate in a physical and social world. Without emotional expression we would be as robots. For this reason, if for no other, medicine has to start with affect: "how are you feeling" is as important as "where does it hurt". Can there be any scientific data that are independent of human utterance, verbal or otherwise?[140] So the medical conversation is a transaction that starts with communication before it can move to interpretation and an offer of assistance. It is a form of education—in its original sense of drawing out—where the physician does not teach but facilitates the patient to learn about self.

---

[140] Expanded in Barker 2013, Section 9.

Then the nurture

During the next stage, the practitioner should reflect back to the patient what she or he has understood to have been presented. This may overlap with clarification of medical history, of clinical details, if these have been a large part of the patient's primary expression. They are often not separate.

Before expanding on the patient's narrative and taking a full medical history, it is helpful to explain your therapeutic approach and to express, on the basis of what has been said so far, of how you use medicinal plants. Giving a realistic, down to earth appraisal of their usage in your experience (and that of others) sets the stage for a practical, egalitarian process. Usually, it puts the patient at ease and levels any incline between the two of you. Like plants themselves, you become their ally.

Nurture comes before treatment. It is not unusual for patients to alert previously that they are looking for advice or informed support about their way of eating and living, so it is often expected. Only after these stages have been fully considered should medicine be formulated as an agent for change and then only as an adjunct to these two primary agents: the attentive listening cure and the advice.

What I choose to call nurtures went by the name of "the six non-naturals" in the Galenic tradition of Western medicine. This did not at all mean that they were unnatural but referred simply to those things one would do well to manage well as their regulation was learned, not innate.[141] As such, they sat at the heart of "The Art of Physick". This phrase, a translation of Galen's *Ars medicinalis* (technè iatrikè in Greek), was in common currency for English herbalists John Parkinson (1567–1650), John Pechey (1655–1716)

---

[141] The "naturals" referred to the elements of physiology in the sense of temperaments, humours and faculties. Contra-naturals (sometimes Preter-naturals) meant pathological states. Vivian Nutton (2013) provides a most helpful overview of Galenic medicine in a single volume. He commends the very readable biography by Susan Mattern *The Prince of Medicine: Galen in the Roman Empire* OUP 2013.

and Culpeper (1616–1654) but also the title of a work translated from the French.[142] The linguist David Crystal includes the word *physic* in the section Frequently Encountered Words and shows that *physic* makes an appearance in a dozen of Shakespeare's plays.[143]

The six items, in modern parlance, concerned:

1. Fresh air
2. Exercise and rest
3. Sleep
4. Food and drink
5. Bodily excretions and evacuations including sexual function
6. Healthy affection and emotional equilibrium—all of these can be connected with respect for seasonal change

I consider that numbers five and six belong more properly to physiology and emotional and mental health. They can hardly be considered as habits over which we exercise conscious control and any advice will be more medical than advice over habits. Item five invites us to prescribe. Item six is surely a matter of empathic discussion.

Though these items concern everybody, they are much influenced by local ideas in place and time. The first temptation for those who give advice is to air their prejudices.[144] Let us hope that herbalists are alert to this danger and want their recommendations to follow best practice, best evidence, or common sense. But even these three notions are subject to wildly differing notions of what is or is not good advice. Culture, ethnicity and social background may give very different accounts of what is considered good and normative and what kind of advisor is most trustworthy. So, a gap between giver and receiver may have to be bridged. In any case, when telling people what to do, always question your inner tyrant.

A consumer culture will promote advice that is commodifiable above all else. A culture such as ours that makes a fetish out of information will want that information to be connected with a commodity, usually with some point of sale. Turnover of ideas promotes anxiety and anxiety is good for business, so fashions must change rapidly for profits to be maintained.[145] Fashionable advice often comes with a strong infantilising message, as if one cannot be trusted to conduct one's daily life without expert advice. "Natural health" remains profitable because it consolidates fashionable advice for those who are fearful or phobic, fastidious to the point of squeamish. What would "unnatural health" look like? Herbal medicine is native and natural in a sense that does not need scare quote-marks.

---

[142] By Nicholas La Framboisire, physician to King Louis XIV of France.

[143] Crystal, D, Crystal B: *Shakespeare's Words: a Glossary & Language Companion* (Penguin 2002) xxvi, 326.

[144] If it looks as if I am about to air mine, I am only joining forces with those who want to resist received wisdom.

[145] If you think I exaggerate, this notice came today from the American Botanical Council: Sept. 28–30, 2022, Las Vegas, NV. This business-focused event will bring together brand representatives, retailers, and investors to meet, network, and initiate collaborations with the intent of expanding their footprint in the cannabis market. "Expanding the footprint" does not sound like a therapeutic strategy.

My own approach to offering advice to patients about these questions of fundamental importance is first to diffuse any patient anxiety. This can come across as dismissing their fears so it is most important to avoid being just as strident as those dictators of fashionable obsessions. For example, in certain situations, hydration should be a primary concern but for the most part, if you are not in an extreme weather event or crossing a desert, just rely on your sense of thirst. The unspoken message currently suggests that you and your sense of normality cannot to be trusted and you had better cling to a bottle of expensive water in single-use plastic.[146] Fortunately, there has been some sensible debunking from those opposed to this kind of highly profitable myth-making.[147] If a person's urine is dark, it is a good sign that their kidneys are doing their job of concentrating wastes efficiently.

Everyone would agree that some conditions like gout, kidney stones and urinary tract infections call for a very attentive and quantitative approach to drinking water so in such cases thirst may not be adequate and needs to be actively supplemented. I am perhaps overstating the issue and can recommend instead of constant sipping, the habit of drinking a pint or more of water at one go mid-morning and again mid-afternoon. Makes a good pick-me-up, especially if followed by a cup of tea. Another benefit of drinking a large glass of water all at once is that false hunger pangs may be allayed, reducing the urge to snack.

To give advice is a human temptation, even when none is solicited. There have always been advisors, some appointed, some self-styled. The very act of offering advice invites hubris. Humility and tentativeness are not considered market strengths compared to brazen self-promotion. This is where the Hippocratic oath stands our patients and ourselves in good stead. It has stood the test of time.

Coming, then, to the first four of the "nurtures" which overlap with one another and are the basis of the good life:

Exercise in fresh air
Rest
Sleep
Food and drink

To advise on these has always involved opinion and debate but opinion and debate—now democratised and therefore crowded and noisy—has become fractious and not necessarily pluralistic. Here goes:

1: Take gentle daily exercise in open air and natural light

This—my first item of advice to most patients—I used to think was universal and uncontroversial. Now it has to contend with the notion that only strenuous exercise can keep you "fit" as if fitness were the only measure of health and as if strenuous exercise can

---

[146] In this approach, the mains water is not to be trusted even if it does save you from the cholera that plagued our great grandparents and many people in parts of the world today who cannot rely on clean water. If you don't like the chlorine that saves lives, you can always put a jug of drinking water in the light for it to evaporate.

[147] Listen, for instance to *Inside Health* on BBC Radio 15 February 2022 where hydration myths are explored by a GP and by Professor Neil Turner, renal specialist.

have no unfortunate consequences. Fit for what, exactly? It makes healthier sense to think of a benign ratio between movement and rest rather than exercise and rest, so that getting up from sedentary work and moving about frequently is as important as pausing to rest from intense physical work. Walking can resolve inertia. Rest conserves calories for movement, for useful activity. Rest leads to refreshment, inertia to depression.

Health has more to do with co-operative harmony than with competition, against self or others. Athletes were fêted in the Athens of antiquity because the likely brevity of their lifespan made them martyrs to triumphalism.[148] There is also the contemporary desire in those who run regularly for the rewarding buzz of one of the hormones of gratification. But hormones never operate in isolation so while I would not want to say anything against gratification, and raised dopamine levels may be just the thing the patient needs, it is possible that other underlying tensions are not being addressed. Strenuous exercise will affect both the catabolic and anabolic arms of metabolism; the balance of these will have consequences for the four hypothalamic-pituitary axes (HPAs). It is likely that an imbalance in these will have created the problems for which the patient presented in the first place. The drives are complex, may border on obsessive-compulsive behaviours, and a misplaced fear of joining the obesity epidemic. They are poorly researched because governing bodies do not want to diminish the message that exercise is "a good thing" to a relatively inactive population.

The real focus should be on daily movement alternating with rest. Walking—our primary exercise—is rhythmic: it helps establish our range of movement and engage our capacity for paying attention. As I have said earlier, movement generates a charge. A useful aerobic charge can be obtained by getting seriously out of breath twice each day. This can be simply achieved within thirty-seconds, by running up and downstairs, for example.

Walking in open air seems intuitively correct, but if it needs emphasising, the following all provide a free invitation to health: being flooded with negative ions, the pleasure of the air and gentle oxygenation, with enough sun to promote the synthesis of serotonin in the ganglion cells of the retina (convertible in the pineal to melatonin), and of vitamin D in the skin without burning. Probably everybody appreciates all those things but need encouragement or practical help to overcome their constraints. We would not have had Wordsworth's best work if he had not taken so many long walks. Walking connects with other qualities of the good life.[149]

In ancient times, when open fires were the norm, fresh air as an absence of smoke would be clearly perceptible.[150] Although we have currently reduced from very high levels the amount of large and visible particulates from smoke (>2.5 micrometers) and hope soon to phase out diesel vehicles, amounts of tiny particulates are rising.[151]

---

[148] Hippocrates was not an Athenian.

[149] These have been cited as: "the practice of affection, physical exercise and the acquisition of knowledge." Though I cannot recall her name, I bear the words of this wise woman always in mind.

[150] The first part of the Hippocratic corpus considers "Ancient Medicine" from *their* perspective now some 24 centuries in *our* past. The treatise that deals with Air is really about winds over places.

[151] Air Quality Expert Group: Fine Particulate Matter (PM2.5) in the United Kingdom, Department for Environment, Food and Rural Affairs et al. 2012.

These can enter the blood stream from the lung and accumulate in organs and blood vessel walls. It has been estimated that such particulate pollution (30–100 nanometres) contribute to 21% of deaths by strokes and 25% by ischaemic heart disease.[152] So be careful where you get your fresh air and how you use heat to cook.[153]

Alternation—between activity and rest, between focus and distraction in a relaxed, musing kind of way—provides one of the keys to health. Alternate rather than fixate. None of this moderation is likely to persuade marathon runners away from their obsession. Addiction to strenuous exercise is just that: addiction.

2: Balance of work, rest and recreation

This second nurture follows from the first. As life is movement, so is rest but at much reduced frequency and amplitude. Activity and movement are as essential to life as rest—the autonomic nervous system is structured to that alternation—we are designed to move. Work, by contrast, if only to secure food, is as much a social as a biological necessity. Work has been a controversial subject historically and continues to be so because justice in its organisation has never been guaranteed.[154]

Temperament comes into it: idlers and dreamers, while letting the chores slip, often work very hard in their thinking, practise the arts of life and contribute a model contrast to the ever-busy. Work can be one of life's great blessings when it contributes to a person's sense of purpose.[155] Purposeful work engages the whole person in the cycle of tension and relaxation. As Wilhelm Reich put it succinctly "Love, work and knowledge are the well-springs of our life. They should also govern it".[156] For those who are excluded from such benefits, burden and drudgery results. Paradoxically, passive consumer culture has converted preparing and cooking food from an essential art into a chore, easier to watch than to do, even if the spectator obtains less satisfaction than the cook. Each nurture flows into the others.

The ratio between work and rest even within a single task depends upon circumstances and cannot be fixed or counselled. In my stints of digging ditches as a manual labourer when young, the older man would often stop and say, "take a blow", which occasionally called for a cigarette. I was surprised at the frequency of these pauses to wielding pickaxe and shovel but then I was young and had to do this for weeks or months not the decades that lay in wait for him. The ratio is really a question of respecting the rhythm of

[152] Global Burden of Disease Study 2016 Institute for Health Metrics and Evaluation, Seattle, USA.

[153] I have recommended in my cookbook to be published by Aeon Books in 2024 (*eat well~feel well*) to braise in heavy pans over low heat instead of frying or grilling.

[154] Rest may be constrained by external forces but gentle herbal intervention can at least help with the internal constraints.

[155] Vicktor Frankl explores this basic human need in Frankl (2004). Paradoxically, this need may be most stimulated by the ludic impulse against boredom rather than industriousness for its own sake. There is a tension between creativity and doing nothing which may reflect the oscillation between dopamine and the regulatory hormone prolactin (Section 3.6). Social creatures may cultivate lazy individuals as energy reserve: no living system supports energy expended for nothing.

[156] The epigraph to his 1961 work *The Function of the Orgasm* (Bibliography).

the tasks. Modern indoor commercial work implies that rest—complete rest away from the desk—represents a reprehensible diversion from the core ethos, the deadline. Whose line is it, and who will be the sooner dead?[157]

The work ethic—the spirit of hard work and progress with contempt for idleness—provided Europeans with a restless, endless goad which they took to all continents, a burden that continues to be reexported.[158] It created much of the modern world and may indeed have had net benefits to human prosperity and health for a certain majority.[159] Those benefits, alas, have entailed atmospheric and oceanic pollution and the despoliation, even destruction of so many terrestrial habitats, as everyone knows but not everybody acts upon. They also entail much insecure work that enslaves by failing to cover the financial cost of working.

The normalisation of consumer materialism discourages us from doing less and wanting fewer things: setting a trap from which exodus may not be easy. As ever, many problems of ill-health are not medical but societal and political. The mental, emotional, and physical consequences of such illness (they come usually to the same thing) can be eased by nurture and ameliorated by a skilfully chosen course of medicinal plants.

Mindfulness in its contemporary manifestation is perhaps an exhortation to reconsider our priorities and may be taken as a technique to mitigate the harms caused by the way of life to which we may have become acclimatised and in which we may be complicit. Although self-employment often entails the very overwork we might disparage, and though it is self-inflicted, it does at least allow for self-agency. Agency and earning the respect of others are powerful indicators of good health and longevity.[160] As a herbalist, I have chosen to overwork, but I thought I had the choice. Even so, I am fortunate never to have lost the instinct for contentedly doing nothing for long stretches; not so easy to *sell* as the contemporary rush towards fretful busyness precisely because no buying is involved. Rather than being taken to task by mindfulness, we could embrace *dolce far niente*!

Maria Montessori was not the only educationist to suggest that infants work at something just for the sake of it.[161] The work of anthropologists who have studied the few hunter-gatherer societies that survive leads us to conclude that adults are inclined to do no more than is necessary to provide food. When this is accomplished, they do nothing very much, or turn to engage in something just for the sake of it.[162]

---

[157] For a comprehensive account of the relationship between exercise, rest and health from an evolutionary perspective see Lieberman (2020).

[158] Max Weber (dubbed 'the father of sociology') ascribed the work ethic to the Protestant, especially Calvinist, Reformation. McGilchrist (2019) Chapters 9 & 10 gives a helpful historical purview. The work ethic is not just of human interest but an engine for environmental destruction.

[159] Taking the cue from Benjamin Franklin: Remember, that *time is money*. In case you think I exaggerate, a fuller text given in the Postscript at the end of Section 3.8.. By his time, religious zeal had been replaced by a kind of mechanised servitude which Weber calls Rationalisation.

[160] As are the same determinants of health for employees in a large organisation: cf: The Whitehall study (1985–2020) led until recently by Sir Michael Marmot. See also Sapolsky in bibliography.

[161] She was a doctor of medicine before she turned to the education of small children.

[162] See Lieberman (2020) again; also, though not their primary focus, Graeber & Wengrow (2021).

Agonies of work and meaning are a frequent cause of illness, especially in earlier critical stages of adult life. I have been privileged in my practice to witness and reflect some of these crises of direction with positive resolutions for those patients. As Galen put it in his *Art of Medicine*: "When the body is in need of motion, exercise is healthy and rest morbid; when it is in need of a break, rest is healthy and exercise morbid".

Doctors rarely give themselves the time to consider how the qualities of work and rest and the ratio between them creates the illnesses that present to them. They have compressed "first the word, then the treatment" into a very short time, sometimes less than a minute. They may offer social prescribing if they have the time and inclination and if services are locally available but these posts are "non-clinical".[163] If time and attention are the resources needed, then we as clinicians should offer them because the "system" apparently cannot afford them.

I have talked more of problems than solutions because formulaic ideas work only for a short time, if at all. There is no shortage of generalised self-help advice on how to relax. Relaxation has spawned its own industry. The ability and capacity to rest, to find stillness and pleasure in stillness is tied up with each person's nature and biography. Although exercise at some point earlier in the day, some of it vigorous, will contribute to sleep and good health, the precursor to sound sleep is rest, not exercise (and respite from bright light).

Careful listening during a full biographical consultation may give you the cues to provide some personalised responses; the patient listening to themselves in a therapeutic space is where they may come to the knowledge of it themselves. This is where and when resolution and healing takes place.

3: Sleep hygiene

Blessings on him who invented sleep, the mantle that covers all human thoughts, the food that satisfies hunger, the drink that slakes thirst, the fire that warms cold, the cold that moderates heat, and lastly, the common currency that buys all things, the balance and weight that equalises the shepherd and the king, the simpleton and the sage.

Cervantes Don Quixote Part 2, Ch. 68

Cervantes did not exaggerate. Sleep and digestion are the primary enablers of life, generating the metabolism by which we build our tissues. Without them we cannot reproduce our own self, let alone that of a newborn. They are fundamental to human survival, let alone flourishing. They belong with the circadian cyclicity of all life. Sleep repairs the preceding day and prepares us for the following one.

The important point to make is that good natural un-fragmented sleep is a product of circadian regulation, which depends upon many enabling factors, principally good digestion. Medication of any kind has only indirect and temporary effects, and may induce a hypnotic state but not the benefit of natural sleep. Relaxant herbs taken as an infusion in the evening will calm the digestisome and so may promote natural sleep.

---

[163] From the NHS England website viewed in October 2022.

There is a wide range of plants to do just this with chamomile, lime-flowers, lemon balm, hawthorn, verbena, peppermint, orange flowers perhaps at the top of most lists.

By contrast, potent hypnotic herbs will favour only Hypnos and so are there to fall back on in the short term. The distinction is not hard and fast and so others, such as hops and stinging nettle, will often help with digestion and restful sleep but here we enter the territory of personalised remedies which feature in Part Three.

There are some habits that facilitate sleep. A summary of suggestions I pass on to patients or even those who seek an appointment for insomnia is found in Appendix I. Shiftwork and crying babies make nonsense of these, as will sleep apnoea.

When treating insomnia, you need to establish a full history of recent sleep patterns but also those in infancy, childhood and adolescence. If there is initial insomnia, is it associated with hypnogogia? If there is middle insomnia, it is probably associated with hyper-vigilance so the alpha-sympathetic will need to be addressed (Section 3.6), assessing whether it is reactive or constitutional. If the waking hour is 2 am consider the stomach, duodenum, and a difficult maternal relationship. If 3 am, calm the liver with gentle tisanes. If there is late insomnia, is it associated with dread or depression? Fear is difficult to contain—its many metabolites will put pressure on the kidney to forego its diurnal bias, it will fail to adjust diuresis to accommodate sleep. If there is late hypersomnia, is it associated with lucid dreaming or hypnopompia? If so, such a deep constitutional vagotonia may not really be a problem to be solved. As well as kidneys, the respiratory tract and colon are permissive of sleep. Improving their function will give leverage against insomnia. In summary, sustain hepatic and renal controllers of sleep as well as improving digestive and eliminative function.

Some insomniacs may (half consciously) prefer thinking over sleeping, others too alert from fears that steal their sleep. In any case, an unsettled digestion will keep anyone awake, with transit managed by bile and the autocoid team HaNDS[164] in conjunction with the microbiome. See Bile, Gut Motility, Mood and Sleep in Section 2.5c where I try to reinforce the idea that fragmentation of bowel habit leads inexorably to fragmentation of sleep. So, if you want to treat insomnia, this is the place to start.

While it would be derelict to overlook the emotional life of a patient, prolonged attention to the psychological foundations of insomnia may be in danger of amplifying and entrenching those psychic assaults.

The architecture of a night's sleep is modular, with each episode lasting about ninety minutes and consisting of a regular repeated sequence of five phases, each characterised by different types of brainwaves. The first four are Non-REM and the last a phase of REM sleep. After three or four consecutive modules have elapsed, phase architecture and overall length tends to alter. There is mounting evidence that 'high functioning' short sleepers pay a high price in later years with shortened lifespan and a greater risk for dementia. Fewer than four consecutive modules a night constitutes absolute sleep deprivation and is a major threat to health. Fewer than five consecutive modules constitutes relative sleep deprivation. Absolute deprivation for much more than a week leads

---

[164] My acronym for the autocoids: Histamine, adrenaline (from the adrenal medulla), Noradrenaline, Dopamine, Serotonin.

to irreparable damage. Chronic relative sleep deprivation reduces life expectancy and causes deterioration in all bodily systems and makes psychiatric and neurological illness and cancer more likely.[165] Pharmacological interventions do not induce normal healthy sleep but promote temporary narcosis. Their progressively shortening half-lives induce dependence and addiction; when these shorten critically, they create the very insomnia they were intended to remedy.

I have probably underplayed the ancillary role that autocoids, which double as central neurotransmitters, play in the maintenance and disturbance of sleep. Histamine and noradrenaline are arousing. Serotonin, as precursor to melatonin, is best stimulated in the retina by sunlight. I recommend patients eye-bathe early in the day from October to March by looking at the sun directly with eyes firmly closed. Luminosity is all that is needed and is quite adequate in other months provided we get out of doors into the fresh air. A bit of vitamin D wouldn't go amiss, either.

It may be that the meta-organiser of sleep is adenosine, the nucleoside that puts the 'A' into ATP—energetics again.[166] Poise as a clinical approach sets out to consider how available energy is distributed and how reserves are sequestered in the patient. In the clinical consultation, we are faced with a culmination of metabolic and endocrine processes in a person and must consider them all together. At the back of your mind, you might try to conceptualise their daily and seasonal excursions between GABA and glycine but the systemic review and history analysis is practical and detailed, involving observation and examination.[167]

State cycles, discussed in Section 1.8, mediated by the ANS (Section 3.6) emerge in personality (Section 1.9). The tabulation of discharge in Section 1.8 fails to accommodate the range of agitation, excitement, enthusiasm and delirium that invests the display of human creative variety. We try in vain to reduce it to the elements we can helpfully treat.

The historian Roger Ekirch has argued that biphasic interruption was the norm in times before the advent of electric lighting.[168] The psychoanalyst Darian Leader applauds his cultural history of the varieties of nightscape and chides us all for our overly medico-biological reverence for nocturnal hygiene. He considers that we have lost the pleasures of un-regimented slumber to the industrialised consumerist world.[169]

A small number of patients seem to behave like Ekirch's pre-industrial citizens. They do not at all consider themselves middle insomniacs, but experience nonetheless a prolonged gap—what I call a hypnopause—between the third and fourth modules of sleep as a normal intercalary epoch in their sleep before embarking on a second sleep period. I notice the hypnopause especially in older patients who, owls by preference, are trying to alter

---

[165] Walker (2017).

[166] These molecules are closely linked to information and structure as they are to energy. Adenine and adenosine are involved in the syntheses of DNA acetyl Co-enzyme A, NADP and the vitamin nicotinic acid.

[167] Just as you can fully understand music by listening without necessarily being able to read the score.

[168] His research is fascinating and challenges many contemporary assumptions: see Ekirch (2006).

[169] Leader (2019).

the habit by going to bed early. It seems that they awake more abruptly from their earlier epochs than in the later, second part of their night that gives them deep but intermittent sleep with vivid dreaming. So, their nights come in two panels, joined by a hinge. This may be their response to ageing and a way of receiving some benefit from the inevitable process.

And what of "perchance to dream"? If we try and interpret them, we may be trying to replicate a process that has already taken place—I shall try to explain what I mean next.

Dreaming

The process of dreaming (based upon what the science suggests and on my own think-ing, and dreaming), whether it is perceived or not or remembered or not, is a function of both hemispheres of the brain in a resolution of their dialogue and necessary collect-ing together of all the percepts, events, responses and thoughts of the previous period of waking, usually (and preferably) a day. The mind matches this assemblage of recent events with prior events and previous attempts at resolution. The reverberatory nature (to use McGilchrist's term) of brain circuits means that they resemble turns of a kaleido-scope and not at all the running of logic boards.[170]

This process exports its activity to all parts of the brain and therefore also sends mes-sages to the prefrontal cortex which decodes them in the only way it knows how—in dramatic imagery—where drama simply means "the thing done". The rest of the brain has no need of "interpretation" because the process is the best attempt at resolution, of reconciliation: it is the interpretative function itself.[171] Dreaming happens each night whether we are aware of dreams or remember them or not. Whether deep desires or mundane choices are involved, it is a neural collective faculty, and one that is local, capa-ble of responding to a full bladder.

The "dream" that does rise to consciousness is a summary process made by the pre-frontal cortex and most people experience them. The response to the "dream episode" may vary between people and certainly varies from night to night in the same person. Unless they are horrific, these dreams may be simply baffling or bizarre or, by contrast, leave the dreamer with a sense of import, of meaning, of resolution or insight.

Dreamers, in the sense that a culture might recognise, are people with both hypno-pompic and poetic tendencies. Therefore, they will have strong, deep and sustained operation of their parasympathetic nervous system. Poetry (as distinct from verse) results from the right hemisphere's contact with external and internal reality (McGil-christ again). Hypnopompia is a waking state that is dreamlike and occurs at the phase of awakening from sleep.

Hypnopompic dreams are not only memorable but convey a sense of meaning, peace and resolution. They may relate to the inevitable conflicts in the dreamer's life and to paths taken or not taken. They may present alternatives which it may be too late or impracticable to act upon but these kinds of dream manifest in meditative and poetic terms. They bring peace and a sense of clarity which does not necessarily entail logic or

---

[170] McGilchrist, Iain *The Master and his Emissary* Yale, New Haven and London (2009) New expanded edition 2019.

[171] If I am right, Freud's *Interpretation of Dreams* is in pursuit of a process that has already been accomplished.

call for action. Even so, they will—via the unconscious—modify tendencies and direct choices and actions for the future.

If dreams attempt to resolve the interdictions of the social day, nightmares signal a fracture, a dislocation during the process when dreaming cannot resolve conflicts. Insomnia arising from intrusions by gnawing troubles from daily life interrupt the whole process of sleep so that they do not even reach the dreaming faculties.

4: Diet: food choice and eating habits

Diet is polypharmacy. There are no simples in a balanced diet. Mono-diets and fasting are important therapeutic options but are intended to be temporary replacements for eating well and regularly.[172] Eating well can mean many different things: as everything changes constantly, food being adaptive to changing circumstances makes for better biology than maximising; even optimising may be elusive. Beyond feeding and nutrition, food is a token of conviviality and pleasure.

For the individual, phases of feeding are best regulated by the sleep/wake cycle. I recommend for adults a feeding phase of nine (or at most ten) hours in every 24 which, just by arithmetic, gives you a resting phase for the digestive system to do its work over fifteen (or at least fourteen) hours.[173] I recommend also that the daily food intake be front-loaded so that breakfast (or an early lunch) consist of the richest cooked meal of the day to provide a broad and good amount of protein, complex carbohydrate and fat (rich in herbs and spices), especially for children and adolescents for whom proprietary breakfast cereals or even wholemeal mueslis are inadequate for the developing person.[174]

As a child born during the privations of war and rationing, I was brought up never to waste food. Either because I was compliant or am just greedy, I have never left a plate with food on it. This approach to bringing up children came to seem draconian and bullying, and no doubt it was, but a hatred of food waste runs deep. In eating places these days whenever I see people leave large quantities of good food on their plate (usually salad and vegetables) I restrain myself from remonstrating with them, so I have yet to be ejected from restaurants on these grounds!

My own example illustrates how the times and culture we were born into influences our diet and food choice but also how food—the stuff of life—inevitably becomes part of our moral faculty and a driver of our psyche. Of course, war rationing was limited and often drab but it gave us one great advantage: we were not afflicted with the burden of choice.[175]

---

[172] The Golden Mean divides 24 hours into just over 9 hours and just under 15 hours. As for regularity, this may not be the universal panacea it might seem: we are periodic creatures (Section 1.5); cf Leader above. See dietary prescriptions in appendix I.

[173] This applies to adults especially over the age of 35 or 42. Children's intake should not be restrictively programmed.

[174] As advocated in *eat well~feel well* published by Aeon in July 2023.

[175] Also the Ministry of Health supplemented the diet and ensured that all children and pregnant women were guaranteed a good level of nutrition so some were better fed than they had been before the war. For the adults, coffee was unavailable so they had to make do with ersatz powders made from chicory and dandelion. Heart disease declined, longevity increased.

Choice is currently the premium offered to consumers to make us feel all the more potent and in full charge of our likes and dislikes. In a three-year-old such a stance might have been described as "spoilt". Surely, we can see through this supposedly libertarian bait offered by those who profit from the proliferation of ever-available foods, often processed. Having too much choice is almost as much a burden on capacitance as having none. It implies that we always know what we want and can easily match our desires with our needs.

Familial preferences, early life and culture are probably the strongest influences, but there are some genetic and biological determinants of food selection.[176] Innate and natural biological capacitance means that most people can eat more or less anything they come across unless it is actively poisonous in small quantities. (Any food is poisonous at a certain dose.) Populations have learned to accommodate foods just by dint of their availability and yet also to embrace exotic items when they become desirable to the people of that culture. Adaptability is built into the human omnivore, so globalised food chains do not inherently challenge most people's digestive systems, though appetite and familiarity do. Even so, there are some population differences in the toleration of some foods, lactose intolerance and coeliac disease, for instance, being common and widespread examples of idiosyncrasy. There is, then, some tension between the food choices our grandparents and parents made (or were thrust upon them) and the multiplicity we are now able to make.

Globalisation means that now many people in our culture can obtain almost any food they want; it has also led to some unhealthy eating behaviours.[177] The commodification of adolescence and the invention of the "teenager" as a fixed class has meant that perennial intergenerational conflicts and rebellion has come to focus on food. There are other more potent effects of industrialised food. For instance: inorganic nanoparticles introduced into processed food may be crossing the placental barrier and getting into breastmilk, potentially damaging intestinal regulation and compromising babies' oral tolerance, predisposing them to food allergies.[178]

Leaving aside the ethics and politics of fair trade, (others will certainly have to pay dearly for our bounty), choice makes life more complicated and so adds to our adaptive burden.[179] The suggestion that we are too busy and important to cook for ourselves is hard to miss. Diet has also become medicalised and a source of ideological struggle. Food as simple joy and pleasure may have become a struggle for tribal identity. This serves industrial food producers very well.

Should one be a nativist and eat what one's grandmother ate? Or should one approach food shopping and eating like a fraught nutritionist, bursting with declarations that "studies show…"?

I believe that food and cooking are integral to living well and simply, adopting a cycle variation within one's repertoire. The first mention of "the good life" is found in

---

[176] *Genetic Background of Taste Perception, Taste Preferences, and Its Nutritional Implications: A Systematic Review* Diószegi, Llanaj and Róza Ádány 19 December 2019 https://www.frontiersin.org/articles/10.3389/fgene.2019

[177] Diószegi and Róza again.

[178] Mohammad Issa et al., *Perinatal exposure to food-borne inorganic nanoparticles: A role in the susceptibility to food allergy?* Laboratoire d'Immuno-Allergie Alimentaire, Université Paris-Saclay, December 2020.

[179] Subject of course to food being available, a large presumption in some cases.

Aristotle and is worth reading.[180] As diet is crucial to health, the aim of physic might be to support the best fulfilment our patients can find.

> ## Clinical note
>
> Appetite in all its forms will provide many clues to temperament during the clinical assessment. Variance in mood is often linked with a impaired reward sensitivity and with phobic and squeamish personalities. Inclination to abuse or use drugs long after adolescence often indicates very narrow hedonic interests. In such cases, pay especial attention to the dopamine-prolactin oscillation. See Level Eight in Section 3.6.

I make the following dietary recommendations to patients because—on the basis of practising what one preaches—I observe them myself and hope they will find favour with some practitioners. They make the case that variety without too wide a variance within a cycle favours the microbiome more than unlimited choice with sporadic enthusiasms.

In these days of anxiety when paradoxically we have availability and variety as never before, some of these suggestions may face refusal and strong objections as well as rejection on principle by patients (and perhaps by the reader). Of course, food inevitably has political, economic, and ecological consequences, and is endowed with cultural markers. But for good food to have become a cultural minefield is a symptom of the restlessness of our times. Food choice in some quarters resembles a badge of tribal affiliation, in others an almost messianic discrimination against certain foods.[181] Everyone has to negotiate it as they see fit, but it will help to trust a pilot.

I choose to follow Tim Spector's recommendation of eating thirty different sorts of plant and fungi each week, which amounts surely to the best form of self-medication. Herbs and spices easily give you a dozen plants for starters. Then a variety of whole grains (cereal and otherwise), legumes, nuts and seeds should contribute another ten or so. Leafy vegetables such as brassicas, salad greens and other leaves, as well as roots and rhizomes should give you at least another half dozen. Leaves of chicory make an excellent bitter pre-biotic. Fermented foods make a good addition including some vinegar. Olives and olive oil need to be taken daily or at least more than one day a week. Mushrooms at least weekly (if not most days) help the gut by competing with yeasts and provide good fibre for the microbiome. Bread is best from sourdough, proved slowly. Coeliacs and those who are currently gluten-sensitive are best eschewing highly processed "gluten-free" products, relying instead on polenta and rice.

Three tins of sardines a week will ensure your supply of calcium. Of course, they are polluted—as is the whole planet—but that is not a reason for not using these to reduce your inflammatory load and to ensure good bones and teeth and good amounts of protein. To rely entirely on unpolluted food is to starve.

---

[180] *Eudemian Ethics* 1241b (revised Oxford translation ed Jonathan Barnes, Princeton, 1984).

[181] For example, in *The Plant Paradox* (Harper Wave 2017) Dr Steven Gundry claims that lectins in many vegetable foods are the cause of much modern disease.

Parmesan cheese added to vegetable foods enhance the flavour and texture and contribute a good deal of protein and calcium. For other cheeses (perhaps eaten with oatcakes) I recommend those made with unpasteurised milk from mountain herds that have grazed on herby meadows. Yoghurt makes a good addition—from both a dietary and culinary point of view—to cereals and cooked savoury foods. Milk in small amounts (added, say, to coffee) provides iodine, as does seafood and fish.

Eating large amounts of red meat is unsustainable for the planet as well as an unnecessary burden on digestion and kidneys. Once a week or fortnight of grass-fed, locally-sourced and butchered meat is the most that one could recommend. Fortnightly, liver would be the best choice of offal. Dark poultry meat has some zinc, and turkey a good amount of tryptophan.

Sugar is not a food but a dietary extract and—however it is grown—is damaging to the health of the soil, and that of the growers and consumers. Apart from its current ecological unsustainability (to say nothing of the horrors of its historical production)[182] it contains no micronutrients and brings only disease and ill-health.

Although the feed/fast alternation should be regulated by the sleep/wake cycle, there are also seasonal disruptions, especially in February and August in temperate climates[183] but also according to the individual's terrain and the personal burdens placed upon their capacitance. Whenever a person experiences disruption to their digestion that lasts for longer than a day or two, it is good to recommend a mono-diet for one to three consecutive days or for a longer fast or special diet [see Appendix I]. When I worked in France in the 1960s, the culture of taking two hours for lunch was one of the greatest contributors to public health. I think that practice has now been eroded though I have witnessed some Gallic resistance to the anglo–American business model. Our culture's habit of working through lunch is an insult to the parasympathetic branch and cannot be good for digestion. When I observe people in cafés staring distractedly at a screen as they munch through their sandwich or lunch, I think they have taken food and digestion for granted. There may be more pleasure in eating with others, but to participate fully in a solitary meal is also good for health.

A very simple tip to aid digesting a meal made up of varied components is to put only a single item or at least a single texture into the mouth and to chew it thoroughly before swallowing and then selecting the next one which may be similar or different. Sandwiches, burgers or other composite products undermine the habit of thorough chewing, with all its health benefits.

An extension of this idea would be to adopt meditative eating or to try this occasionally for a whole meal. Such a scheme provides an antidote to the notion that eating is simply the provision of nutrients. Here is an easy and reliable way to calm and relax, therefore augmenting digestive function.[184]

---

[182] As I have personally witnessed in Central America, these are not confined to the past.

[183] Expanded in Barker (2011 & 2016) and shown graphically in my *Photic Calendar* (2020).

[184] Learnt from Dr Kamyar Hedayat during his Courses in Endobiogenic Medicine in Lithuania 2015–2018.

The Eating meditation

1. Place one kind of food or mixed food with a similar texture in the mouth at a time
2. After putting the food in the mouth and before chewing, put down the utensils and place the hands on the lap
3. Chew carefully and slowly until the bolus of food really cannot be softened any more before swallowing
4. Pick up the knife, fork or spoon and move onto the next mouthful

Consistent attention to the nurtures, with their grace and pleasure, repays with good health. Once they are in place, they can be taken for granted, so fretting over health becomes misplaced.

Giving advice that one would not take oneself must count as one of the gravest examples of professional hypocrisy. Encouragement and kindness goes much further than preaching, though if you can make a strong case for the principles behind the recommendations, you stand a chance of being listened to. When asked for advice on the deeper issues, such as "what should I do with my life?" There is only one reply and that is: in your search for a "path with heart" (an apt phrase taken from Carlos Castaneda[185]) "never take advice" especially from someone who thinks they know you. The answer to these questions are found deep within, hiding in plain sight from the self you have covered; there is nothing else for it but deep and relaxed contemplation on the desires at their root; these can often be extrapolated from the things a person did and were drawn to during the early part of their second heptade; age eight to eleven, that is.

The search, then, is a brief silent project, the converse of a talking cure.

5: Bodily excretions and evacuations including sexual function

Excretions are culminations of metabolic processes and so attending to breathing with exercise and all previous nurtures along with care of lungs, skin, bile secretion (with an eye on renal health) calls for clinical vigilance alongside any advice. Just as we cannot live without nutrient as substrate for energy transformations, their products must be removed for us to maintain a steady state. Cycles of evacuation are major indicators of circadian health and is discussed in Section 2.5b, with focus on gut motility. Unless we evacuate carbonic acid in our breath, our kidneys would be overwhelmed and lose their capacity to buffer our systems.[186]

If patients want to talk about their sex lives, this is probably part of their complaint: loss of libido or sexual dysfunction. Here the review of their systemic and organ physiology

---

[185] The phrase is taken from the epigraph to the first of several accounts Castaneda gave of his apprenticeship with the Yaqui herbalist and curandero Don Juan Matus (Univ. California Press 1968). He followed this with a number of celebrated books which some regard as fictional, not the anthropological study he claimed them to be.

[186] See buffers in Section 1.8.

will run alongside hearing about their rhythms and style of life and possibly what they do and don't like.[187]

6: Healthy affection and emotional harmony

In the course of a long and comprehensive consultation, you will surely have picked up something of your patient's mental and emotional health whether or not it forms part of the reason for the appointment.

Many patients will ascribe their problems to their "hormones".[188] Loss of emotional harmony is a strong feature of premenstrual dysphoria, which herbalists can treat somato-psychically just as well as the other way around, unless you are convinced that it calls for a psychotherapeutic rather than an endocrine resolution. Nurtures five and six belong to the personalised medical part of the consultation. Generalised advice has less of a place in the treatment phase.

All six nurtures can be connected with…

Response to seasonal and meteorological change

Temperature fluctuation may well affect the ANS in a chaotic way and sufferers with postural orthostatic tachycardia syndrome (POTS) are prone to feel very unwell when atmospheric pressure changes rapidly and respond badly to squally winds. Humoral theories made much of heat and cold but it is the rate of change as much as the extremes that characterises a person.[189]

Response to weather may be amplified by season. The primary seasonal driver involves the alterations in day length and luminosity that occur in high latitudes.[190] Different terrains respond differently to the hormonal changes evoked by the critical seasonal midpoints and so need individual attention. This specifically requires analysis of the patient's current and historical disposition within the four hypothalamic-pituitary axes. Such an analysis belongs to Section 3.6 that deals with treatment strategies.

Feeling as if one is "coming down with something" is a sure sign of lowered capacitance. Prescribing plants with reputed anti-microbial properties may be the overt strategy but those same plants will help restore capacitance. Patients with meteoropathy and barometric sensitivity can do badly when there is rapid change after a period of settled weather. Often photosensitive, they prefer gentle variance and change and are easily unsettled by weather.[191]

---

[187] See the tabulation of Discharge in Section 1.8. Oxytocin and the beta-sympathetic are the surface drivers of personalities that characterise them as accumulators or dissipators.

[188] The patient might find it unhelpful to learn that practitioners of terrain medicine ascribe *all* problems to hormones!

[189] Refer back to Section 1.9 on temperament.

[190] Refer back to Section 1.5b on seasonal cycles.

[191] See also Recurrent Infections in Section 3.3. Cf. Hippocrates, Epidemics Book 1 and Aphorisms Section III: Lloyd (1983).

Surely this is as good a place as any to quote Hippocrates:

> "Whoever wants to pursue properly the science of medicine must proceed thus. First, he ought to consider what effects each season of the year can produce; for the seasons are not at all alike, but differ widely both in themselves and at their changes… For with the seasons men's diseases, like their digestive organs, suffer change."[192]

Quantity and quality: nurture by plants

These variables are often applied to sleep and to food: not just how much, but how good they were. As sleep is modular, the quality refers to its architecture but then the *number* of modules refers us straight back to quantity. The vexed contrast (at least in science and philosophy) between quantity and quality seems to me as futile as that between nature and nurture. We cannot do without both at the same time, context deciding which is of dominant interest.[193] Quality as a perceptual value depends upon the perceiver: for instance the sense of blue-ness means nothing without a viewer, whereas a light wavelength of somewhere between 380 and 500 nm (centring on 440 nm) is the quantity that correlates with that sensation.[194]

Herbal medicine is quality dominant, which is to say that the qualities of the mixtures you prescribe defy easy categorisation and the living plants present themselves to the observer in a most distinctive way, to understate hugely the effect they and their appearance in a landscape can make. So, although dosage does impose important constraints[195] qualities tend to be quite as significant as quantities. In pharmaceutical medicine, it is the other way around: categorisation is imperative and dosage critical on account of the great potential for harm involved.

We should be grateful that we live in a world where potent medication for acute, urgent, perhaps life-threatening conditions are readily available. The value of using such potent remedies in a chronic situation is, however, questionable. Their effects often limited by the law of diminishing returns so that as their efficacy reduces over time, attendant risks increase. The quantification their potency demands becomes overlooked as weeks change to months and years of continued use. There are several candidates for this type of negligence: prominent among them are proton-pump inhibitors, non-steroidal anti-inflammatory drugs (NSAIDs) and selective serotonin re-uptake inhibitors (SSRIs), as well as the hormone replacements of, for instance, corticosteroids, thyroxine, and oestrogens or progestogens. We are obliged in our practices to negotiate these situations and find ourselves treating rebound effects from withdrawal or the noxious effects of treatments that never were intended to address the underlying problems, even if they were so capable.

---

[192] From *Airs, Waters and Places*.

[193] I summarise these as the N and L contrasts, as in quaNtity and quaLity. Steven Connor has an interesting if obsessive take on quantification in his *Living by Numbers ~ In Defence of Quantity* London: Reaktion 2016. A good quirky read.

[194] Physicalist philosophers hold (in opposition to Bishop Berkeley) that the quantity of light exists independently of a perceiver. For a novel understanding and detailed examination of the question of Quantity and Quality I strongly recommend Wolff (2020).

[195] See Section 3.7 Mixed Messages.

The so-called qualities in ancient humoral medicine can be derived from admixtured quantities and so can be measured: blood temperature and haemoglobin estimation (hot, sanguine), the percentage humidity of air (in moist and dry), respiratory reserve, pulse rate. It is true that the character of the pulse is almost as important as its rate but even this can be plotted geometrically or algebraically (as an ECG does). Blood pressure monitoring can be overdone: the very measuring of it influences the measure; even so, such quantities can show up a trend and monitor the efficacy of treatment, herbal or otherwise.

Modern medicine demands statistical analysis of its interventions and calls for quantifiable evidence. None of this can be available for scrutiny unless the criteria to be evaluated become standardised. But here, quantification is replaced by *scoring*, assigning an amount to a subjective account of phenomena perceived by the clinician or reported by the patient, usually under questioning, which I liken to a form of duress. Likewise, the "findings" in social sciences and clinical psychology answer a question in the mind of the researcher and one that does not match entirely—and may be qualitatively different—from the experience of the respondent. Even at a crude level, the scoring or the questions in multiple choice surveys may not contain the appropriate question nor permit the accurate and true answer. It is a short step from designing a questionnaire that matches what the interrogator wishes to show to an article that complacently asserts "Studies show…". Partly as a reaction against the absence of readily quantifiable material in psychological treatments and wishing to distance their psychotherapeutic stance from unfalsifiable theories, clinical psychologists have embraced the questionnaire and the scoring of human behaviour they entail. They wish also to distance themselves from the speculations of Freud who considered himself a scientist and had after all trained as a neurologist.

Modern psychiatric medicine is peculiarly prone to descriptive labelling where the range of human behaviour, emotional response and cognitive styles and abilities has to be enclosed within a name. Many of the contemporary absurdities will no doubt be satirised by a future Molière once the insurance companies that fund in part the pharmaceutical interventions have lost their hold on consumerist societies.

Blaming institutions for bad decisions we all make, however satisfying, prevents us from learning and practising well with the natural qualities at our disposal. Trying to understand the qualities of our work is the work of this book. We all always build upon what came before. I pick up the thread again in Parallel Medicine (Section 3.1).

Dreams are motivational emotional phenomena which does not make Freud's speculations fraudulent. Feeling is the basis of consciousness. Feeling is confabulatory and can be dislocated in time and place, which is one important reason for hearsay to be inadmissible evidence in court. Even though the justice system tries to rely upon facts, not impressions, emotional feelings and motivations trump cognition. A quality is a perception, the feel of a quantity.

And only then the herb

After the word comes the herb. Treatment follows on from the advice about changes in habit. It is unusual to send someone away without any herbal medicine, but sometimes the hearing and the nurtures call for a light touch. More usually, where problems are deeply entrenched and constitutional, medicinal plants may need to be prescribed for long periods, with seasonal adjustments. Here the important lesson, given us by Hein Zeylstra and vindicated in practice, is not to attempt everything in one go.

As for priorities, one seeks first to improve and enhance digestion, evacuations and sleep. This way you avoid some of the fallibility of diagnostic labels. Work with strengths not deficits. Improvements to the other complaints the patient has brought to you will follow on from attention to these.[196]

Still, you might expect that diagnosis should precede the formulation of a treatment plan, that a prescription is invalid without some idea of what one hopes to achieve. Of course; I want only to emphasise that a diagnostic label can easily be a social artefact and a distraction from a careful reading of the physiological presentation. More on diagnosis below.

If you have attended to digestion, evacuations and sleep, you will almost certainly have taken note of the disposition of your patient's ANS. Invariably this will tell you how best to modify it as the first line of treatment. Then their symptoms will also indicate how their autocoid circuits operate with each branch of their ANS and with each of the H-P axes.[197]

---

[196] If your patient has good appetite, eats well, suffers no abdominal bloating or reflux, experiences a regular bowel habit with nothing remarkable about the stools and enjoys sound and refreshing sleep, then you may have a puzzle on your hands! The sources of the presenting complaints of this unusual patient will eventually reveal themselves, probably through the maternal line.

[197] See Level Seven in Section 3.6.

While you are devising strategies to modify the patient's dispositional response to these, you then go on to consider the organs and bodily cavities and how best to support their function and drain any congestion.

Just by looking carefully at your patient and from clinical examination, it becomes clear whether their metabolism is overall in an anabolic or catabolic state or in balance. Current weight, height and morphology need to be matched against birth weight.[198] How childhood physique changed at puberty and whether growth stopped then, or how much of a post-pubertal growth spurt was experienced will all give you some indication of the relative dominance between the two anabolic axes: the gonadotrophic versus the somatotrophic. This assessment has to be seen against the level and character of physical activity of the child and adolescent. The easiest opener is to ask "Were you sporty?" If so what kind of sport: teams, hand-to-eye, endurance? The catabolic axes will influence the age of menarche and adrenarche, which may also indicate pheromonal influences in the home.[199]

You want to analyse the patient's terrain, to elucidate the disposition—first imprinted in the womb—to help throw light on their current and recurrent problems. This is what we are aiming to understand with the history of early life, of the first three heptades: the conjoint working of the major H–P axes. These give you the most reliable cues to the patient's metabolism. These clues need to be integrated with your understanding (mainly from digestion—see above) of the bias within their ANS and the capacity of their digestive organs (with their small intestine and colon microbiome always in mind).

These levels of treatment are tabulated and summarised more fully in Herbal Treatment Strategies by Levels in Section 3.6.

Communication before interpretation

People are understandably queasy about artificial intelligence (AI) in medicine but, as the distinguished psychologist Daniel Kahneman documents in great detail in his latest work,[200] we should be more concerned about the misjudgements we and others might make. He and co-workers document disastrous outcomes that have flowed from flawed opinions in criminal law, medicine and forensic science. The authors argue that we have less to fear from errors that robots might make than the actual harm caused by bias and confusion in decision making

The surest way to optimise your strategies and to avoid errors is to dedicate the amount of time to the patient that she/he needs and to make contact with their feelings rather than their thoughts and secondary opinions (by which I mean labels attached by self or others).

---

[198] The importance of the relationship between current morphology and birth weight is developed in a variant of the *Thrifty Phenotype Hypothesis* developed by David Barker. It may be a powerful predictor of cardiovascular risk and the development of Type 2 diabetes. Barker, David (1998).

[199] *A hypothesis on the role of pheromones on age of menarche* Burger, J Gochfeld, M 1985 https://doi.org/10.1016/0306-9877(85)90018-0 *Family composition and menarcheal age: Anti-inbreeding strategies* Matchock, RL; Susman EJ Am. J. Hum. Biol. 18:481–491, 2006 See also: Barrett and Dunbar (2007).

[200] *NOISE ~ A Flaw in Human Judgement* Kahneman et al. (2021).

Feeling is the reliable diagnosis of the self.

Put simply, the quality of your attention, the fastidiousness of your process and the time you give to free and open communication leads to your better understanding, to the patient's experience and the best possible interpretation of their situation and how best to modify it with medicinal plants. Bandying about a handful of labels cannot compare with this summative interpretation. It replaces a jargon-laden process with great benefit and leads on to efficacious treatments, once the nurtures have been fully detailed.

So, medicine should be communicative before it is transactional, educative before it is interpretive. Education is a leading yourself out of where you are to a better place.

Diagnosis

Don't rush into it. Avoid labelling in personalised medicine. Diagnosis may serve as shorthand but best to think carefully about the individual and their history before generalising. The patient may have arrived bearing a diagnosis (or even clinging to one). It is your duty to modify it gently, unless it gave them comfort.

Your treatment strategy will need physiological names and pointers. How else would you go about choosing the plants that you do? How else would you explain to the patient and other medical professionals what you are trying to achieve, or to yourself when you come to clinical audit? But if you want to practise personalised medicine, avoid tagging the patient with a syndrome. Give them a paragraph or two, not a word or two as a label. The generalisations you will have to make belong to physiology and the naming of parts will of course be anatomical. It is too easy to reach for ready-made ideas and presumptive labels like irritable bowel syndrome (frequently called by its acronym IBS). Some labels are serviceable, but think it through before falling back on untestable ideas like "leaky gut" unless you know how to stop the leak.

This does not mean that you reject medical diagnoses brought by the patient, providing they result from imaging and other investigations, from clinical methods and not on guesswork. Even in such cases you need to review the medical record with a critical eye. I am told by a doctor in an Accident & Emergency department that unexplained vomiting and diarrhoea is invariably labelled as "viral enteritis" and respiratory distress given some presumptive diagnosis in the absence of findings.

The deeper criterion is that the diagnostic label—the attempt to explain briefly—needs to satisfy the patient's sense of themselves as much as it serves the clinical communication. It should not diminish or reduce them. Shorthand is all very well for professionals but encompasses the patient experience very poorly. This is where the educative empathy of the therapist comes to help the process of healing and acceptance.[201]

Having said all that, I did not resent being labelled a "spasmophile" by Dr Lapraz (along with a characteristic Parisian shrug) as it perfectly explained my default physiological response to reduced poise.

If you will recall from 'Impediments to Recovery' in Section 1.1 (and 'Hot and Cold' in Section 1.9), spasmophilia is a brake—an impedance mechanism—that slows up a person whose immediate energy is not supported by adequate reserve.

---

[201] Cf. Montague (2022).

If the person overrides this impedance and carries on disregarding the impediment afforded by their symptoms, (and spasmophilia is rich in symptoms), their terrain may invoke the second level of impedance—the 'histaminic'. As we shall discuss in Sections 2.5a and 2.5a, such irritable, agitated states provide a strong motive to find peaceful rest so that energy may be replenished.[202]

The third lowest level of impedance—the 'arthritic' usually serves to limit movement and normal function and so is very difficult to ignore.

So, when you are faced with these clusters of symptoms, it is more helpful to think of them as responses to loss of poise that have become entrenched rather than fixed diagnoses. They are stages of impedance acting in physiological defence of the integrity of the terrain. You want to encourage mobility in your patient's terrain, raising it to a higher level of capacitance. Your treatment will aim to make these losses of functionality temporary, to move upwards.

Before discussing what your therapeutic plan might be, first best ask how the patient frames their situation. Is their complaint a question or an attempt at an answer? Sometimes the problem is cut and dried or at least presented as such. You do not have to question their self-assessment or probe for deeper currents. If some kind of grief is beneath the physical complaint, it will surface given time and over a long and thoughtful documentation given by the system review of medical history and physiology of general health. If some kind of grief surfaces, the psycho–social mind is involved whether or not it comes with a label. Each case of depression is unique: an outcome of the terrain intercepting its world. "Anti-depressant" remedies do not have to be reached for: the terrain will respond to any prescription that supports or supplies what is needed. Physical pain in a joint or on a limb that is visible and palpable may be associated with a collection of griefs just as much as may visceral disturbance, distress or discomfort.

This is not to say that all physical complaints are in the mind but the mind is always involved, as much in physical states as any other. The mind has visited arthritic changes in hand and wrist or an inexplicable rash. Lack of anguish at such changes, apparent to any observer, may be a sign of stoicism but that itself is a mental or temporal disposition. What we call stoicism may be no more than the normal melancholy that can attend all conscious beings. Only social or pack animals display joy or exuberance. For the rest, consciousness of the immensity of the world looks like the melancholy of acceptance. Though we cannot ask animals, sometimes there may be little more point in asking humans: sadness may simply be the default position of a thoughtful mind. To feel (*pathos*) is to suffer. Witnessing it may be the required remedy.

All I would suggest is that you not arrive too soon at demarcations that are too definite. The deterioration in the structure and function of a small joint points not to lack of poise in the present but its loss in the past. By great contrast, intractable clinical depression, suicidal ideation, complete inability to operate in the world (which might come on in stages) present families with great challenges, overwhelm general practice, and belong usually in a psychiatric hospital. If they do well and are discharged well, they may be grateful. But there are disorders of affect and delusional states that have

---

[202] Histamine provokes an irritable mood but also irritates surface membranes in the upper and lower respiratory tract, the alimentary tract, and the skin. Treatment strategies will be found in Level 7 in Section 3.6.

to contend with the clumsy affectless diagnoses of that profession and treatments that are either harsh or ineffective, or both. I have seen my fair share of psychiatric cases and claim no special insights but did notice that a few simples were often able to take the edge off the suffering.[203]

If all experience registers in the adaptive body and if mental illness has its basis in a reactive physiology, all ailments are invested in the tripos of domains (see Figure 12) from where they reemerge for us to look and listen before presuming to act.

Brooding and rumination are connoted negatively in our culture, equivalent to or a presage of "mental illness" as if illness were anything other than a subjective state. One that we would dearly love to objectify with the unspoken suggestion that the "sufferer" is failing as a productive market agent. This is not new: *accidie* was seen as a sign of lack of grace if not sin in the middle ages: the agricultural labourer John Clare was committed to an 'asylum' against his will though his poetry now is celebrated. Brooding and rumination bring the poet in us to the poetics of our reality.

Poetics find equivalence with the melancholy of perception, a lowering sensation, floating downwards. Shakespeare's Merchant of Venice opens with Orsino broodily listening to music that "hath a dying fall".[204] As wave forms characterise biological phenomena, what goes down will eventually rise up just as day follows night. Joy is the rising, metallic counterpart to melancholy, trumpeting a rising above all gloom. Joy as an expression of unity and connectedness may be found in nature as may sadness at separation and inevitability. A sense of humour depends upon both. The move towards the top and bottom of the wave are expressed globally in the duality of glycine and GABA, operated on by the autocoid hormones. Poetics offer a version of reality and, when truthful, avoid sentimentality. Medicine, like poetry, witnesses the reality of the patient.

---

[203] One notable case, who was the subject of a BBC television documentary, would not submit to coercive treatment until she had "spoken to my medical herbalist". The staff eventually conceded (for a quiet life presumably), because she always did comply after talking to me. They made her use the coin telephone in full view of everyone but this perhaps suited her theatrical style. This was before mobile phones and may have given her some sense of agency.

[204] Act 1, scene 1 in Complete Works, Clarendon Press, Oxford 1988, p. 693.

The consultation

The singularity

As statisticians are fond of broadcasting: association is not the same as causation. In the stream of life, all things are connected. In its maelstrom single agents do lurk but only because the system has woken them from dormancy. Cholera becomes a pandemic when previously separated waters meet.

The whole point of systems medicine is that a problem with a single cause is a rarity and not routinely seen in clinic. If a child falls off his bike and breaks a bone, the cause may seem to have identified itself and so it may be, but his levels of attention and physical agility may also have played a part. I was an accident-prone child and you can see me projecting male gender, so let's move away from the individual to the singularities we call pure accidents. Herbal medicine first aid may have a place in recovery: comfrey and calendula, yarrow and arnica but herbalists routinely treat quite a different kind of singularity.

The differences between all people are genetically much smaller than they appear. The phenotype may be unique but the human genotype is essentially the same with minor differences (with occasionally major outcomes in rare disease). An individual is unique in that no-one shares experience and epigenetics exactly (and one's microbiome becomes especially one's own). An individual's uniqueness is not an entity but a nexus of relations and feelings about those relationships. For example, the relationship of each of my two brothers with our maternal uncle differs from each other and from mine. Yet they started as similar and shared then diverged so that they are now quite different in character: different routes share common roots. The divergence also reflects difference in our characters, part of which stems from our birth order. Divergence and convergence characteristically occur within families, often manifesting at births, deaths and marriages, then they may retreat into quietness between these events. Friendship—convergence outside the family—is a most precious gift to health. Capacity for friendship perhaps improves the chances for successful love matches.

In the clinical situation, the practitioner is invited to the singularity of a person in a certain time and place and alters and expands it by becoming involved in its intimate details. Medicinal plants may further alter the terrain: that is the point of their prescription. The hippocratic ethic reminds us, however, that we remain outside the singularity except within the confines of the consultation.

The consultation

After the first observations, do not shorten the initial phatic phase too soon: it gives an opportunity to display a bit of your hinterland and yourself as worthy of trust. As a cultural trope, it reverses symmetry in the encounter in the patient's favour, so do not "get to the point" too abruptly except with brisk and impatient persons.[205]

Once the important phatic phase of the conversation is over, I explain and hope the reader will follow me) that plants as remedial agents are often quite effective but, when effective, only for a short time.[206] If that sounds like faint praise, the following is quite the opposite: what plants can do more remarkably, consistently and predictably—I quickly go on to reassure the patient—is to modify the relations within the neuroendocrine system, to nudge the terrain into a more harmonious state. I reassure them that we will not overlook the current complaints, but these started longer ago than might be assumed (as will always be the case).

Was the current predicament inevitable? Could not their terrain have resisted it? What caused it to develop? Was it just contingent life factors that led to this lack of capacitance, or were changes in season, or even heptade to blame? Or all of the above in combination?[207]

These precipitating factors will emerge both for practitioner and patient as the phases of the conversation unroll. The internal narrative the patient has been carrying for a while may fixate until it is spoken aloud; then it alters at each externalisation and the alteration is entrained by the listening environment.

Towards a profile of the patient's terrain

After the presenting complaints have been given due airing, and I have explained the concept of the terrain and some of the background, I ask the patient whether I might build a profile of their terrain, which inevitably starts with the past and current state of health of the mother. This starts the ball rolling.

---

[205] In Japan, at least in the past, taking the longest time to get to the point is considered an art in allowing understanding to unfold.

[206] I exclude from this the great perennial efficacy of *complex simples* but these are widely available; nobody needs see a herbalist for them.

[207] For capacitance, see Section 1.1; for rhythms, cycles and seasons, see Sections 1.5 and 1.6.

Of course, you will match your enquiry to the character and style of the patient, as they start to connect their present predicament to past events which may or may not require a prompt or cue from you.

It will go smoothly if you are relaxed and practiced—that is how performance flows and improvisation works. You will need a good system that you have internalised, with an unfussy but comprehensive record sheet that suits your methods. You will need one even if you have a prodigious memory because the patient needs to know that events are being registered and externalised. Even patients who profess to be rebels will expect their practitioner to be ordered. But there is an important middle point between recording and eye-contact. To be forever writing will greatly resist to flow, distract your concentration and interfere with the eye-contact conducive to therapeutic engagement. It also implies that you are taking dictation. Especially when the material is most sensitive, the sense of it being taken down verbatim (which may be appropriate in a court of law or police custody) would be unsettling. On the other hand, if you write nothing at all, the patient might wonder what you have managed to retain.

The design of the record sheet lifts you out of this dilemma. Make it large enough to be scanned at a glance (I use A3 landscape) so that you just put a tick or a shorthand symbol against the answer to your question. Nothing does more to dissipate trust and attention than fumbling or ruffling through sheets of paper. When it comes to sensitive material, I write it up in a little more detail when they have, say, gone to the loo or are rummaging in their bag or are otherwise distracted or a natural pause comes in the conversation. Blood test results and medical reports are usually printed on A4 paper. They can therefore slip inside your A3 master sheet without the need for fumbling with pins or clips which fall out anyway. By folding the whole document in half to A5, it makes a convenient handful and can be stored in an A5 box or cabinet. You may prefer some other system but have one that displays the salient facts at a glance and doesn't rely upon reading copious notes. Don't underestimate the importance of the art of documenting the case. I shall return to this later on in the following section in a segment on case records. I presume that even the youngest reader will accept that the ancient technology of paper and ink from plants will be less intrusive than an electronic machine.

After you have together established the important nodes of the terrain and once you have chronicled the medical history (including their experience of menstruation and obstetrics, if relevant), and know something of their familial and social arrangements, it will be time for a systemic review. One way of embarking on this would be to talk through their day which might start with "what did you have for breakfast"? However, you do it, you arrive at some notion of diet and sleep, the two critical functions of life and an opening to embark on the nurtures, discussed at length in Section 2.2. Exercise can come out of the musculoskeletal enquiry and you need to know if there is a history of tobacco use and the current intake of alcohol.

After a full enough discussion of the presenting complaint followed by explaining carefully[208] that you wish to explore and develop a profile of their terrain, you go

---

[208] The explanation is usually met with enthusiasm and gratitude that someone at last is willing to seek the root cause of their problems. Health tourists and consumerists will, however, need further reassurance that you will not overlook their current predicament.

on first to understand the health of the patient's mother and then proceed with the scheme that follows:

> The critical features of a life: mother, her pregnancy with the patient, birth order and siblings, maternal grandmother, (and birth order of mother and her siblings) will emerge once you start the conversation.

According to one variant of the Thrifty Phenotype Hypothesis,[209] the birth weight is predictive of adult cardiovascular risks and gives an insight into the somatotrophic axis.[210] As does early or belated delivery, or to term. This information is not always available with younger patients—a call to a mother's mobile can provide it quickly.

Then, when the earliest phase of life has been considered—sleep, evacuation and digestion—together with the nature and experience of feeding, the period of weaning needs to be considered. Whether these phases were disturbed or unproblematic are likely to influence sleep and digestion later in life. If problematic, they often submerge and seem to disappear altogether only to reemerge when an analagous crisis hits later in life. If the patient was adopted, a separate and parallel constellation of relations, entailing a pluralised whole where the seams may be entirely or only partially restituted.

After the weanling comes the toddler. An important question to ask is whether a diagnosis of asthma was ever suggested. Infants are structurally prone to congestive states especially in cranial and thoracic cavities and asthmatic diagnoses are often made uncritically (especially as the prescription of an inhaler will seem to resolve the situation or at least to remove mother and child out the door) but, by default, file mentally as vagotonia until further tales tell otherwise. An ancillary question settles whether a tonsillectomy was considered or performed, or any other surgery. Surgery may save a life but always at a cost.

Life's first heptade of eighty-four months is developmental and its evolution is too complex for critical facts to be established in general practice. We can at least establish whether the patient was active or studious or both, and their memory of their general shape and size. The clinical point is that you are comparing current presentation with previous stages, at least as far as memory allows. You are comparing morphology, physicality, mentality and other dispositions with the backdrop of familial and social events.

Age of menarche and adrenarche is the juncture to explore the health and circumstances of the father and his family, including his birth order and siblings. As for adolescence itself, the absence or presence of acne establishes the strength or weakness of gonadic androgens respectively and the corresponding reliance on androgens of adrenal origin, the principle one being DHEA.[211] This type of hormone alters the

---

[209] Barker, David (1994) and (1998) in bibliography.

[210] Somatotrophic means growth of the body. This is the second of the two anabolic axes, (the other being reproductive) and features Growth Hormone and Prolactin. Anabolism featured in The nodes about which the tides of life swirl in Section 1.6 and will be dealt with from a therapeutic perspective in Levels 3 and 5 in Section 3.6.

[211] Dehydroepiandrosterone.

constituents of the cutaneous lipid film and so allows the microbiome on the sebaceous areas to proliferate. Indeed, the adrenal axis cooperates with growth hormone and prolactin towards a proliferative state.

Try to establish whether limbs lengthened gradually through adolescence: a growth spurt at the end of puberty signals a reemergence of growth hormone after the dominance of the reproductive hormones.

At the end of the consultation, as a seemingly idle question, you might ask if the patient resembles any one of their relatives who have been mentioned. The answers may give an insight into the symmetries at play within this informatic constellation with the patient at centre. Often a split between physical appearance and temperament is disclosed or a very strong feeling of connection with one of the personages, a grandmother for instance. For quick reference, here is a checklist of items you really do have to know to form a coherent picture on which to base your assessment and formulate your treatment plan.

Consultation Checklist for Establishing the Important Nodes in the Terrain

- Patient's date of birth; this is not a mere formality: birth months correlate with health outcomes to some extent[212]
- Mother's health and year of birth; her experiences of pregnancy and labour with patient
- Patient carried to term or early/late for dates (EFD or LFD)?
- Birth weight [see the Thrifty Phenotype Hypothesis, referenced above] mother and baby's experience of feeding, digestion, sleep and weaning[213]
- Birth order and spacing in patient's natal family and health of siblings, if any
- Comparative obstetric experience of mother with birth of siblings, (if any); occurrences of miscarriages or terminations
  - Maternal grandmother's health and year of birth; order and spacing in mother's natal family and health of her siblings[214]
- Extent of upper and lower respiratory problems during infancy

---

[212] The effects seem to differentiate between mental and types of physical disease. As important will be your patient's mother's pre-conceptual and perinatal experience.

[213] As the maternal environment during gestation directs the nutritional status of the child, there will be some relationship between birth interval and child birth weight and growth. The mother will need a reasonable amount of time for the restoration of reserves to provide optimum nutrition for a new gestation. Well-nourished women will require less time for maternal nutrient repletion than poorly nourished women. When there is inadequate time between pregnancies for the mother's reproductive system to return to optimum biological functioning, the foetus may not receive adequate nutrients and may make it more difficult for the pregnancy to carry to full term.

[214] Maternal, grand maternal, and great-grand maternal nutrient echo down the generations. Also instructive to know whether female relatives were prescribed DES or Diethylstilbesterol, a dreadful miscarriage of medicine which will ripple down the generations. During one of the early compensation cases, this scandal was called the 'silent thalidomide' according to a report by Sarah Morrison and Jaymi McCann in the *Independent* dated 22 January 2012.

- Any surgery, or strong diagnosis of infantile asthma?[215]
- Current height and the age they reached it, trying to find out whether there was a growth spurt after puberty (to assess relative dominance of gonad axis over growth)
- Current weight and their morphology in childhood
- Health in childhood and infancy, levels of activity, and tendency to engage in sporting activity and of which type (hand-eye coordination and their preference to work in teams or alone)
- Age and experience of menarche
- Father's health and year of birth with paternal grandparents' health; birth order and spacing of father's natal family and health of his siblings
  - Then to the present and health of children or others cared for; the health of their partner indicates whether they sustain or drain your patient

Vertical and horizontal axes

You will see that horizontal and vertical axes[216] are as important to the data collection as they are to the treatment plan. As the family history is recounted, affections and identifications may emerge along with anecdotes. It is worth asking the patient almost as an afterthought whether she or he strongly resembles any of the characters mentioned, distinguishing between physical appearance and dispositions. Even a mixed picture may throw up a strong physiological tendency to help with your deliberations.

But there will be horizontal branches on every vertical tree. It is difficult to understand the influence of the grandparents on the current terrain if you do not know anything about the world was like during their formative years. The wars and displacements of the twentieth century affected those people powerfully. It is unlikely that you will treat many centenarians but they will have grandparents too. If you want to find out about an old person's terrain you will have to go back a long way. When it comes to the older generation, you need to be able to understand the world as it was during their formation.[217]

> The point I want to emphasise strongly is that a good general knowledge of human geography and the history of at least the past hundred years helps you understand the situation faced by the women with whom your patient had to negotiate in formulating their terrain. When they perceive that you have some appreciation of what they and their ancestors experienced, their trust in you will deepen. Medicine is a humanity as much as a science.

After exposition and analysis comes reflection and a synthesis, a plan to move forwards. This is when the practitioner thinks everything through and is seen to do so. It is not

---

[215] Bronchodilators and steroid inhalers are routinely prescribed for persistent cough.

[216] Discussed in Section 1.5a.

[217] I have treated only two centenarians but my grandmother was born in 1884 in the west of Ireland. I spent time in her village in my teens when it was more like the place she knew than ever it is now, a few decades on. These facts and experiences affect my knowledge of the people I treat now and feature in my own epigenetics.

an abrupt stage but a culmination of observations made throughout. There is a marked difference between confidence and certainty. The former comes from experience, the latter from lack of it and the humility we all need in the face of the unknowable.

It may seem like an elaborate courtesy but I think this plan to move forwards needs the patient's explicit agreement. Surely their presence is tacit commitment to the process? I know, but commitment comes in stages, so I ask them whether they would like me to put my mind to a prescription. Then I tell them how many preparations I plan to dispense, just so that there are no surprises. I have been caught out before when the cost came as a shock, but it is not just about money. Generally, I dispense enough tincture to last forty or sixty days, depending upon the case and the season.

When you deliver your preparations to the patient, rehearse the labels and present the bill, they will generally ask what comes next: how do we proceed?

Strategies: follow-up

Writing a prescription is rarely a one-off event (though I have written these from people who are about to disappear and those who are about to die a good death). For reasons of cost or difficulty in making arrangements, I recommend that some patients let the preparations run out and then (following a fortnight of reflecting on life without herbs) arrange to collect a repeat of the treatment, which they may suggest needs tweaking on the basis of that reflection and their experience of the process.

Others, though, will want and some will need a follow-up consultation. This gives an opportunity for you to reassess the long-term strategy in light of their response to treatment. Some will be engaged with adapting to disease and so your witness needs to be extended, perhaps for some time. Hypertension in those over sixty need at least eighteen months for the process to reach a desirable plateau. Hypertension in those under sixty may be transitorily associated with one of the endocrine pauses and that may need rather more than eighteen months for the process to play out fully.

Three time aspects also concern how you develop strategies for the long term:

1. Season
   As discussed in Nurtures (Section 2.2) and Temperament (Section 1.9), some people are more sensitive to seasonal change than others. The season at which a person first presents may give a clue to how seasonal change is embedded in their terrain, reinforced by annual returns for the same or supposedly "different" problems. In such cases, it might be helpful to suggest pre-empting trouble *before* it happens by inviting them for an annual appointment ahead of their troubling season.
2. Stages
   If the first visit coincides with an *early* developmental stage at heptade or other critical juncture,[218] one treatment should suffice to set them on the right course to complete the stage without further difficulty, indeed with enhanced understanding and scope for health. A later heptade usually requires reinforcement of the treatment, but not necessarily continuously so but by seasonal adjustments for some portion of the heptade.

---

[218] Such as a prime number age: see Sections 1.5, 1.6, 1.9.

3. Phases

This is just a shorter version of the Stage (as above) and though one treatment may be sufficient, the phase may recur in similar fashion at another critical place in the same heptade.Another way of looking at phases is that they occur—reliably but irregularly—in cyclothymic individuals. In such patients, phased or pulsed treatments are generally to be preferred though the phase may be as long as a season of three months.

Before, during and after consultations

L iving systems are relational: about events, not things in isolation. Personalised medicine is not individualism but treating each person within their unique relational system. A person's physiology is equivalent to an ecosystem but one that is inherently psychosocial. Rehearsal of its whole extent leads to therapeutic realisation. Life is physical, relational and informatic.[219]

Working in this way and especially if you have a well-stocked dispensary to run, professional life alternates between extensive detail and intensive therapeutic work of the heart. These are complementary: managing nitty-gritty physical systems gives you the platform for your clinical work, which—with respect for your patients, colleagues and the reputation of herbal medicine has to be well documented, with ease of retrieval.

Case records

I am surprised when a patient is surprised that, even a decade on, I still have their records and can access them in less than a minute. Who did they think I was, a hobbyist?[220] Professional life is an archival store, a repository of knowledge and relationships of trust. Before you see your first patient invest in a record system that suits you and,

---

[219] Although we consider infectious disease as an assault that is worthy of remedial attention, from an ecological point of view it is a meeting of informatic systems. Even though the introduction of medicinal plants into a body is not a live event, the plants had once been fully alive and so we profit from the products of those informatic systems.

[220] I have been sent some case records that didn't even look as good as that, which shocked me in a profession that takes itself seriously. I hope rolled up handwritten narratives on scruffy lined note paper belong to the past: NIMH is an institute because it has a documented history.

however idiosyncratic, will be consistent across the decades even though it will develop and evolve as you do. As explained in the preceding section, I strongly advise against recording narratively during the consultation. Afterwards, copies of letters, emails and synopses can fit within and alongside the consultation record.[221] Even in a digital age (or perhaps especially now) paper records provide overall greater security and legibility and are less prone to breaches of confidentiality.

While you need to keep medical and dispensary records together, they need to be capable of being separated so that you can, with the patient's consent, transmit a prescription record to another professional, without compromising the confidentiality of the initial consultation.

I recommend a card system that holds all the personal identifying details. If you ask them to fill out a card in their handwriting, it implies that they consent to treatment. Don't ask them to fill any other disclaimers or put their name to any horrid legalise. Just a small card to which you can later add a numerical code. Then the medical notes that make up their main record contain only name, sex, and date of birth with the numerical code; the prescription record will have only family name, sex, and age and the numerical code. File the cards in alphabetical order and the records in numerical order. It may not be a very sophisticated system but, simple and robust, it defies casual snooping.

Before and after the diagnosis

Your patient will notice and appreciate being the subject of astute observation and the clinician's ability to remember and marshal a great deal of complex information, bringing all that to bear upon a summary diagnosis and treatment plan. They will come to trust you if kindness and patience always accompanies your curiosity and good will. In human interaction, two people in a symmetric conversation try to attune with the speed of the moment. Kindness is this attunement because no conversation can be perfectly symmetric and the therapeutic relationship cannot be, because it is staged, not casual. Neither party wishes it to be casual as that is not how healing comes about. Both are aware that there is life outside this moment but wish for a while to be separate from it.

It all takes a great amount of mental and emotional stamina, so come prepared with the biggest meal and the right amount of sleep behind you.

Once you have emerged from the educational cocoon, try to move towards your own approach, your style, the demeanour that is comfortably yours even though everyone borrows and imitates from all sorts of places. Being your authentic self will always be more interesting than being original.

"Chance favours the prepared mind" but it does not favour a mind lumbered with preparations. These, once completed, are left behind so that the emptied mind can respond with heightened awareness. This is the developmental path a new apprentice might take towards becoming a seasoned clinician.

---

[221] An A3 model of the consultation sheet is offered in Appendix III.

Clinical sense

This is not about which herb to prescribe. It is not utilitarian, not about grasping every hunch that surfaces. It is about creating a space for the patient to fill and for you to sense a gap in the narrative and to have the patience to allow the patient to fill it without prompting or probing. This permits the lacuna to be willingly fulfilled.

It is a sense of the dramatic and narrative fabric being unfolded for the first time. It is born of not doing not seeking but seeking all the same. I can say what it is not but cannot frame what it is. I can say with certainty that it comes only to the prepared mind whose preparedness are left outside the door. The prepared mind attends to everything that can be anticipated then leaves it to the event.

The event is a meeting between the known and the unknown from which both you and the patient should emerge having learnt something they did not, could not, have known. Your panoramic clinical record sheet, however you design it (and I refine mine every few months) will tell you what you have established and what you do not (yet) know about your patient.

Inevitably, you will have to ask some questions. Even if you think you can tell their bowel habit from the look on their face (a notion I don't subscribe to), you will have to ascertain not only the facts but how the person feels about them. Questions, questions, replies, responses. But even in our all-knowing liberal televisual world, now complacent, now anguished, for all its inquisitiveness, a peaceful acceptance of the unknowable can emerge. If we exclude the sense of chance, not knowing how things are going to work out, we also exclude the therapeutic moment. We also limit our capacity to develop the *clinical sense* necessary for an enduring practice.

There may come a moment in the therapeutic space where an answer emerges without a question having been asked. The lacuna in the person's narration has revealed itself.

Narrative, legend, myth, parables, oral history, stories, anecdotes, version of events, testimony, confessionals, knowing, and unknowing

Every culture has myths that tell of its origins and some foundational story speaking to the strengths and special character of its originating heroes and, by implication, bestowed on their descendants. The myth-maker is not lying or dissembling. As in literature, the truth behind the words does not belong to the author. Myths may help a person mediate between contradictions in their life, say between desire and reality. In medicine, the patient's meaning involves a re-imagining of a buried event. Mythos is the Greek for story. History writing in contrast to myth-making is supposed to have begun with early Greek historians Herodotus[222] and Thucydides in the fifth century BCE. Both relied heavily on oral testimony.[223]

---

[222] He invented the name and the genre. Good translations with interesting introductions are found in de Sélincourt and Burns (Penguin (1954) 1972); Waterfield and Dewald (Oxford 1998).

[223] While narrative may be universal, styles and forms are culturally specific as I discovered from Shinobu Hashimoto; see the segment entitled n = one in Section 3.2. Also the style of Herodotus—polycentric and paratactic—was considered old-fashioned by his contemporaries.

Oral History as a modern movement grew out of a desire to record the testimony of people whose contribution to a culture was interesting and deemed important but somehow never seemed to figure in the pages of academic history. The advent of sound recording helped develop what is now an enormous archive.

Every individual life has the makings of a biography which is not really a story but a crafted presentation of the self.[224] Biographies of prominent figures, contemporary or historical, have a certain following but by their very selectivity may almost count as works of fiction. Confessionals only entertain if something that was previously hidden is revealed or that the celebrated star author turns out to be beset by human foibles, after all.

Story-telling has civic agency and, along with genealogies, are of great political importance. The story of our age is that we are all story tellers. Everyone does have their story, of course, but it seems to me important not to conflate narrative interest with the liberating world of conversation where each participant has an equal interest in each other. Otherwise, the narrator is in danger of becoming a self-promotor, part of a world-wide vanity project. I bought a book recently to find out how to make fermented food. It started declaratively with a section called *My Story*. Somehow the author's story managed to permeate the entire book making it difficult to know exactly how best to make fermented foods. I bought another that was content simply to explain how it is done.[225]

In case my meaning in this segment should be misconstrued, everyone's story is interesting, but I want to differentiate between conversation and self-presentation, between self-declaration and self-discovery.

Since the creative writing movement took over from positive thinking in the United States, academics coined the term "narratology" perhaps tiring of the postmodern "discourse". Now that academia has become a business, its terminology has entered the public sphere and so has been commodified.[226] By a bizarre twist in this puritan world, 'dreams' (a euphemism for desires) are not to have limitations. This is energetically improbable and forgets that limitation drives inspiration. While every mention of the word "anecdotal" is tinged with apology, it is naively assumed that the narrative cannot be confounded with propaganda.

Staging the therapeutic intention: the patient as personality in time

Stories (like dreams, but with less superposition) tell of how things might be so depict hypothetical outcomes. As a reflection on causality, they situate us in time.

---

[224] By chance, the week I write this, I am invited to present an earlier (pre-phytotherapy) part of mine to a company meeting to celebrate its fiftieth anniversary. I happened to be part of it, but it might as well have been someone else.

[225] Just in case someone spots it, I do tell some personally deprecating anecdotes in my cookbook *eat well~feel well* but only to reinforce notions about cooking.

[226] If the reader is interested in the debate, Peter Brooks gives a good succinct account in *Seduced by Story: the Use and Abuse of Narrative* NYRB 2022 (a worthy follow-on to his *Reading for the Plot* NY Vintage 1985). He takes on the objections of the British philosopher Galen Strawson whose *Things That Bother Me: Death, Freedom, The Self* (NYRB 2018) is also well worth a read. I suspect it is no coincidence that Strawson (in common with the great Argentinian fabulist Jorge Luis Borges) has been a lifelong insomniac with a consequent deprivation of REM sleep.

The physical present as the source of our sensory inputs is but an episode, typically lasting a few seconds, a moment. So, time seems to pass from moment to moment. The moment gives us our current coordinates but is an extensible unit into which the most physical unit—*the day*—is divided. Lunar and terrestrial tides wash about each of our days. The so-called present, which we try to envisage as a point in time no more exists than the gap between two waves on the sea. In this sense it is no less abstract than the past or future.

The past is a storage system for events and also for what we think of as important events. Not so much a narrative as a bundle of connected episodes, roughly reassembled on demand.

The future is predicated upon the past. In childhood it is barely formed, in youth, tantalisingly open, in middle and old age, rather too formed, not to say predictable, though predictability is one of the great blocks over which humans may stumble. Our sense of the predicate has been mapped out by our circumstances and the degree to which we can prospect for change.

From the practitioner's perspective, patients divide largely along a line separating those who seek results and those who seek explanations. Not that they are mutually exclusive but the former are impatient with explanations while the latter patiently await good results.

The terrain responds and adapts to events but tends to return to a previous conformation. Life may take a random path but is equipped with a temporal compass which coordinates physical events with biological timers.

Yourself in the consultation

For it to be a sensory and pheromonal process, virtual consultations will prove inadequate. Make sure first that you have provided a therapeutic space and that, having slept well and fed and watered, you are at your most relaxed and capable. This is your preparation. A full consultation, painstakingly conducted, requires a great deal of stamina, but looking as if it is effortless puts the patient at ease. The best form for it to take is the most natural: a conversation. To converse values the ordinary against the technical and while great shared stories might belong to literature, everyone's story is interesting. Literature, after all, is technical recounting. Like medicine, it is an ethical exploration.

Conversations belong to no-one. There is neither script nor scripture. The play opens upon a fresh scene. Your knowledge base and experience wait in the wings. You and the patient are co-authors, equal but with different roles, with a theme in common: the human experience both conscious and, till that moment, hidden.

Healing may be hoped for but, as often as not, better habits for a future daily life with greater ease and comfort may emerge.

How to start up in practice

You have to announce yourself: people cannot know of your good intentions without mentioning that you are available. Advertising is proselytising: at odds with Hippocratic medicine. Besides it mostly tries to interest people in things they don't want or need or are not good for them, so that is out, and so is standing on street corners with a placard.

The more virtuous way is to speak about culinary and medicinal plants and not about yourself, except with a leaflet or card, almost as an afterthought. Once you have done this for two or three years (a realistic foundation for a successful practice) and have acquired a reputation, you can leave this good work to newer entrants to the profession. Do this to anyone who will listen but prompt groups with wildlife, gardening and child-rearing interests to invite you. The social wing of schools, colleges and churches often like to have people speak, especially if there is vocational or health interest.

Perhaps people will expect you to have a website but these are mostly vanity projects which is all very well if you are going to be a hair stylist or a life-coach. Listings—local or national—remain an important reminder that you are available however long you have been in practice.

Avoid business plans. Rather have enough people dependent upon you for failure to be unlikely. If you fail to generate enough interest in your practice, have a second best arranged: it might even have been always the better option.

Be empathic with advice, understanding how easy or practicable it will be to follow and never recommend a course that you would not take yourself.

> Best to avoid what I and others have done: to be a sole practitioner. Instead, get together with a few colleagues (seven is probably a good number) and form a collective partnership. The group practice will generate more interest more quickly than a single person can. More importantly, you will be able to draw upon a wider range of skills, aptitudes and interests. Some will prefer dispensing in some moods and others being in the clinic; at least you will be able to share the rough with the smooth; you will also be able to roster the administrative drudgery.

Dispensaries are time-consuming and expensive. Grow herbs in the garden when the medicines run out. But to have the time and energy for this hard but enjoyable enterprise, you need to feel part of a team working with and for people.

How a person or body might complain?

Central versus peripheral

After a lecture given by Dr Robin Royston at the School of Herbal Medicine, one student asked him whether he thought there was anything in the conjecture that having a problem in the periphery (such as osteoarthritis) at least protected the sufferer from cancer. As he was pondering the idea, I interjected that my favourite aunt, who had recently died from breast cancer, had to give up playing the piano on account of arthritis in her hands. I think he felt let off the hook by this contra example but it made me wonder if certain trends tend to make others less probable. Cancer was a poor choice for such a conjecture as it starts locally in a cell, then a tissue and takes so many diverse forms that though it might have a single origin it can scarcely be thought of as a single disease. Over the years, I have noticed that patients with osteoarthritis, especially in the hands, seem to be spared from cardiovascular disease, and to some extent the converse. I am half-tempted out of curiosity to search my records more systematically to see whether there are any such correlations. The other half of the thought sees this as pointless as, if validated, it would only establish a piece of lore and not really direct treatment because both central and peripheral conditions make themselves known without prompting.

In neurology, by contrast, distinguishing between central and peripheral drives the diagnostic process. So, it is with the autonomic nervous system: although the peripheral manifestations produce the symptoms, the cell bodies originate in the CNS. Although medicinal plants do not always distinguish between central and peripheral, we need to appreciate that our choice of herbs—and the dosages and mixtures we employ—do.

The terrain might withdraw from the periphery to protect the centre or, with a different centre of emphasis, the centre cannot extend its full reach to the periphery in the sense that the heart knows its own capability, or so the vagus outflow would direct it. Life flows always in a circularity, a loop that is never fully closed.

Central : peripheral | Hot : cold | Joints : vessels

Is there any truth to the old adage "cold hands, warm heart"? Osteoarthritis in peripheral joints involves inflammation so is not "cold" as used to be thought but the person suffering from it might well feel the cold. Feeling the cold—assuming thyroidism is excluded—implies that the centre has held onto the blood or that spasm in digital arteries (as in Raynaud's phenomenon) has resisted its flow (or the other way around where spasm manages a response to scarcity of blood). Chilblains, though painful, are transient, not considered serious and affect only a minority, and consequently have received little attention. Yet if there is a microcirculatory component of osteoarthritis—which has been researched extensively—peripheral joint conditions might be aided by research into vascular conditions considered minor. Cold hands implies a retentive centre, a beta-sympathetic not fully discharged. In old age, a failing heart must be considered.

For peripheral conditions you can use anti-inflammatory plants like *Boswellia*, *Guaiacum* or *Harpagophytum* (all from hot countries) or *Apium* (which originated in the Mediterranean), but you will have to keep on using them whereas if you use plants like *Achillea* you will modify the vagal tone and so ease relations between central to peripheral towards greater equivalence. This approach will need the addition of *Tilia* (to relax arteriolar spasm) along with vaso-protective plants and a diet rich in vitamin C and bioflavonoids from paprika, lemon, buckwheat and chilli.

Ageing probably affects tissues more or less equally but may tilt in some towards the centre and in others toward the periphery. More certain is the increasing resistance to anabolism during late middle age. This "sarcopenia of age" becomes inexorable at some point, resulting in the loss of muscle bulk. Given that the small joints in the hands and writ depend upon shoulder muscles, this loss of strength will put strain on these joints on which so much depends. The same could be said for knees and ankles with the muscles clothing the femurs. Pain is not just debilitating, it increases uncertainty of proprioception and reduces the capacity to exercise for the benefit of both centre and periphery.

Local treatments work well in peripheral problems: soaking hands and feet in warm oil infused with aromatic oils and anti-inflammatory plants, such as *Arnica*[227] and hand or foot or body baths in Epsom salts with sea salt for twenty minutes give a great deal of relief. An adjunct to the management of osteoarthritis would be to focus on a high protein, high complex carbohydrate diet accompanied by lashings of butter and olive oil.

Pharmaceutical treatments for osteoarthritis are generally toxic. Taking them is like throwing a spanner in the works, the opposite to the lubricant offered by herbs. Treatments like NSAID's have no long-term future, subject as they are to the law of diminished returns as well as revenge effects. This is how nature responds towards toxic agricultural products. Antibiotic resistance becomes inevitable when these potential life-savers are used in industrial nutrition, let alone in hospitals.[228]

---

[227] Just as effective and cheaper if you have a lawn full of them is to infuse in warm daisy heads (*Bellis perennis*) in a big jar of oil.

[228] See Tenner (1996).

When it comes to the systemic review, by all means have a checklist so that you know what you have yet to cover but do not follow it slavishly.[229] Rather be guided by the patient's symptoms and points of emphasis. This way you move fluently between central and periphery.

Mapping the body

Learning to examine the body does not belong in a book and certainly not in one that tells more about how to approach than how to do. Learning to read a face with all its micro-expression began in babyhood. The quality and dynamic production of a patient's voice let's you into the working of their ANS. The musicality of speech is as revealing as a person's posture and may give us a glimpse into the metabolic centre of gravity.

Looking at the abdomen is the very least you must do to assess this particular example of regional anatomy. Palpation of the abdomen will help make an assessment of the viscera. Refer pilosity (to include the eyebrows) and altered pigmentation to your assessments of the adrenal, gonadic and thyroid axes. You will have taken in texture and density of scalp hair at first glance.

The chest and areolae will exhibit the endocrine drives behind structures. Surface structures can locate vents to inner function and so offer you clues to treatment. Petrissage below each clavicle will relieve not just muscular tension but liberate energy to deeper structures and energetic function, a performance mirrored above the scapulae.[230] Broad shoulders in both sexes witness strong androgens.

On the back, tenderness at the bronchial point of T4 speaks of unmanageable pressure on that pivot. Tenderness on the scapulae and their medial borders suggests an overcharged liver on the right, pancreas on the left. Below them, if rolling the skin produces a bright pink flare and exquisite tenderness, the adrenals have long been overtaxed. The technique taught by Dr Lapraz involves raising the whole thickness of the dermis and pushing this roll with its fascia firmly with both thumbs; it is not pinching as one of my patients used to dolefully call it.[231]

Immediately below the knees medially, if firm thumb pressure elicits a brisk pain, on the right indicates gallbladder congestion on the left pelvic congestion and an overtaxed thyroid (even if biochemically euthyroid). As for the feet, refer to Balance and Proprioception in Section 1.3.[232] Cracked skin on the sole and foot edge implies strong growth hormone, but you could probably tell that from long bones and a strong chin. If the top of the foot is chubby and soft, prolactin will be strongly expressed.

Always look at the tongue if only to assess the degree of yeastiness in the colon (and recommend mushrooms to lower it). If the size is large for the mouth (growth hormone dominance), the teeth will leave indentations on the margin. If bright, central perfusion

---

[229] I have offered mine in Section 2.4a.

[230] Petrissage is a kneading massage technique that applies pressure to deep tissues and contrasts with the slow, smoothing stroking of effleurage.

[231] But he really did appreciate that the pain produced gain. The technique is as much treatment as diagnosis.

[232] See also Figure 7 in Section 1.5a.

is high, if light, peripheral perfusion low. A bright red tip is supposed to indicate hepatic congestion. Take the radial pulse at the very least though why not auscultate when looking at the chest? It pays to invest in a cardiology stethoscope as I did as a student wanting to minimise my natural limitations. You can listen to the music of all that activity.

Mental illness

Not so easy to map the mind as the body, not just because of the brain's complex microstructure but because the products of the mind—speech and imagined worlds—are intangible even after they have been communicated. "Medicine is too narrow" would say one of our lecturers in medical physiology at the School of Herbal Medicine. Dr Robin Royston had been an anaesthetist at a London hospital and was undergoing therapy and training as a Jungian analyst at the time he was teaching us. He adopted a tone of wry worldliness as perhaps a way of inducting us herbal idealists into a state of greater realism; he went on to become a consultant psychiatrist. When it comes to mental illness, I would charge modern medicine as being also too knowing, as if it concealed within its narrowness a lofty sense of broad understandings, as if medical doctors really believed that the term psychosomatic could really explain anything. All illness comes from a state of personal consciousness that has to face the world and its history of doing so, whether you have lost a leg or your 'head'. Literature, broader than medicine, can give us a body of case studies of individuals and of cultures, a set of examples, for which we could reasonably use the word paradigm. Mental disorders are real enough but states labelled as mental illness can sometimes medicalise reasonable unhappiness or associative distress, they also testify to and police social norms.

The industrial medical systems in industrialised countries attempt to nail down all manifestations of human consciousness and behaviours by a comprehensive system of labels, the most egregious example of which is the *Diagnostic and Statistical Manual of Mental Disorders* (DSM).[233] This attempt is not new: Avicenna did it in his *Canon of Medicine* and so did Burton in his *Anatomy of Melancholy*; Hippocrates outlined causes and mechanisms of disease; Galen tried to reconcile his observations of dissected or wounded bodies with humoral theories of cause and effect.

Because herbal medicine is marginalised as much in countries that are striving towards industrialisation as those who are already industrialised, we have the opportunity to offer something new and different, without plant labels. Instead of competing with a narrow medical model, seeking to find, enthuse and celebrate plant-based remedies which can compete with pharmacological drugs, we can both reaffirm some ancient truths and create a modern synthesis. One that remains happy with longhand, that does not favour fashion in diagnosis over an understanding of process, one that refuses to label human illness and suffering. Personalised, patient-centred medicine does not revere the individual but rather places each uniqueness in our familial, social, economic and political context. The where-ness of contextual somatopsychic medicine situates the patient within her or his biological and psychosocial history over at least three generations and over several boundaries of affection. This is the terrain: relational

---

[233] Diagnostic and Statistical Manual of Mental Disorders written and published by The American Psychiatric Association (APA). Insurance costs cannot be calculated without labels.

structures that are both external and internal to the person at the same time. Once this clinical situation is fully perceived and documented we can go on to use plants and fungi (facets of our coevolution, that is) to biologise rather than psychologise the patient: this one particular manifestation of the human condition that seeks our help. The physician and the plants can then present them with two teams of allies.

Mood

Mood is a mode or output state of consciousness, arising from the psyche but delimited by bios (Section 1.1). Watching, and seeing through the world may just as well initiate sadness as well as gladness but a vanished contentment characterises flat or absent mood. Mood, like any other state has its own natural cycle.[234] Mood can be observed as the amount and quality of movement in a person. Gladness may increase with movement and the climbing of the sun. These are just notes on a scale and hardly call for medication except for a brew of some sort: a cultural variety to which medicinal humans gravitate.

Beyond mere mood, depression shows a self that is unable to fuse with the objects of perception so that, for instance, a sunlit rural scene usually evoking pleasure, can be seen but not fully entered. The limbs can move but as if not fully engaged in gear, or engaged robotically for whom energy is locked in a warehouse for which no key can be found.

Anxiety and depression

By contrast, anxiety is a high energy state but the movements do not engage with purposeful movement or repose. Motion and drive are unconjugated. Agitated states can certainly be helped by medicinal plants like *Tilia* and *Matricaria* without the risk of dependence posed by potent anxiolytics. Psychological causes may be identified but that process alone may provide understanding but little relief. Physicalist theories like the poise hypothesis may explain but such explanations do not always help. The cause may really be the burden of consciousness for which remedies quite outside medication can offer relief. Animation stands in great contrast to agitation. Both are states of excitability and high energy but animation shows someone in continuous controlled effective discharge, with effective beta-sympathetic operation coupled with an efficient response from the thyroid axis. Oscillations are controlled because of smooth flow from good reserves, with no need to call upon impedances.[235] Agitation, by contrast, is dominated by alpha-sympathetic discharge with an ineffective beta response. It leads inevitably to exhaustion.

Arousal without discharge characterises irritable, histaminic states. Managing poise with particular attention to how autocoid hormones play out in the terrain has more long-term benefits than just dispensing anxiolytics. We may know about the parts GABA and glycine and glutamate play in agitated states, but these are players in a causal cycle. Terrain medicine looks at the whole picture, vertically in time, horizontally in the current environment, and how energy is conserved and managed.

---

[234] State cycles and cyclothymia have been discussed in Section 1.5a.

[235] As first discussed in Section 1.1). Other aspects of discharge are tabulated at the end of Section 1.8.

Tension is costly, so undischarged states of arousal will result in fatigue and anxiety. If prolonged, depression may follow on as depletion passes a point of low reserve, low poise (Section 1.7). The influence of bile in depression will be discussed in Section 2.5b on gut motility. Figure 18 suggests how a simple treatment can be help fearful and melancholic states. Emotionally, depression is felt as a loss that cannot be filled, even if named; anxiety is a state of surfeit with no place to put it, no name to attach it. Mental pain needs no name to see it and try to understand and help it. You will need to keep your own spirits up if you are to lift others from dismay. I think you will find that the term nervine is as unhelpful as the word 'neurotic'. Systemic thinking is needed. The terrain is in continual movement and process, so defying attempts at static categorisation.

Anxiety and depression may just as well be physiologised as psychologised as the peak and trough of the wave. Alternating between peak and trough is how cycles work and how prescriptions can be framed (see Section 3.5). Being marooned or fixated in one state defines both highs and lows. Discord signals will intensify anxiety and blunted responses figure in depression. As herbal medicine is biological, we might resist turning over the entrails of the psyche to the point of tedium. Speaking of which, I have heard psychotherapists opine that boredom usually masks depression, but there are reasons enough for it to be the other way around. Energy flow describes both states and we can do something about energy flow. Boredom may be described as a state of one's desires being poorly recognised or, if recognised, unfulfillable or when the fulfillments on offer are inadequate to mobilise the flow of reserve energy into availability. Inflammatory states will confuse the terrain and make boredom or depression more likely. The singularity of the consultation combined with attention to the levels of herbal therapeutics (Section 3.6) offer good chances of resolution.

Pleasure and contentment: being content to be in the world and more or less pleased with our lot, is surely a prerequisite for mental and physical health. Anxiety and depression—major disruptors of sleep—offer resistance to pleasure and result in nocebo, its opposite. The modern fetish of seeking proof about being pleased is one of the drearier aspects of medical scientism.

Placebo

All physical events are real. We step or do not step off the pavement. The pencil falls to the floor or we catch it just in time. Physicality bypasses belief. Our limbs are the closest we get to certainty. Mental events try to catch up and match but approximate them at best. These mental events make up fully linguistic humans with an eye on the future with possibilities, shadowed by a replete past. Our sense of our inner state is our repository of belief. It stands like a gateway into the feeling of completeness, integration and wellness. All enterprises have to pass through this gateway and consumption of pharmacons is a human preoccupation. When the "effect" on our well-being feels positive, the gateway has been opened; when negative, it has been closed. Both are real, one pleases us, the other not: the placebo and the nocebo are as much part of our mind as the nature of the pharmakon, whether with k or with c, whether morphine or *Melissa*. Pain, as a mental output, can itself be a barrier to relief, generating a tightening cycle, not loosened by feedback.

Clinical overview of the body

The unique trajectory of each self with its populated companions cannot be thought of as a completely random path through a field of incidents and accidents. All the "determinants" will themselves be modified by experience. For example, birth order: our position as conceptus in the womb of our birth influences our psycho-social setting. We are to a great extent created by the experiences of our mother during pregnancy just as her mother when pregnant with her necessarily responded in turn to her world, its events and behaviours. The previous inhabitants of her womb will influence the terrain of the incumbent just as that one will influence later siblings, as will birth spacings.[236]

The full family history—populated by companions and trajectories—taken during the initial consultation will draw attention to these critical influences and will help evaluate the patient's terrain from the metabolic and endocrine point of view, which is surely the deepest for the physician to take.

Even the supposedly deterministic genome provides no more than a range of possibilities and probabilities, rather than certainties (rare monogenetic and unusual chromosomal abnormalities excepted). No wonder humans need help with negotiating their state of body and mind!

As to human physiology

Relationships between the systems rather than within them give us a more coherent picture of the dynamics. We separate only for temporary focus but keep the parts always together in mind. Especially unhelpful to think of immune responses as autonomous:

---

[236] See L. A. Gavrilov and N. S. Gavrilova, *The Biology of Life Span: A Quantitative Approach* Harwood Academic, New York 1991; L. A. Gavrilov and N. S. Gavrilova: *Early-life programming of aging and longevity: the idea of high initial damage load (the HIDL hypothesis)*, Annals of the New York Academy of Sciences, vol. 1019, pp. 496–501; also, D. J. P. Barker, *Mothers, Babies, and Disease in Later Life* Churchill Livingstone, London 1998.

surely they are both responder and organiser of others: the kidney as an organ of last resort is the first to stimulate the bone marrow that in turn populates the circulation and peripheral tissues where immune responses may be initiated.

The alimentary tube provides a parallel sensory and executive operation that is primordial, parallel also to the neural tube and the skeletal structure that houses the stem cells of the marrow. So, the municipality (as I prefer to think of the "immune system") unites all domains. Keeping a tissue focus always in mind, remembering the distribution of the three germ layers into these eventual structures gives you a unitary view.

Thinking of the intermediates between the domains in the figure below, especially the movements of the ANS, will enable a practical, clinical approach:

	Skin microbiome and pituitary	
Central	Nervous domain	Peripheral
Hypothalamus	↑↓ ANS ↑↓	
Mouth primary sensory modalities	Alimentary domain and microbiome	Anus
	↑↓ ANS ↑↓	
Converge to thalamus	Musculo–skeletal domain and blood	To PNS

Gastrulation distributes tissue between these three domains

Figure 12: The domains of the municipal system

The municipality

Just as a municipality looks after public spaces and regulates their use, we must orchestrate tissue states in the body with its myriad of local concerns, and also protect vital structures. A domain, then, to provision and inform, with a finger in every pie. It makes us feel at home, informs us of good governance, occasionally of a threat. Deeply connected with temperament, it may in some cases be more averse to risk than alive to opportunities. When it comes to perceived threats it can become overbearing and pompous, declaring that some of our own tissues are out of order and may even send round officious operatives against innocent tissues in other domains such as the alimentary tract and our own thyroid gland, ignoring local expertise. Information loss is communication loss.

Disinformation

This so-called auto-immunity requires a very literal understanding of informatic rules and a conscientiousness on the part of the municipality in applying them. Ambiguous information may pose a threat or present an opportunity. Knowing the difference confers huge adaptive benefits.

Hyper-vigilance is not necessarily the same as hyper-sensitivity though one may lead to the other. We see a great deal of both in practice. States of heightened arousal are not always associated with histaminic symptoms: overthinking may lead to fatigue and sleep disturbance but may coexist with good appetite and digestion. As shorthand, high cognitive speed needs alpha-sympatholytic plants like lavender and melilot, while hypersensitive digestions call for astringent, cooling (because draining) remedies with agrimony taking first place. Matching plants carefully to the patient and not the named condition is the herbalist's art. For instance, if you wanted to prescribe liquorice to a patient with disturbance of the digestive tract and dietary sensitivities, you need to understand the situation of their adrenal axis (thinking of peripheral tissues susceptible to aldosterone), their gonadic and anabolic status, with an eye on their blood pressure. Even here, what you might prescribe in the short term to encourage immediate improvement might not suit a longterm strategy. The past is always as long as the patient's age plus nine months in utero, whereas the future course is amenable to successive light touches on the tiller.

Foliae provide us with the elements of the folic acid cycle without which cell replication would be faulty and scarcely possible. Without the cell cycle our municipality could barely function.

Excretory function

Poise stands behind every case but available energy can be swamped by poor rates of excretion. The patient's face is usually the first and sometimes the best clue to poor function. The consultation and examination will evaluate the four major routes even if they are not the manifest complaints. Lungs, biliary duct to colon, kidney and skin in order of volume need to be assessed, as much by observation as systemic review.

A primary question will be about ask about asthma, then bowel habit and digestive function. Ask always about cramp, easy bruising and itch, with or without rash.

Skin

This border municipality—highly invested with blood vessels from the centre—calibrates our reactivity to events. It communicates through its sentinel outpost of the ectoderm—the pituitary—thence to the CNS. Communication with pacemakers in the liver by the hypothalamus continues the loop and so provides several nodes for therapeutic intervention.

Peripheral heat coupled with a disturbed microbiome manifest in the skin. As dermatitis is inflammatory and blood temperature peaks at 6.30 pm, it is good to encourage sufferers to drink hibiscus tea an hour or two before that time. Eczema, psoriasis, and acne may be different conditions but they have in common a tendency to dwell in hypersensitive and hyper-reactive terrains. Even in the absence of any dermatitis, constitutionally high levels of cortisol show up in translucent skin, best seen on the abdomen, clearly revealing pale blue veins.

For this reason, essential oils and strong aromatic plants will generally be ill-advised in eczema and it may be that the recommendation that sufferers resist putting spices in their food (turmeric and cinnamon excepted) may meet with some resistance. Astringent and antihistaminic remedies (notably from Rosaceae) are mostly indicated as we shall note in Section 3.6. Organ drainage needs to be gentle otherwise the discharge of metabolic waste will exacerbate external affronts and make the condition worse. Tisanes offer the best route of administration though aromatic waters of rose and lavender (and even thyme and angelica) offer very pleasing and effective remedies. All inflammatory skin conditions will be helped by an anti-inflammatory diet—as in Appendix 1. Neural impulses if persistently hyper-elevated will put pressure on the cations zinc and calcium, and so double as irritants. The nerves can be soothed and the ions increased with a dish, such as whole sardines with potatoes, leeks and tomatoes.

Aggression—whether from within or without—evokes heat without light (if you want to be humoral about it) and most psoriasis is improved by UV light. Fire drives *chole* towards choleric. Proliferative hormones produce a lot of heat. Thyroid hyperactivity operating at the level of the skin must be reduced in psoriasis whatever the levels of serum TSH. *Lycopus, Zea, Fabiana* and *Leonurus* will be called for. Plants like *Borago* will also diminish FSH (responsible for the heat surges in menopause) and ACTH (also high in acne).

Acne results from a combination of metabolic and endocrine dysfunctions in vagotonic individuals. Congestion in liver and pancreas leads to impaired excretion and a consequent deterioration in the microbiome, setting the stage for a concomitant deterioration in that of the skin. Congestion there makes the pilosebaceous unit more susceptible to changes in the skin's lipid film. The liver makes many of the binding globulins, which regulate peripheral hormones. So, when a surge in proliferative hormones from the pituitary (as at puberty) couples with a diminished peripheral response (as in hepato-pancreatic congestion), the stage is set for acne where the commensal bacteria thrive on the lipid film.

Growth and reproductive hormones are rivals for the anabolic programme of adolescence. GH (with high prolactin) dominates in acne; neither is switched off by insulin, which enriches the lipid film for bacterial overgrowth. The stimulation of the gonads by LH is not switched off by progesterone and androgens (liver again).[237] Without the dampening effect of gonadal androgens, ACTH is activated to secrete a compensatory rise in DHEA but this detracts from the maintenance of anti-inflammatory cortisol. Acne represents a diminished response to an increased demand at a time when emotional certainty is sought in a field that shifts constantly. These are insights from Endobiogenic medicine.

Treatment calls for at least one of the following overlapping strategies:

Table 1: Treatment strategies

Treatment strategies	*Some examples of useful plants*
Hepato-pancreatic drainage along with appropriate nurtures	*Arctium, Dulcamara, Fumaria, Rubus fruticosus, Agrimonia, Olea*
Maintain cortisol	Buds of *Ribes nigrum* do this better than anything; also *Thymus, Calendula*

(Continued)

---

[237] The surge in LH at puberty and all luteal states parallels the surge in FSH at menopause.

Table 1: Treatment strategies (Continued)

Treatment strategies	Some examples of useful plants
Reduce FSH	*Borago, Vitex, Lycopus*
Reduce hyper-vigilance	*Lavandula, Melilotus, Menyanthes*
Reduce LH	*Achillea* and *Alchemilla*
Reduce TSH with brassicas	*Zea, Leonurus, Convallaria*
Taper the androgen surge	*Salix, Foeniculum, Salvia, Angelica, Hedera, Humulus, Anthriscus*
Yet prevent its free-fall	*Trigonella* (and reduces ADH)
Reduce prolactin	*Rubus idaeus, Anthriscus*
Also paradoxically helpful	*Lamium, Sambucus, Vinca*

GALT

Birth launches the alimentary domain. The experience of the developing foetus (and its ordinal place in the mother's womb), the character of early feeding, sleeping and evacuation will profoundly influence the infant's future as its three domains develop in unison. Congestion in all cavities, but especially the cranial (given the anatomical unfolding) and thence the airways, make inflammation and infection of ear, nose and throat commonplace in early years. Histaminic states can mimic bacterial and viral infections.

Gut-associated lymphoid tissue (GALT), the acronym for the surveillance signalling tissues that invest the alimentary canal—from tonsils to vermiform appendix—are thus hyperactive and so tonsillitis can be expected. Gentle but effective interventions with medicinal plants and practical unfussy dietary measures will avert any routine prescription of antibiotics, steroids or bronchodilators. The coincident beneficial action of herbs on the autonomic system will dampen incipient asthma. All of these measures must be associated with attention to nurturing the development of a healthy microbiome. This is easily done by avoiding baby food and eating what everyone else is eating.

Tonsillitis is debilitating for parents and child but removing the tonsils (the forward sentry of GALT) is like removing the battery of a smoke alarm. If you shoot the sentry, everything will undoubtedly go quiet. But for how long? With diminished surveillance, peace in the alimentary tube may have come at some cost. The appendix (the rearguard of GALT) may have become more vulnerable.

In early years and certainly well before the end of the first heptade, if all is done with due care (without undue attention) and if surgery and over-medication has been avoided, the risk of a sudden appendicitis at the onset of puberty will have been much lowered. Although there comes a point when the only safe answer to peritonitis will be surgery, preventive measures are always to be preferred. As with the tonsils, green plant and fruit fibre will be protective to the caecum and its part in the municipality. Don't reach for cleavers every time the lymphoid system is mentioned: think it through. Agrimony, thyme and lime-flowers are liver-sparing and protectors of the gut.

The axial skeleton

The spine has to mediate between the vertical axis and limbs, between locomotion and the cavities. Although they are married seamlessly, plenty of seams stitch the axial cavities together, but that is not what you see at first glance.

During the conversation, you will be facing a face and chest and see most of the person, presumably seated. You will form impressions bit by bit of the hidden structures of spine, limbs, and the four cavities as the discussion unfolds. Your systematic review will of course consider all of them. Noise features in the head, grief is felt in the chest, disturbance in the abdomen, congestion and tension in the pelvis. Even before any clinical examination, the sense of each emerges in the posture as much as the voice and the words spoken.

The clock on my desk records the room temperature. Before you have to ask how the patient responds to heat or cold, whether they feel either intensely and declare a preference, watch how they respond to the environment you have created, depending on the season. So much is common-sensical as much as clinical.

If the patient complains of pain in knees, hips, shoulders or neck, ask first (before any methodical examination) if you might see the bare feet (or the left at least). Even if the arch looks high, ask the patient to slowly put weight on them and stand up. Often the arch disappears if it was there in the first place. Like tyres on a wheel, feet bear the brunt of contact (we are not hovercrafts) and send their shock upwards. I have found from experience, that many pains in knees, hips or neck can be resolved by a nurture: recommending strong shoes, supportive of ankles and cushioning the shock[238] and, almost as important, thick weave hiking socks. Health comes before fashion! Observe from the outset movements of hands, fingers and gestures but I usually leave looking closely at the hands till last as, combining it with taking the pulse, I want to evaluate it after all is said and done.

Even if you do not perform a complete examination (in defiance of your teachers), if you leave out the abdomen, you miss out on so much information but also touch to the abdomen can be a form of treatment and a way of building trust. Always examine a man's chest to see hair distribution and the shape and size of the areolae. If they are large, they suggest high prolactin and strong oestrogen. If they are elliptical, what tension, you may ask, stretches the elongating circle? I see this often seen in boys at puberty where the anabolic drives of growth hormone and prolactin are due to be replaced—for an interval at least—by reproductive hormones. This competition for resources between these two anabolic axes are at a critical stage during puberty. There may also be conflict between parental expectation, societal clues and inner doubts. Distribution and amount of chest and abdominal hair provide other clues. Whatever the presenting complaints, reducing prolactin with raspberry leaf tea and supporting with fenugreek are usually starters for a treatment to enable the release of a resisted or conflicted process.

---

[238] I recommend Mobils by Mephisto. Unfortunately, I earn no commission!

Physiological systems and organs from a clinical perspective

Though this overview may look like a diagram and an excuse for making lists it hopes to provide indicators for the places where herbal medicine can realistically make a difference. As medicinal plants work more subtly on the systems level than abruptly at the cellular and tissue level it helps to have an overall perspective and checklist. Lists are just aids to thinking and depend upon arbitrary separations to replace the actual connectivity. Clearly acute emergencies need to be differentiated from chronic states but in practice herbalists more often treat complex chronic multi-system problems rather than the emergencies seen routinely by paramedics.

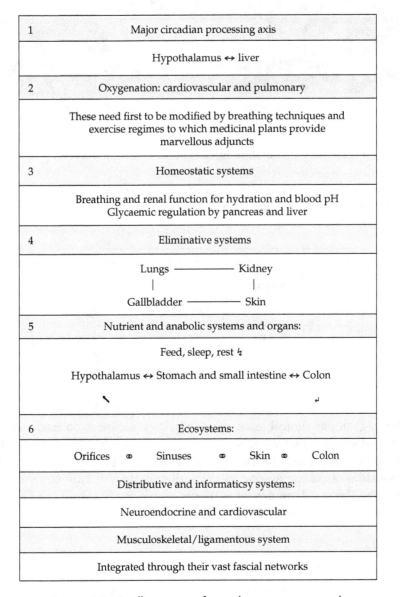

1	Major circadian processing axis
	Hypothalamus ↔ liver
2	Oxygenation: cardiovascular and pulmonary
	These need first to be modified by breathing techniques and exercise regimes to which medicinal plants provide marvellous adjuncts
3	Homeostatic systems
	Breathing and renal function for hydration and blood pH Glycaemic regulation by pancreas and liver
4	Eliminative systems
	Lungs ——————— Kidney | | Gallbladder ——————— Skin
5	Nutrient and anabolic systems and organs:
	Feed, sleep, rest ↳ Hypothalamus ↔ Stomach and small intestine ↔ Colon ↖ ↵
6	Ecosystems:
	Orifices ∞ Sinuses ∞ Skin ∞ Colon
	Distributive and informaticsy systems:
	Neuroendocrine and cardiovascular
	Musculoskeletal/ligamentous system
	Integrated through their vast fascial networks

Figure 13: An illustration of a multi-system approach

This approach outlines the various meta-functions that systems perform but belies the differential quantities involved. Without chlorophyll, there would be no free oxygen in the atmosphere, and without haemoglobin, its sister porphyrin, there would be no way of sequestering it and so prevent an oxidised world. Without its cousin cyanocobalamin, our cells including pro-erythrocytes could not replicate. To ferry enough oxygen to mitochondria to release potential chemical energy within substrates, red blood cells numerically dominate all other cell types as the figure below demonstrates. Muscle cells, by contrast, account for 0.01% of the totality of 10^{13}–10^{14} cells.[239]

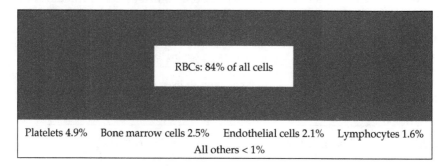

RBCs: 84% of all cells

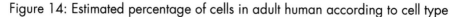

Platelets 4.9%   Bone marrow cells 2.5%   Endothelial cells 2.1%   Lymphocytes 1.6%
All others < 1%

Figure 14: Estimated percentage of cells in adult human according to cell type

With numbers in mind, it is worth reminding ourselves of how critically our essential needs depend upon time duration. These are the upper limits for the life of most adults to be sustained:

Breath	4 minutes	Loss of breath = death
Water	40 hours	Thirst for life
Sleep	4 days	Saves previous day to 'hard-drive'
Food	40 days	Keeps adult body and soul together

Figure 15: Time criticality

They remind of us of our fundamental needs, putting all else in proportion. Also, during the stage of our clinical assessment, it helps if we focus on tracing the origin of the tissues and systems that we wish our treatments to influence.[240] The endoderm of vertebrates produces tissue within the lungs, thyroid, and pancreas. The mesoderm aids in the production of cardiac muscle, skeletal muscle, smooth muscle, renal tissues and red blood cells. The ectoderm produces tissues within the epidermis and contributes to the formation of melanocytes and neurones within the brain.

---

[239] Figures derived from Milo et al. (2016).

[240] Concurring with the remarks of the evolutionary biologist Lewis Wolpert: "It is not birth, marriage, or death, but gastrulation which is truly the most important time in your life".

Organs organise and even direct systems. Let us look at them from a clinical perspective:

The heart

The heart contains emotion and lets blood go on its way. It serves the circulation as do the emotions. The heart needs sustenance as much as treatment. The five foods for the ageing heart (from the sixth heptade onward) are: lemon, parsley, garlic, buckwheat and hawthorn. As we add very little to the total number of heart muscle cells we are born with, we need to treat them with the respect they deserve by taking pressure off them and feeding them properly. Most of the herbs used to treat the heart actually treat the circulation it serves. Dietary protein needs to be sufficient to sustain muscle bulk to protect cardiac muscle from strain.

Congestive cardiac failure presents an enormous challenge because treatments that benefit hypertension by dampening cardiac output (such as the potassium in the plants we use all the time) are entirely counterproductive when the heart starts to fail. Other herbs directed towards making the myocardium more energy-efficient are diluted out of efficacy by oedema in all the tissues. Although *Convallaria* does play a part, it makes more sense to focus on reducing systemic inflammation and supporting adrenal function (with plants that are not usually associated with cardiac function, such as *Thymus, Rosmarinus, Calendula*) the better to help the kidney regulate fluid balance.[241]

The blood

If your patient has a copy of their Full Blood Count, it is always helpful to be able to see the ratio between three primary elements: the counts of red cells, white cells and platelets. Figure 14 illustrates the numerical importance of erythrocytes. Platelets play a core role in coagulation and are a major reservoir of serotonin, which no doubt contributes to vestibular symptoms and to migrainous states more generally. *Zingiber* has clinical benefits in reducing the opsonisation of platelets. The effectiveness of the adrenal medulla in releasing platelets from the splanchnic circulation and spleen in emergencies shows a poor state of poise.[242] Of course, alacrity of adrenaline when *not* called for ushers in a whole range of crises, with many physiological effects and calls for physic.

Total white cell count can tell us about underlying inflammatory tendencies (even with a low CRP or raised ESR) and the ratio between red and white cells indicates the global disposition between androgens and oestrogens.[243] According to the Endobiogenic Biology of Functions model, normal range is 0.8–0.95 for men and 0.75–1.15 for women. The ratio between lymphocytes and neutrophils is discussed in Section 3.6.

---

[241] See Hedayat, Lapraz et al. (2018).

[242] For their margination in the splanchnic circulation and sequestration in the spleen, see Figure 7 in Section 1.5a.

[243] Lapraz et al. (English version 2013).

Full oxygenation of tissues is a critical factor influencing health and even survival: strokes come at a stroke, often with catastrophic consequences. Viscosity of blood is a crucial factor in the likelihood of internal bleeding or coagulation. The flow characteristics—rheology—of such a variable emulsion as blood in tubes of such variable dimensions—are affected by the autocoid hormones—especially histamine and serotonin—but also vasodilators and constrictors: kinins, tensins, and several types of eicosanoid as well as nitric oxide. Plant polyphenols and foods like beetroot are necessary to the health of the blood vessels.

The blood vessels

As life so depends upon them, for protection, add paprika to most foods to aid both flow and endothelial integrity; plenty of ginger to correct opsonisation of platelets. Ash leaves may enter your prescription to prevent platelet clumping. There are many vasculo-protectors but bilberry leaf (and berry) stands out as does *Ruscus*. Venotonic and anti-thrombotic plants will be listed more fully in the materia medica summaries in Part Three.

If so important, why say so little? The complexity of flow of composite fluid materials through tubes is beyond computation so let's not pretend we know more than we do!

Lungs

Most herbal remedies towards ease of breathing act indirectly, to reduce bronchospasm or reduce mucus secretion, for example; or to limit the cause, by reducing the effect or a bacterium or virus or host sensitivity to them. *Equisetum* is credited with strengthening the connective tissues of the lungs; to that end I use the juiced fresh plant (in conjunction with *Plantago* leaves) but it needs to be done for a long time for good effect.

The state of gums and teeth and the nasal and sinus cavities which feed into the throat and lungs depend to a great extent upon the digestive tubes and its organs. There are hundreds of astringent anti-microbial agents. Sage, thyme and rosemary are standbys.

Asthma as the major, often constitutional, condition to show up in the lungs is principally an energetic one: an attempt by the terrain to slow up carbonic excretion and improve oxygenation of tissues. It needs always to be approached as a dysregulation of the ANS (see Section 3.6).

The alimentary domain

Much initiating gear clusters about the head of this tube: hypothalamus, olfactory bulb, tongue, lips, parotid and salivary glands. We'll look briefly at the glandular organs that serve the tract but most therapeutic aims will pick up these clues in Section 3.6.

The stomach

Relatively low gastric acid is more of a problem than an excess and leads to poor absorption with a risk of low vitamin B_{12}. If there is pain, think not of reducing acid (though this can be done with *Solanum dulcamara* and a diet rich in potatoes) but of protecting the mucosa with emollients such as marshmallow leaves or slippery elm and of stimulating pepsin. Low levels of acid are often associated with slow gut motility and, if recalcitrant, merits investigation for gastroparesis, especially in young people following a viral infection.

As for reflux, most often this is a function of strong alpha-sympathetic tone which, once reduced, will stop the peptic contents going the wrong way. Loss of height in the spine with age has the unfortunate effect of thrusting the abdominal viscera up against the diaphragm, abolishing the competence of the sphincter and is more complicated to resolve. Older people with reflux are more in need of high pillows or even an orthopaedic back-stretcher[244] than they are of medication. In any event, good massage with lavender oil over the breastbone offers some relief. As with the pancreas, replacement therapy with betaine hydrochloride before meals is not a bad option.

The pancreas

Insufficiency of the exocrine pancreas is common in vagotonic individuals, which the compensatory engorgement of their parotid gland does little to correct; indeed, it rather contributes to the upper respiratory complaints to which they are prone.

Correcting with digestive enzymes (betaine, papain, bromelain with or without the addition of acid) seems to me one of the more benign examples of replacement therapy. The foods that contain them—beetroot, papaya, pineapple—can be recommended for their nutritional benefits. Of course, overeating is disastrous for vagotonic individuals with poor pancreatic response, as is the consumption of starchy or sweet food.

It is important to not over-treat pancreatic insufficiency, as it may exhaust and exacerbate the function: one of those rare conditions when it is best to treat only symptomatically. An exception is when alpha-sympathetic drive is strong and congestive; then the frequent addition of *Lavandula*, *Melissa* or one of the chamomiles will reduce both alpha and vagal tone, as will *Thymus*, with its relaxant effects on the alimentary tract. Also, in small doses, *Fumaria*, *Rosmarinus*, *Salvia* and species of *Mentha* support the exocrine pancreas; both *Agrimonia* and *Arctium* support exocrine and endocrine pancreas. *Sambucus* facilitates the drive from the pituitary to pancreas.

While the bitters are directed towards gastric and hepatic function, they complement herbs given for pancreatic support. The polyvalent nature of herbs cautions against being too categorical with their application. Digestive problems are rarely confined to a single organ or tissue which is why herbs, with their overlapping tropisms, are so beneficial for them.

The liver

As the liver occupies the central nexus of metabolism, sits at the core of the enzymatic matrix, sets the timing of so many rhythms, and modifies anabolic and catabolic drivers, herbalists may veer towards it as a favoured location for their treatments given that so many plants are reputed to do well there.

In hepatitis and other liver disease, the recommended diet is "liver sparing", which is to say low in protein and not high in fat so that the organ is spared the difficulties with

---

[244] These are simple frame with struts that, when lain upon, helps release the diaphragm.

catabolising such large molecules. The same goes for herbal treatment—spare the liver by not using plants that stimulate a liver that already has too much to contend with. A "liver sparing" regime for patients with hepatitis or other liver disease is outlined in Appendix I.

The safest and most reliable herbs for long-term liver drainage are agrimony, German chamomile and lime-flowers as tisanes and olive leaves as a decoction. Lavender may be added in heartache and distress. All bitters stimulate liver function. Many plants that are used for other indications are also bitter, so it is quite difficult to avoid the liver in herbal treatments. However, the use of cold and hot macerations of the mallows including hibiscus spare the liver and soothe the digestive and respiratory tubes.

As for bitter remedies that are used primarily to stimulate the liver, for short term usage, gentian is obvious; the following herbs are very potent: and have many main effects which you may or may not wish to obtain: *Artemisia absinthium* and *A. vulgaris*. Cooking occasionally with French tarragon (*Artemisia dracununculus*) will help with digestion of a rich dish. Its essential oil has effects beyond the liver, though. Russian tarragon (not favoured in cuisine for its coarse flavour) actually does more than the French variety to drain the liver.

As for bitter remedies that are used primarily to stimulate or to drain the liver, or both, perhaps *Taraxacum* radix is the most favoured; the leaf is less bitter and, with its high levels of potassium, is diuretic and tends to reduce diastolic pressure. *Stachys betonica* offers a most useful cholagogue that is not too imperative and gently tones and relaxes.

Agrimony and fumitory provide the best hepato-protective tisanes. *Menyanthes*, an excellent bitter tonic to be taken after breakfast, has broad effects upon mood and the ANS. Perhaps the most versatile aromatic bitter is *Achillea*.

The gallbladder

This organ can be thought of as the excretory arm of the liver and so is dynamic, potentially overworked and so is vulnerable to tissue change, usually hypertrophic. The same could be said for the colon and may initiate or mimic changes in other excretory tissues in the skin, respiratory tract and kidney.

The vulnerable sites are the wall, the duct and the sphincter of Oddi.

The vulnerable processes feature hepatic waste-products and dietary inputs, notably starchy, sugary food; composites like pastry are particularly to be avoided. Apples (which tend to mitigate metabolic effects of peripheral oestrogen), pineapple and berries are helpful in chronic relapsing cholecystitis, as is cold-pressed olive oil as salad dressing or used to braise foods slowly in a cast iron pan on the lowest heat. Large amounts of ripe fruit will certainly exacerbate cholecystitis once a person is afflicted and so will a lot of fat but these are not causative and mask the real culprit.[245]

The aqueous components of the bile are absorbed and may maroon the micelles in a hypertonic medium, becoming a focus for the formation of stones. This risk is perhaps complicated by the gallbladder's involvement in the metabolism of cholecalciferol.

[245] Yudkin, John (1972) (1986) (2012) Reading his book in 1973 coupled with my experience of the political effects of sugar production in Guatemala led me to stop buying or adding sugar.

This large steroid vitamin sits at the core of the calcium economy, so gives an over-worked organ an extra task.

As illustrated in Figure 14, 84% of the number of cells in the human body are erythro-cytes which contain the large haeme molecule. This and other porphyrins, cytochromes and catalases are excreted in the bile along with other complex metabolites. The traffic is voluminous and constant.

A diet overly rich in animal fats and sugar predisposes to gallstones. Once cholecystitis establishes itself, fried foods and animal fats become provocative. Such items increase risks in those with high levels of circulating oestrogen and cortisol. These steroid hormones are constructed from cholesterol. Endocrine and metabolic disturbance will influence the consistency and constitution of the bile with an inevitable risk for cholesterol mixed with other bile components to come out of suspension, creating stones that then may calcify.

In a sense, one could visualise the liver as the much larger, well-resourced organ with plenty of slack and recuperative potential and the gallbladder as its underfunded annexe with little room for manoeuvre.

If an inflammatory state in the gallbladder becomes infected, a medical emergency is triggered. If ignored and badly managed, a surgical emergency may ensue.

High alpha-sympathetic tone targets all smooth muscle but particularly sphincters in the alimentary tract, notably in the cystic and common bile ducts.[246] This chronic tone can be effectively reduced with *Lavandula, Melilotus, Leonurus, Angelica* (and where appropri-ate with *Vitex*). Antispasmodics like *Tilia* and *Achillea* are usually indicated. *Rosmarinus* improves the flow and processing of bile and should be valued in particular for its reduc-tion in tone of the sphincter of Oddi.

Bile partakes in two out of the four humours of ancient medicine. It is intricately con-nected with gut motility, general digestive health, and with mood and sleep. It deserves a segment to itself.

Bile, gut motility, mood and sleep

The fact that oil and water do not readily mix directs the partition in all organisms between an aqueous medium compartmentalised by lipid membranes, all enclosed by and separated from the outside world by fatty composite barriers. So, this structural con-trast leads to metabolic differentiation. Fats are absorbed into lymphatic ducts to preserve some separation from the predominately aqueous blood. Hydrophobic and hydrophilic polarities in lipids allow cytoplasmic environments to be meshed with their membranes.

Bile—a double-agent—acts in a predominantly aqueous medium to emulsify fats. Without it, we could not absorb fat-soluble vitamins. Second, it is an excretory product removing the breakdown products of large molecules such as haeme.

The recycling of bile in the enterohepatic circulation allows for a second attempt to pass excess wastes. In passing, its alkaline pH tends to quench any gastric acid remain-ing in the duodenum and is bacteriostatic. This movement favours gut motility, along with serotonin. It is a cycle within a cycle: if the flow of bile is diminished or held up by tension in the ducts, the movement of digestive products from food to faeces is slowed.

---

[246] For further detail, see Section 3.6 Level One.

In this way, it does operate as the ancient humour *kholé*. An exaggerated flow will correlate with an aggressive impulse: *choler*, as in choleric. A sludge from diminished or retentive flow will correlate with a darkened, thickened *chole* or melancholy, from the Greek for black (as in melatonin, melanin, melanocyte).

> Fragmentation of flow will fracture the smooth movement of semi-solid liquids throughout the alimentary tract. Fragmentation of digestive flow will disturb the microbiome and fragment sleep. *Chole* is the collection of excretory products that most determines the restorative quality of sleep.

The brisker the flow, the brighter, more metallic the mood. The slower flow will lead to a slower, darker mood, even depression and what psychiatrists call "psychomotor retardation". Improving the flow of bile, reducing tension all the while, will reduce this abnormal sluggishness. There are so many remedies to choose from but *Stachys betonica*, *Hypericum, Verbena, Thymus, Melissa, Rosmarinus, Salvia, Marrubium* may be among the first to come first to mind, depending upon the individual circumstances. Here you need to have in parallel mind the levels and foci of treatments as set out in Section 3.6.

Bile flow modifies gut motility, which in turn is modified by the autocoid hormones, especially serotonin and histamine. Serotonin is an ancient molecule, found in insects, amoebae, and fungi. In plants it stimulates birds to rapidly excrete and so disperse seeds. Most of the body's serotonin occupies the enterochromaffin cells found between villi of the small intestine. Eventually serotonin will be absorbed and migrate to platelets in the bloodstream where its vasoactive properties will, under appropriate circumstances, induce migraine in susceptible individuals.

If serotonin induces expulsion of the content of the gut, it may act with histamine and noradrenaline in reverse so that migrainous individuals will be prone to nausea and vomiting as well as diarrhoea. Abrupt bowel movements can be the discharge of an underlying constipation: tonic if spastic, atonic in serotonin delay. Irritable bowel syndrome (IBS). may then be seen as a variety of migraine, alternating or cycling between high and low states of activity of the five autocoid hormones, or in differential states between them.[247] Migrainous episodes of any type are downhill events: a culmination of stress that was waiting for an opportunity to discharge, like a tanker entering port.

The gastro-colic reflex occurs with the stomach filling with food. It is a normal signal to the caecum to contract, moving the contents along. When, unusually, it results in an urgent need to empty the bowels even before the meal has ended, it is a sign of acute arousal in a person with constitutionally high alpha-sympathetic tone. This hypersensitivity to ACTH (which has receptors in both caecum and rectum) discharges noradrenaline which then co-opts serotonin and histamine. As the rectum alternates between congestion and rapid discharge, it is prone to inflammatory changes. With or without haemorrhoids, this terrain—often accompanied by a deep fear of conflict—presents with periodic anal pruritus.

This is painful and debilitating and usually part of an irritable bowel in which a mismatch between the enterohepatic circulation of bile and portal venous drainage back to the liver. Rapid movements when not enough bile is resorbed (altering the pH of the rectum and the stools) alternates with a retentive phase when the stools become compressed

---

[247] Details in Section 3.6 Level Seven.

like pellets, often covered in mucus and sometimes stained with local blood. Although treatment for such a situation needs to be personalised, vagal and alpha-sympathetic tone needs to be reduced along with appropriate liver remedies such as *Menyanthes* and *Agrimonia* with a gut relaxant like *Thymus*. IBS is misnamed as a syndrome. The bowel cycles reflect a highly personal response to the world. In spite of best efforts, sufferers have been unable to comfort themselves.[248]

Many years ago, a patient who was a merchant banker came with a terrible rash spreading over his buttocks and thighs from his anus. In desperation, he had visited a consultant dermatologist weekly with poor results until one week, as the doctor reached for his BNF to select yet another corticosteroid, the patient snatched it from his hands with, reportedly, the words: "No, let *me* stick a pin in the book and see what it comes up with"!

The doctor had treated it primarily as a skin disorder whereas it was clearly one of motility of bile within the alimentary canal, debouching onto the delicate skin of the perineum.[249]

Bile circulates between liver, gallbladder, duodenum and ileum where more than 90% is resorbed and returned to the liver. It makes about six circuits in every twenty-four hours. If, as seems to be the case, these roughly correlate with mass movements, the colon could be blocked out into modules of four hours each, as in the figure below:

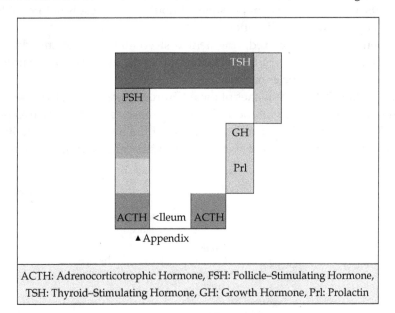

ACTH: Adrenocorticotrophic Hormone, FSH: Follicle–Stimulating Hormone, TSH: Thyroid–Stimulating Hormone, GH: Growth Hormone, Prl: Prolactin

Figure 16: Matching bowel transit with hormonal sequence
in the pituitary gland (after Duraffourd)

The correlation between transit through the bowel and the distribution of receptors matching the horizontal sequence in the pituitary gland (which itself follows circadian

---

[248] Often cyclothymic, they oscillate between the two poles of spasm and release, rarely regressing to the mean. See Ballast in Section 1.8.

[249] Another patient of mine had consulted this same consultant over a long period for the itch of solar keratosis. He was incurious and dismissive when she reported that her long travail had been eased by chickweed cream.

and seasonal sequences) provides us with many useful clinical pointers.[250] For example, alpha-sympathetic driven individuals will be prone to appendicitis during liminal phases (notably puberty) and to proctitis, especially if of high birth weight and any other sign of GH dominance. Biliary problems are more likely to show up at the top of the ascending limb close to the hepatic flexure, especially in the sixth heptade. Adenomas will need, whatever other measures might be taken, reducing the proliferative effects of FSH with the appropriate use of *Vitex*. Disturbance located at the splenic flexure will need thyroid support (perhaps with *Avena sativa* and *Salvia*) and tempering of LH with *Achillea* and *Alchemilla*. GH dominance calls for complex carbohydrate and resistant starch in the diet with herbs like chervil and raspberry leaf to curtail prolactin.

In summary, although mass transit of faecal matter from zone to zone will respond to diurnal and nocturnal contingencies—especially diet and feed\fast phase lengths—conditions in the terminal ileum and the entero-hepatic circulation of bile will strongly influence a person's mood and energy. As will fatigue and stress influence bile resorption.

Fragmentation

Ripples in the alimentary tube move according to the rhythms of life, orchestrated by the hypothalamus. Just as music is not possible without silence, rest is not possible without exercise nor appetite without digestion.

If movements become fractured, fragmented sleep and fractious moods usually follow. The core function of nurture and gentle medicine must be to integrate all these rhythms. Capacitance will be enhanced.

Alternations between the branches of the ANS are both responses to events and initiators of daily rhythms. Herbs with no influence on these cycles are rare exceptions. You will see in Figure 17 that the cycles match those of the alternation of activity and rest, catabolism and anabolism as in the cycling of the autonomic nervous system.[251]

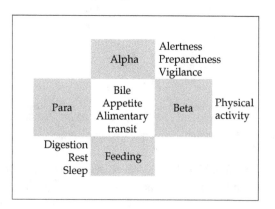

Figure 17: Daily rhythms

---

[250] Dr Duraffourd did not give any references during his seminars. The foundational work on endocrine cells in the alimentary tract is referenced in the chapter on Splanchnology in Gray's Anatomy 37th edition p. 1379; see bibliography.

[251] See Tables 3, 4 and 5 in Section 3.6.

The urinary bladder

Like the mouth, it is vulnerable to infection. Many astringent herbs help by dissolving the colloid coating of bacteria, and there are plenty of demulcent herbs to soothe. As I always have *Calluna, Agropyron, Alchemilla* and *Althaea* in stock, they are the first thoughts in cystitis along with *Agrimonia*. As the neck of the bladder is particularly innervated with alpha-sympathetic fibres, *Lavandula* is particularly indicated along with *Thymus* for its anti-infective anti-spasmodic activity.

Treating cystitis well usually means looking beyond treating an episode of infection with all the means at our disposal. Congestion of organs that occupy and pass through the pelvis play as great a part in this common debilitating condition as the bladder itself. Often managing the microbiome of the colon will have the greatest benefit and softening stools with demulcents and osmotic agents like psyllium husks will be necessary adjuncts to treatment of cystitis.

The kidney

Leaving this organ till last makes sense because it is in effect the backstop to life, stabilisers to internal change, and close companion to the heart.

The most important consideration is to spare renal function and get over any obsession with treatment. A very helpful exception is the dissolution of calculi by plants such as *Eupatorium purpureum*. Otherwise, even more than with the liver, you can best support this precious organ by closely monitoring its function and leaving it alone. I use the singular because renal agenesis is by no means uncommon and even with a pair, one does much of the work.[252]

The use of diuretics in essential hypertension has its place, (dandelion leaves as a morning tisane for instance), but they may eventually become counterproductive in congestive heart failure. In fluid retention, members of Boraginaceae can be used to oppose mineralocorticoid activity. Plants which are uricosuric—like *Solidago* and *Urtica*—are important adjuncts to the management of gout.[253] Oedema in surface tissues will probably mimic internal states, so consider the great dilution effect this will have on the absorption of herbal remedies, especially important in congestive cardiac failure. Differentiation between different sources of any oedema—metabolic, lymphatic, cardiac or renal (or mixed)—needs to inform the direction of treatments. Oedema in the eye-sockets usually points to the kidney though bags under the eyes is seen commonly in vagotonic individuals. Aldosterone and ADH must also be considered.

Although we cannot be regulated as Earth's oceans are by thermo-haline currents, we have always to recognise that life is made possible by powerful "adversaries" like oxygen in the mitochondria and sodium in the kidney. Plants invariably contain an

---

[252] Having no license for human dissection, our cohort at the School of Herbal Medicine were permitted to observe the pathologist at Croydon morgue. Much of his teaching about organs and tissues, especially the kidney, have been confirmed over the years in practice.

[253] Uricosuric agents promote the renal excretion of urate from the blood and should be distinguished from drugs like allopurinol which reduces the formation of uric acid in those with high turnover states or prone to gout.

abundance of potassium, the partner electrolyte. Inorganic chemistry behaves somewhat as homeostasis: belligerent elements like the metals calcium, iron and zinc collaborate with other bullies like oxygen to render them all as inert chalk and rust. The wonder of life is that it resurrects the power and manages to limit the damage. For a time.

Common complaints in search of repair

There are so many ways of feeling unwell. Searching for labels to identify them may be a kind of illness in itself and while that ailment of ailments is prevalent, it is certainly not new. We have lost the meta-labels of religion and wander into a mirage of postures claiming and clambering towards lost certainties.

When does a complaint become a condition? The therapeutic intention is to dissolve the complaint so that the condition becomes a faint memory or remembered with satisfaction after its demise.

Aches and pains are almost part of the human condition. To banish them utterly would be associated with a kind of rabid perfectionism that might also like to see an end to humility. The constant furnace of inflammatory states represent the urge to ascend and against the inevitability of gravity. This fire is ubiquitous. If we can dampen it, we can improve the quality of the lives of our patients and even extend them. It is not a question of making extravagant claims but of fulfilling the nurtures and applying physic to physiology.[254]

Against that heroic aspiration must be countered the structural states that can only compromise firmity. Of these, perhaps the greatest and most prevalent is hyperlaxity of ligaments. This causes a profound and extensive drain on energy, which drains capacitance and resilience. As a somatopsychic consequence, the structural load on mental and emotional coherence is immense. To understand the constant strain involved, imagine having to lift and push a loaded wheelbarrow, the handles of which are highly elastic. Leverage, which fundamentally saves effort, is unavailable. As it is almost certainly pre-congenital, affected individuals have had time to learn to adapt and these adaptations may form the structure of presenting complaints. There are many degrees

---

[254] The nurtures play the second note on the tritone scale. The levels of phytotherapeutic intervention are concentrated in Section 3.6.

of hypermobility, many not conforming to a diagnosis of the genetic Ehlers-Danlos syndrome. Some are supple, others brittle, perhaps showing a predominance of metabolic oestrogens over androgens. Oestrogens soften connective tissue and allow it to absorb fluid, fat and nutrient. If peripheral oestrogens of metabolic origin dominate central drivers of gonadic oestrogens, some of these connective tissue effects will dominate over reproductive health. A holistic approach will want to reduce excess drives in the corticotrophic axis of the anterior pituitary while supporting gonadic oestrogens and thyroid function and, most important, to dampen oxytocin and ADH. You will see from the Tables in Section 3.6 that *Melissa* and *Levisticum*, *Thymus* and *Calendula*, *Borago* and *Salix*, *Salvia* and *Zingiber* already make strong candidates.

As components of the migrainous state, vestibular sensitivities relate to the digestive organs, notably stomach and gallbladder. Ways of managing these presentations, which are intrinsically structural, is to manage the architecture of the ANS and to reduce hypersensitivities (see Tables 2, 3, 4) where *Agrimonia*, *Ballota* and *Olea* make good first choices. Vestibular troubles may show up for the first time as a sign of ageing.

Fatigue is the first impedance to loss of poise. It becomes an illness when chronically disregarded, though should be expected in hyperlaxity as mentioned above. Fatigue is a kind of pain that should not become entrenched. Support over the long term with nurture and nutrition towards rest that is restful and sleep that refreshes can be accompanied by vagomimetic and sympathomimetic and alpha-lytic plants with gentle sympatholytics like *Olea*, *Lavandula* and *Tilia*.

Cough is to be expected in young children. Inhalants and chest rubs, infusions and oxymels along with nurture (and the nurture of their long-suffering parents!) should see them through it. Histaminic states can mimic bacterial and viral infections. For adults, see my approach to infectious illness in Acute Attacks in Section 3.8.

Most problems with a 'wandering' quality may belong to creative individuals whose circadian entrainment tends to wobble.[255] To relate these to oscillations and Discharge, see Section 1.8. Most symptoms originate from our handling of signals.

Signals

In the broad sense of signals as information coming both from outside and from within the processing organs of the body—brain, liver, kidney, endocrine organs—if this composite information is too powerful for the receptors, then they are likely to provoke the opposite from that expected. Receptors at cellular level are measured by their density and receptivity, a function of their threshold for stimulation. Receptors at the level of an organ or even organism rely on the systemic availability of energy to process the incoming signal. If the herbalist provides information from a medicinal plant that is generally stimulant to the sympathetic branch of the autonomic system to a person whose receptivity is high but energy low and poise chronically challenged, the effect of this herb, say *Salvia officinalis*, may in such a case induce the very lethargy the herb was chosen to address. Much will depend upon the dose of the stimulant and the other plants in the mixture and on the stage in the course of treatment and the length of time the person has

---

[255] Refers to diurnal fluctuating proprioceptive stability. See 'wobbly states' in Barker (2020) p436.

been depleted. The choice of plants may be appropriate at a different dosage or at a later stage. When seeing a patient for the first time, the advice to bear in mind is not to attempt to do everything at once but to devise a treatment strategy that has clear stages. In this way, abreactions may be reduced and poise gradually established. This must be communicated clearly to the patient and a realistic time frame offered which may, sometimes, be as long as eighteen months. Much depends upon the season when the first consultation occurs and the seasonality of the patient. This may be flat or spiked and may be at least in part related to their birth month; good statistical evidence shows correlations with month of birth and health.

If the signal strength of a plant prescription matches poorly with the patient's organisational strength and receptivity, plants that modify the ANS will be the first to manifest this disjunction. Plants that modify the posterior pituitary hormones—oxytocin and vasopressin—or the autocoid neurohormones—serotonin, histamine, dopamine, noradrenaline—are also prone to induce a brisk responsiveness. Anterior pituitary hormonal effects are more likely to be delayed. Effects in the short-term are, therefore, possible from a huge range of medicinal plants. The advice has to be "if you are faced with a very complex symptomatology and history, keep it simple". Conversely, if faced with a single stubborn symptom (and presented stubbornly) then the advice is "make it (i.e., the prescription) complex" but keeping in sight a clear (even simple) treatment plan: the complexity comes from the many angles from which you address the so-called "singular" problem. Complexity does not equate to muddle.

The multiple pauses

The menopause is composite and does not revolve simply about a single hormone such as oestrogen. Hormones themselves do nothing unless they are delivered to a receptor in the same way that a key is just a chunk of metal until it is fitted into the appropriate lock. The other important thing about any peripheral hormone is that it responds to a stimulating hormone from the pituitary and that in turn to a pulse from the hypothalamus. The secreted peripheral hormone switches off its stimuli by feedback loops.

The threshold at which the response fires changes with age, season and circumstances. When the stimulating hormone receives no feedback instructing it to switch off, it redoubles its effort and amplifies its effect—so levels in the blood rise. This increase gives rise to symptoms. Androgens and oestrogens switch off their respective stimuli—the hormones FSH and LH within the vertical gonadic axis— at different rates in different people.[256] Each of us has different thresholds and these alter—narrowing or widening—every seven or so years for the rest of life. So, I don't think any trajectory is at all predictable given all this complexity with horizontal within the pituitary gland and transverse effects between its four main axes added in, to say nothing of the aromatisation of oestrogens and other local effects within the reproductive glands. Levels of hormones may be measured in the blood but that tells you little if anything about the receptor density for that hormone sit on or within which cells.

---

[256] The decline in androgens is more gradual than that of oestrogens. A sudden drop in oxytocin often signals the commencement of a decline.

Peri-menopause is a term that is less useful than understanding that all four pauses have different and mixed characteristics in both sexes:

Gonadopause	From infancy to puberty
Menopause	Cessation of menstruation with a surge in FSH
Luteopause	Erratic menstruation with a surge in LH
Andropause	Loss of drive yoked to energy and stable rhythms.

They all need to be assessed in relation to prolactin. This hormone determines the pattern of fertility and the menstrual cycle, along with the need for TRH to make an appearance at ovulation (and keep out of the way for the rest of the month). It may seem odd that this is about the only mention I make of the menstrual cycle, but it is a vehicle of procreation, not an illness. As the long-suffering wife of the diarist Samuel Pepys would complain: "not everything in life can be laid at the door of my monthlies". Menstruation is a reset, a kind of monthly pause.

In short, if you focus entirely on a single H-P axis and ignore the posterior pituitary hormones, you will classify each pause as a singularity when, more realistically, they are all in it together. So, rather than focus on "herbs for the menopause", consider that particular pause as part of an entire endocrine life, part of the ageing problem, which we come to next.[257]

---

[257] All post-pubertal people will eventually see a diminution in their sex hormones, their binding and the receptor density for them. But the steroid hormones of the gonadic axis cannot usefully be separated from the steroid hormones of the adrenal axis nor with steroid agents, such as vitamin D and with cholesterol the precursor to them all.

SECTION 2.7

Ageing

The primary goal of the zygote is to reproduce itself in measured, ordered ways to produce a person, the person maintaining itself all the while. The invariant cell cycle produces all the differentiation. Building is more complicated than destruction[258] so anabolic processes outnumber the catabolic. All of this is production and reproduction of the self, but the more specialised role of meiosis is afforded a restricted number of years (usually heptades, often more) after which the anabolic processes lose their grasp on energy reserve as their mission has presumably been fulfilled. Only social animals live on past the decline in anabolic hormones to help with the grandchildren. The world is biologically and socially sensitive to age, with the energy of youth and the understanding of age.

While feeling unwell always signals a failure of capacitance measured by poise, disease and ageing applies the greatest pressure on our capacitance and so are universal sources of illness. After our physical peak, we begin to lose the strength and capacity to maintain the energetic ratio of poise and interval timing. If we manage circadian regulation well, we may down-regulate the speed of ageing as measured by the Horvarth clock, which assesses the rate of methylation of base pairs in the nuclear DNA. Additionally, the constant negotiation between chromosomal and mitochondrial DNA (enforced upon all eukaryotes) can probably either reduce or accelerate health as measured by the decline in capacitance that ageing entails.[259]

Calcification of vessels and the failure of calcification in the skeleton are entailed in the depredations of age. Of all the griefs that ageing brings, loss of height is surely the

---

[258] As will be seen in Figure 21 in Section 3.6.

[259] The latest biological revolution was initiated by Carl Woese in the 1960s, developed by Bill Martin and extended in current times by Professor Nick Lane at UCL. Steve Horvarth, Professor of human genetics and of biostatistics at UCLA, has used techniques of statistical analysis to generate this index of time in the lives of cells and tissues.

greatest. Accidents aside, ageing in bipeds entails the inevitable reduction in the height of the spine which in turn reduces the capacity of the lungs, the functionality of the digestive tract and exacerbates the congestive blockade of redundant generative organs. Destruction of the structure in the ageing brain, while less inevitable, is even more devastating. The attempt by any kind of therapy to defer these reductions when they make their appearance is far too late for remedial medicine. Embodying medicinal plants into a younger life provides a more realistic alternative, and brings learning and pleasure. They will ensure a less steep, more delayed decline in anabolic yield. Old age comes a bit late to fret over antioxidants: all that and the power of the nurtures should be in place at least by the fifth heptade so that the decline in anabolism will be slowed.

Osteoporosis is more likely without the anti-inflammatory calcium-rich diet of oily fish in earlier decades, if not in infancy. Many even quite active people move about indoors without getting enough vitamin D. Reducing catabolic dominance and increasing nutrient extraction by supporting digestive organs with medicinal plants will gradually counter the trend of bone loss, providing exercise and protein intake are maintained.[260]

If resources have retreated to the centre as discussed in Section 2.5a, pain in small joints will be the common complaint. Increasing protein intake and facilitating its absorption and reducing stress in the corticotrophic axis, and so in the alpha-sympathetic, will reduce the inflammatory load and the burden of fragmented sleep.[261]

If resources have been maintained in the periphery and anabolic function retained, the stress on the centre will be greater. Supporting cardiac function and ensuring (by diet and herbs) the integrity of endothelia in small blood vessels will lower the risk of stroke and infarction which mount with age.

> In all cases, calm the heart and reduce the risks associated with fibrillation. *Melissa* should be the mainstay of most prescriptions. It is a difficult herb to extract and preserve well so nothing less than the very best quality will do.

Bowel habit becomes critical in the aged as the colon becomes prone to folding and to diverticula. Transit of faecal matter from zone to zone depends probably upon diurnal and nocturnal contingencies, especially diet. Length of feeding and fasting phases will help regulate the entero-hepatic circulation of bile and the efficiency of its resorption in the terminal ileum.[262]

Supply massage oils to elderly patients with diverticulitis or problems with bowel habit. A simple fixed oil in which you infuse volatile oils of (at least) lavender, lemon and thyme and others you deem appropriate. Show them how to start by generously filling the palms with oil and applying it first to the left and then to the right iliac fossa then drawing the oil up each flank in turn with smooth strong movements of their hand. If you are able and practised, roll the skin in areas highlighted in Figure 18 with the Lapraz

---

[260] See Tables in Section 3.6.

[261] For plants to use, see the Tables in Section 3.6.

[262] To recap from Section 2.2, advise a feeding phase of nine (at most ten) hours in the 24.

technique mentioned in Mapping the Body in Section 2.5a. This is painful if there are kinins and histamine to release but the reward will come as a night of deep sleep.

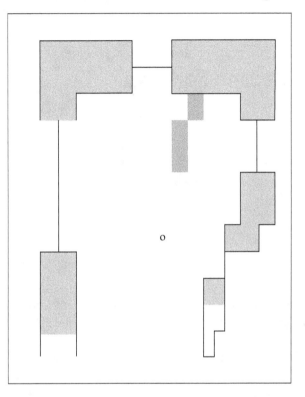

Figure 18: Anatomical intestinal areas show where abdominal massage will offer most benefit

As for fatigue and stress in the older person, use herbs like *Melissa* and *Levisticum* to dampen the intensity of fears, including the fear of losing function. Reducing catabolism is safer than forcing anabolism—careful what you build. Best from diet high in protein, good fats and complex carbohydrates with plenty of nuts and seeds for minerals.

Résumé of ideas in Part Two

Listening is a biological activity. In Shannon's Theory of Information, effective communication requires an open channel where the signal is larger than the noise, not the other way around. The action of a medicinal plant is a spurious signal: it is very noisy. This allows complex signals to enter the terrain surreptitiously where they can nudge at pivots, ballast S-O-R thresholds and buffer nodes without creating disturbance. Secondary effects permit organs to organise more effectively with less energy.

Don't work to a script. If the consultation is an open but guided conversation, not an interrogation, the personality of the patient reveals itself and therefore the constitutional sources of their current problems, which may be said to have started yesterday but actually started when they started. Improvisation takes courage, openness and the preparation that study and reflection has provided the practitioner.

As herbalists we can modify the assaults of pathology but mostly focus on preventative medicine, improving the capacitance of our patients. We can be more the catalyst for change than its fighting agent.

- Human need for an interpretive scheme for our individual and collective ills is universal—therapeutics in other words. Particular therapeutic styles and operational modes may be historical, geographical and cultural. However, especially in urgent cases, certain approaches are found everywhere—the empathic impulse is relatively, but not entirely, free from local variance, at least in peacetime.[263]
- Built upon our physicality, we humans are linguistic and technological: we verbalise and make things. Accordingly, the components of human medicine always involve communicative domains—tactile and verbal—but also recommendatory with respect

---

[263] See the Pharisees who crossed to the other side of the road in the parable of the Samaritan. See Graeber & Wengrow (2021) for what is, in effect, a history of empathy.

to regimen and medicament and, if the need arises (and often it does), technical. As for technics with a therapeutic aim, we have massage and manipulation, restorative exercises, surgery, medicine and regimen, with good nursing (trained or natural) taking primacy.[264]

- A primary requirement of good medicine is to know which of these modes are most appropriate to a case, and to know that communicative skill will improve any outcome. Accidents and emergencies require urgent application of physiological and anatomical knowledge, as everyone surely understands. An aortic aneurysm, for example, may have been precipitated by unhelpful life choices but this life-threatening situation cannot be resolved by medicinal means or change of habits. Even so, good recovery from surgery may be aided by medicinal and pastoral care. Physical therapies may offer temporary respite from a great deal of apparently musculo-skeletal problems, but they will be helped by pastoral and medicinal interventions and also by physical therapies and acupuncture—a combination of technical skill and the kind of wholistic acumen that herbalists learn to deploy. The majority of cases are not emergencies and calming the drama is a constituent part of therapy.
- Culinary and medicinal plants in the right hands associate well with medicinal interventions of nearly any kind, which need always pastoral care in the broader sense of the nurtures.
- Self-care requires energy and so depends upon poise.

The clinical relevance of all this I hope is now obvious. Beyond repairing short-term injuries or mishaps (and even these may turn out to have a deeper hinterland), using medicinal plants well is to situate the patient in the therapeutic environment *care*-fully provided by the therapist.

This is the fundament of physic: empathy combined with curiosity and a desire to offer helpful service in the most detailed and careful way possible.

By extension, I would advocate that allowing the patient to witness the exploration of their own psycho-physical and psychosocial lives is the prerequisite. Situating it in their ancestral and contemporary lineage, they will be best prepared for the integrating effects of a carefully personalised prescription of medicinal plants following the appropriate advice on nurturing relations with the self and others.

---

[264] Expanded and summarised in Barker (2013) Section 2.

PART THREE

PHYSIC FROM THE ELEMENTS OF WATER, SUN,
AIR AND EARTH—NATURE IS OUR NURTURE

Where to begin again?

Zeaxanthin and lutein, we are told, may protect the musculoskeletal system; pomegranate extract could indeed improve skin; walnuts may combat side effects of stress; extra virgin olive oil could combat cognitive decline; blackcurrant may mitigate bone loss in older women, and a mediterranean diet could reduce the worst viral symptoms ...

So they say: a trawl through reports of studies make these and so many other announcements. Who do they wish to inform or impress? Zeaxanthin and lutein and the rest surely do us a lot of good but note the subjunctive mood, the "may" and the "could": better make no assertions lest the puritans think we get above ourselves and come after us. Or better to live well with plants and not have to endlessly proclaim the benefits.

Everybody attends to themselves every day (no citations needed), which is to say that they practice first aid when they are unwell or, when well, think or feel about their fortunate state, feed it, or pay it no attention, according to their disposition or mood.

You might think first aid would be error resistant because it is instant: there is no time for you to think of doing things differently. Even hardline empiricists who repudiate ideas have to start with an idea or hunch. These are open to change, even improvement. As a child I was taught to spread butter immediately on to a burnt hand without stopping to think. Nobody does that any more but rather dunks the hand into cold water and keeps it there. This is where science—stopping to think—comes to the rescue of bad ideas, like butter which should be put on bread, not burns.

Empirical medicine develops from the observations and techniques of first aid and elaborates a whole body of techniques, a whole corpus of practice so that practitioners can intervene effectively without having to stop and think. This is where holding on to traditional ways of doing things (as if traditions were immune from evolution) may lead us to doing things without thinking because surely the authoritative works only recorded their successes. In ancient medicine, Galen expressed contempt for Empirical medicine for their having no theory of practice, no philosophy.[265] As Robert Winston said of contemporary fertility treatments, "I tried not to do things just because that is the way they had always been done". Pondering a question holistically deters you from using or avoiding a medicine just because it is novel or just because it is ancient. Speaking of which …

Hippocratic medicine takes a more long-term view than first aid and asks physicians to position the patient in their whole environment and history, to allow space for a more interpretive view of the self, to take, what today we would call an anthropological approach. This involves looking at things through the eyes of the patient and allows the patient to see things from, if not the physician's perspective (which should involve knowledge, skill and understanding), at least an altered point of view. This takes time and appropriate space, quite unsuited to first aid.

The intention of terrain medicine favours a hippocratic approach but is not slow or averse to recognising useful heuristics for which a perfect theory has not emerged (and perhaps the better for it). Although terrain medicine is addressing the singularity of a person's life it has nonetheless to draw on generalities. Without generalities, we would not have any written materia medica. We would have to rely on the words of others, and they would have to be present or nearby. We test these generalities in our practice and modify our ideas with experience where experience is a singular experiment. If the generalities harden into a theory, they lose the specificity of time and place and harden so that their message becomes distant, puzzling, or even absurd. Of course, scholarship tries to unravel the social realities behind the indications of Dioscorides but a more singular herbal medicine is passed on by living apprenticeships so that the past indication is modified, not revered. A clinical trial fixes an idea as inflexibly as can a hallowed text.

So, writing and making up a prescription in the dispensary juggles the theoretical and the practical, moving ably from generality to singularity. The deft medical plant anthropologist shifts from one to the other as occasion arises. Work with the particular and be slow to generalise. Your materia medica needs to be questioned after every prescription is reviewed in the follow-up appointment.

Plants also practice first aid. We not only eat them as food for our primary care but we also scavenge the products of their self-medication to help us digest that food and even extend it to a life of being well rather than ill.

---

[265] Galen mocked doctors who did not know their plants (Morton 1981) yet there is another layer of confusion in that Dioscorides has been called an Empiricist because he allegedly *did* know his plants (*Dioscorides' Botanical Legacy in the Medieval Mediterranean Critical Practices of Botanical Illustration*: lecture delivered by Professor Andrew Griebeler to British Society for the History of Pharmacy January 2023).

Plants, people, process, the natural world

Herbals in history have put the plants first, as agents of the natural order, perhaps of the divine. They sat alongside textbooks for doctors and apothecaries when most medicines were plants. The recent past, at least in the anglophone sphere, has seen books and papers that use plants as exemplars of process. The process has been to place together plants with a fully modern understanding of human physiology and asks to be treated as respectable science, even with a well-argued heterodox twist. While the handful of such works have been adopted as medical textbooks by most phytotherapists, they have not entered into mainstream medical training and have met with some reluctance and misgivings from some herbalists who hanker after a deep past where herbals would have put the plants first as supreme agents of nature.

Culture and cultivation emerge from our deep need for plants. Beauty has always been figured into the natural world but has had to contend with utilitarian concerns, such as eating. Horticulture and visual arts have in common the desire to tame or placate or respect nature while exploiting it. Artificial or artful ideas present nature to be rather disorganised and dishevelled in detail, hence the charm, but beautiful and harmonious at both very large and microscopic scales, hence the awe.

Science is intensely competitive. Competition tends not to induce humour except among actors and comedians. Religion, once it wields power cannot contemplate humour with its subversive suggestion of ridicule. Religion when it is non-conformist is too attentive to resistance to be funny. But you do not have to be an ascetic to appreciate at times that the facts of life possess an austere beauty. Medicine has ousted organised religion as a primary cultural force.

Humour, as comedians like to remind us, is a serious business. Humoralism takes itself too seriously and literally in modern times but when such ideas were conceived, they were philosophy, that most serious subject of all. Today, the humours, when taken literally, entail a certain religiosity. Pharmacists and other medical scientists are nervous about humour and aesthetics. Media medical pundits, by contrast, have to be endlessly jokey and chummy for fear of seeming too serious, though I can't see why this inspires us to take them too seriously. I think responsible herbalists can relax and just get on with helping the people who ask for help and not fret too much which side of which divide they are supposed to be on.

It is supremely human to take sides even when there are really no sides to take. Without people there is no discussion to be had, without the natural world there can be no people. Plants and our other eukaryote allies figure at our scale and vision, but insects and their prokaryote prey outnumber us and may come to inherit the world which we have done so much to alter to what seemed at the time to be for our own convenience.

As for practitioners of herbal medicine, we are probably better off being marginalised rather than being symbolically and superficially endorsed. Although in recent decades I joined enthusiastically in the campaigns for us to be granted statutory regulation in Britain and would continue to do so if the political climate were conducive, cultural directions in the age of the internet move towards fragmentation and the threats from consumer capitalism and commodification of health operate at both large and small, even individual scales.

The celebration of plant-based medicine can best be conducted by practice, by suggestion rather than by strident claims; by being an integral part of a local community. An interest in historical uses of plants is always instructive but I think reverence is misplaced. Why is 'traditional wisdom' considered superior to modern wisdom? We have primary evidence of today's human follies, why should we suppose our ancestors did not have their own? I am grateful to Mrs Grieve for having notated so much material from the past but much of what she talks about does seem like tales from a foreign country, fascinating as they are, delightful as they may be, and as prone to error as the rest of us. The criticism the Eclectics and Physiomedicalists made of orthodox medical practice was no doubt salient at the time. They made knowledge of plants from America available to a wider audience some of which have become mainstays of contemporary practice. We should be grateful to them for that service alone but I think it better to see how we can adapt their therapeutic ideas (which to me seem dogmatic in tone and narrow in focus) to our own in light of recent not earlier physiological understanding. I wonder whether we maintain respect for these in the sense that we do not wish to speak ill of the dead rather than believing literally in their biological merit. Even so, if you have the time to be a jackdaw, there are gems within many elderly texts and even from a few decades ago. If the ideas seem arcane, some germ of them or some detail of a herbal preparation can be adapted to one's own purpose.

For example, *Herbal Medication* co-authored by husband and wife A.W. and L.R. Priest contains many useful therapeutic ideas expressed in an admirably concise and lucid style.[266] The second paragraph of their Foreword states a clinical ambition with which surely no reasonable clinician would disagree. Yet, their Introduction declares from the outset their firm adherence to "the vitalistic philosophy", which by the mid-twentieth

---

[266] Subtitled *A Clinical and Dispensary Handbook*. Reprinted by NIMH in 2005. *Herbal Thymes* of December 2004 carried an obituary of the Priests to which an eulogy was added by one of their unnamed children.

century had become discredited as superfluous, if nothing else. I have discussed this with some practitioners who, though they hold the Batchelor of Science degree in herbal medicine, find nothing anomalous in this position. However apt the 'vital force' may sound, it does not have the explanatory power of biological energetics and so makes vitalism superfluous, even as metaphor. Unless it is simply a question of faith.

From the clinical point of view, I have yet to understand how you apply the physiomedical contract-relax axis in practice. Their book repeats the assertions from first principles without explaining with which physiological observations they correlate. The authors were naturopaths and osteopaths so their focus on physical structure may have contributed to the astringency of their style.

I think John Fletcher-Hyde[267] summarised better what I am trying to say: 'don't venerate any therapeutic measure just because it is very ancient or very modern'. Our style of expression reflects our generation and milieu—also our political orientations. Herbal medicine in Britain reflected a subculture that felt comfortably besieged because it had right on its side, much of it explicitly religious. In America in the 1970s, herbal texts seemed to be dominated by the Christian Right. Even when not overtly religious, the books and articles and events I attended were evangelical in tone. This conflicted with my own view of nature, which stands for itself and has more need of our care and respect than for our enthusiasm. Enthusiasm often bestows virtue on the enthusiast rather than the object of affection.

I have certainly found naturopathic practices such as compresses and massage helpful and many herbalists will make them an integral part of their practice. They are so natural and empirically useful I cannot see that they are in need of much flag-waving. One notion that sits strangely with biology concerns the notion of purity. The whole point about a medicinal plant in the raw state is that it is impure: made up of complex mixtures. We want them to be pure only in the sense of being unadulterated and free of harmful substances, whether natural or not. Rules of hygiene insist that our medicines are uncontaminated by unwanted materials but being pure in this sense does not mean simple. Purified single substances belong with pharmaceutical and homeopathic products.[268] Purity in the sense of unmixed has many puritan antecedents, one of which dates back to the naturopathy of the 1930s which, coincidentally or not, is associated with the notion of racial purity. Apart from the horrors (as if one could forget them) of this culmination of eugenics, they are scientifically wrong. The creativity of biological form tends always towards admixture and hybridisation, the better to adapt to a changing world. There are no pure essences: to quote Heraclitus, "there is nothing permanent except change". A small exception to this in our ever-changing bodies occurs in the iris. For just this reason, it finds use as a biometric marker. This makes the practice of iridology particularly absurd, yet Bernard Jensen is still celebrated among some herbalists in America, even though his ability to diagnose from the iris was demonstrated beyond doubt to be

---

[267] He was the son of Fred Fletcher Hyde (an Emeritus President of NIMH) and grandson of Jesse Hyde who in 1908 founded Hydes Herbal Clinic in Leicester, which has seen continual practice since then and prospers to this day. It was on their premises that I was inducted onto the NIMH Tutorial Course in 1976.

[268] Standardised herbal extracts take an intermediate position.

flawed.[269] During my training in herbal medicine, I found myself tacitly acknowledging many ideas and practices that I have since found to be without merit.

My point is not to debunk them but to suggest that students and apprentices of herbal medicine retain their critical faculties, something I failed to do. The power of criticism is not to disparage but to protect your future patients from ideas insufficiently thought out or just plain faulty. At the School of Herbal Medicine, I think we felt like a besieged minority (at times besieged by other herbalists), so it felt disloyal to question anything that famously challenged mainstream thinking, or at least that is how I excuse some of my uncritical thinking at the time. I urge my herbal readers to be remain sceptical of all assumptions in medicine, alternative as well as mainstream.

Parallel medicine

The archaeological record shows that long before the invention of writing we have practised some form of medicine. The style, form and character of the practice emerges from social norms and environmental needs.

In classical times, only that envisaged by and for the middle and upper echelons of society, made its way into writing, be that in pre-Columbian Mesoamerica, India, China or the Greece of Hippocrates.

Folk medicine is much less recorded though many of its useful remedies no doubt leaked into written medicine or inspired it without citation.[270]

Hippocratic medicine excelled at being environmental and personalised in the sense of seeking to match remedy to constitution but also to widen the horizon of diagnosis from the present peril to health, to lay emphasis on nurtures.

Galenic medicine was more utilitarian but its empirical insights were straightjacketed by humoral theory. As medicine and religion proved powerless against the scourge of epidemics, faith in doctors and their theories of cure turned to derision by writers in the Early Modern Period like Petrarch and, later, the satires of Molière while religion shifted its power base. Modern medicine (eventually) did well out of the scientific revolutions and doctors regained social status, which they would like to retain. For surgery and the management of some diseases, they have earned their trust. For most other illness, they are straight-jacketed by the scientific method and hemmed in by the industrial complex.

The only good medicine is that appropriate to the presenting circumstances. There should be no alternative to good medicine. Medicine of any sort fades beside the pressures of poor housing and other burdens of poverty, accidents and ill-luck, addictions and folly.

---

[269] I read him while I was studying in North America and found him forceful but uncongenial. I do not know how far right Jensen was but Eric Lindlahr, an early proponent of iridology, declared white supremacist beliefs very graphically and explicitly in his textbooks. When he was cited in a presentation in recent years by an acclaimed phytotherapist, I pointed out this connection. The man in question did not know this but did not think it worth retracting as if herbal and natural medicines were beyond politics. After Auschwitz, can anything be?

[270] Cf. Barker (2013) p. 14.

Medicine should not be primarily about flogging you some stuff, which is often allied with an attempt to satisfy some insurance anxiety, as in "Could you be low in zinc? Is your immune system up to scratch?" (as if it were an item of software); the suggestion is that deficiencies can be replaced by a market commodity without necessarily questioning how the alleged deficiency arose.

Alternative medicine sounds like a hopeful (or hopeless) prescription for social dissidents. Well, they need good medicine like anyone else. Complementary medicine is a euphemism: a polite way of saying that it may be used in conjunction with orthodox "proper" medicine and at least will not do any harm.

There may be a wide range of motives for anyone to wish to practise herbal medicine and it may be a dissident voice. But if, like me, you think the patient is more important than ideology, I suggest that herbal medicine should not be celebrated just because it was once orthodox medicine. That it is ancient is reassuring but is not a reason to idealise it. After all, orthodox herbal medicine did little to lower the death toll of the epidemics and plagues that have characterised human history.[271] Parallel Medicine depends upon a coherent body of knowledge, theory and modes of practice that are adequate to treat a range of non-communicable conditions. These, on the admission of the many doctors with whom I have had the pleasure to work, orthodox medicine is less well equipped to treat. There are historical reasons for this, as there must always be, but also the shortcomings of the scientific method for complex psychosocial illness provide a niche in the ecological sense of the word that needs to be well and sustainably filled. Modern medicine, often for good reasons, has engendered rigid protocols by relying on evidence from narrowly defined criteria or stays waiting for evidence to catch up with our practices and modes of treatment. As a medical herbalist, I conduct necessary and auxiliary treatments in parallel with all true and ethical forms of medicine. The practice is alternative only in the narrow and local medico-legal sense. I hope I have encouraged the reader to say so too.

The expression of herbal medicine may have attracted unworthy opponents but its broad, humane properties belong to everyone and no-one so are neither cause for crusade nor a cult, though some may see it that way. Herbal medicine is a major designation not in opposition to anything or anyone and needs to be treated as such.

We can go to the natural world, visit beautiful gardens and wonderful horticultural centres and botanic gardens and take our instruction from the world of plants. Looking and wondering dispels our need of any daft ideas to float our practice. Healthy scepticism sits very well with an observant eye. Curiosity and willingness to change our minds saves us from being dogmatic, too certain. As Britain was the first country to industrialise and urbanise from a relatively small rural catchment area, it lost, except in small pockets, the matter-of-factness about medicinal plants that persisted in populations in other places including countries with an advance industrialised economy and an orthodox

---

[271] The aromatic plants and resins in the nosepieces of those tending the sick or more often attending to the corpses in Italy during the plague of 1643 may have protected the few but did not alter the fact that up to half the population died in appalling circumstances. Medicines were futile. Tibayrenc, M Encyclopedia of Infectious Diseases Wiley 2007.

medicine quite as dominant as our own.[272] Such cultures seemed to be very comfortable with holding two apparently opposed approaches in parallel and have easily shrugged off dismissal and scorn, as I came to know in France, Poland and Lithuania.

Herbal medicine used to be unique in being pan-cultural and even now that modern industrialised medicine has become global, local herbalism may act in industrialised countries as a bulwark against the commodification of life. In parallel with surgery and other technical modalities of orthodox medicine, modern phytotherapy offers a better outcome for many conditions that threaten the quality and productiveness of life.

Herbal traditions travel well and have no need for conflict with other approaches to remedy the human condition. They can create exchanges if they resist the tribalism to which we are all prone. They can integrate treatment modalities like acupuncture that were once exotic without the need for importing the plants from the country in which the tradition first flowered. Localism and exoticism easily hybridise and new traditions emerge. Traditions operate in their patients' better interests if they combine theoretical ideas and practical methods without too many demarcation disputes and banner waving. Being eclectic enriches if one can do so without an enfeebling promiscuity. Economic interests still trawl the plant kingdom for new molecules and colonial powers have appropriated indigenous plants over the centuries. The ancient spice trade has been a cornerstone of cultural influence (and appropriation) over millennia for the benefit, ultimately, of human health.

Flowers are emblematic of love in many cultures. A culture is a consociation of shared values whereas a cult is exclusionary. As herbalists pay due observance—in common with gardeners and naturalists—to the flowers of the field, we are blessed in belonging to such an open culture and saved from being confined within a cult.

Forms and styles of herbal medicine

Like any other human cultural activity, there is a range of approaches the character of each of which depends upon the temporal style of the practitioner and the sub-culture to which they tend to adhere. In contemporary herbal medicine these range from the high-minded—whether philosophical, spiritual or humanist—to the pragmatic and empirical. These in turn reflect the needs of the moment: if you have acute distress you might want a different approach than called for in the case of a chronic ailment. But it goes deeper than that, as evinced by the separation (more like a divorce) of the Society of Apothecaries from the Grocers in seventeenth century Britain. A similar division came about between the pharmacists and *herboristes* in twentieth century France and the hiving off of *heilpratikers* from orthodox medicine in Germany, and the uneasy relationship between medicine and *fitoterapia* in contemporary Italy, to name but a very few and to say nothing about the self-proclaimed "health-food" industry.

It goes back to the distinction between commodity and process. Archaeology supports the notion that trade preceded agriculture so there is nothing new about goods and artefacts being exchanged between peoples. These may be tokens of the reciprocity that lies at the heart of human interaction, even within a family or small group.

---

[272] I am gliding over complex historical and sociopolitical questions that I would love to pursue but they belong in a fat book.

Reciprocity underpins the human need for justice. Empathy and kindness—though they might imply reciprocity—are almost instinctual impulses. The idea is that we respond spontaneously to human hurt before we put a price-tag on to it.

But everyone has to make a living. How rich we become depends upon how society values our contribution or how instruments of power skew that valuation. The industrial-medical complex has become self-sustaining because you could not afford the massive capital cost of hospital building without commanding the budget and whole-hearted support of the majority of the population. The increase in average human lifespan and the rise in overall prosperity has been allied in large part—correctly or not—to modern medicine. Even if agriculture and trade in foodstuffs are also given credit, the political environment in which they operate expects medicine to provide the safety net for those who have become ill, however realistic that expectation might turn out to be.

In Britain and elsewhere in the post-industrial world, medicine and law are privileged professions. In the anglo-Saxon in contrast to the Celtic mindset, education is Cinderella to these elder sisters.[273] The distinction between a profession and a trade can still be made, even if the disparity in earnings is not always as great as in the past. The simple advice given by an aspirational father to his son in the 1960s according to Ian Jack was "Never take a job where you have to get your hands dirty".[274] Since then the situation has become more complicated and differently gendered but the question remains: "Is herbal medicine a profession or a trade"? Or is it some kind of hybrid such as a cottage service industry?[275]

The answer to this question is as varied as the routes practitioners have taken to their practice. Some move sideways from a previous profession or service occupation. Others are born gardeners or else come from families with an 'alternative' disposition. Perhaps all of us are critics of, if not refugees from, contemporary culture. When I decided to become a herbalist, to act upon a buried impulse that I did not know was there, my first instinct (given my cerebral temperament and dreamer tendencies) was to start from the bottom, to get 'my hands dirty'. To that end I became an apprentice herb grower but that decision does not imply that I rejected professional ethos for the subsequent practice. Modern medicine, after all, sits upon the apprentice model and combines it with academic discipline. My view of apprenticeship has more to do with lifelong learning than in the presumption of supposed 'mastery': while respecting experience and acknowledging the benefits of successful practice, it rejects hierarchy or veneration. I find it astonishing that anyone might think that a course of primary instruction could confer the title of 'master'. (Perhaps it is time to refigure the award of MSc!). The professions have always been hierarchical and herbal medicine might show the way in making it more convivial,

---

[273] When I joined the teaching profession in 1965, we had just been awarded an increase but were still paid less than postmen who at the time went on strike for more pay. When I became a manual worker to make a better living, I still managed to evoke respect in rural Wales when it was known that I was a qualified teacher.

[274] LRB 43,14 p. 45.

[275] The distinctions and cross-fertilisation between art and craft, trade and profession is deep within many cultures, perhaps in all. The separation has played out notably in the history of the natural sciences and herbal medicine. For an excellent historical analysis on a broader canvas, historians of our art and craft may be interested in Pamela H. Smith, *From Lived Experience to the Written Word: Reconstructing Practical Knowledge in Early Modern Europe* (Chicago: 2022).

along the lines expressed by Ivan Illich.[276] One obstacle would be the commodification of health which, though not at all new, has accelerated in secular consumer cultures so that every ill has an expectation of a remedy that has been industrially produced or professionally "delivered". This returns us to the question I put to the herbalist: are you plying a trade or joining a profession. Doctors have neatly sidestepped the issue by deputising the trade side of their operation to the pharmacists.

When the National Institute of Medical Herbalists (NIMH) changed its name and charter, it outlawed the selling of herbal products over a shop counter. The provisions of the relative Sections of the Medicines Act of 1969 made specific reference to this by insisting that patients seeking remedies on shop premises were obliged to enter by a door not available to the general public; in other words, a consultation could not be conducted over a shop counter. The driver of this position in the United Kingdom was Fred Fletcher Hyde. The wife of Ernest Cockayne FNIMH who had also worked towards the inclusion of herbalists into the statute told me at a conference in 1980 that in her opinion this was the single biggest mistake the herbalists had made: corner shops, especially in the Midlands and the North but also in poorer metropolitan parts further south and in niche positions elsewhere had been a corner stone of local communities and a major source of professional income. All beside the point, really, as very few herbalists have respected the provisions of the Act in this regard and many do not even know that they are flouting the law. This became ironically apparent in the campaign of 1994 which saw the foundation of the European Herbal Practitioners Association when shops that did conduct consultations over the counter invoked the very act whose provisions they were contravening. In all the many discussions over the years, advocates of retail herbalism have maintained that it is the only way of making a living.[277] My own professional experience contradicts this assertion and when, newly qualified, I was offered a part-time job at a wholefood shop that sold dried herbs where I was to give advice to customers on their health benefits. I was depressed to find that people with chronic arthritis asked in all seriousness whether 25p worth of a common herb could help resolve their problems. By contrast, selling medicinal plants in a tent or the open air seemed joyous because the plants were live and engaged the purchaser actively. But, close as it comes, horticulture is not medicine.

This returns us to the fundamental question: as a herbal physician are you selling a commodity or engaging in a process? My answer would be that my dispensary is not a shop but ancillary to the consultation, part of its outcome.

The problem with going into a shop to seek help and advice is that you have not invested in a planned and purposive encounter. Intimate problems require a private space for an open discussion. Ideally that place feels generous, well-lit and open. The investment the practitioner has made will invite a reciprocal sense of being in the right place. Trust is typically built in and trust cannot be bought and sold

Without meaning we suffer. When between what we want to mean and what we think we have meant are in mismatch, we also suffer.

---

[276] His works—*Tools for Conviviality, Medical Nemesis, Imprisoned in the Global Classroom*—remain fine critiques of the industrial-medical complex and advocated apprenticeship over school learning.

[277] There are a number of herbalists who have recognised the dichotomy and approached it head on by separating their shops from successful practices (though these are often entered via the shop in contravention of the Act).

Philosophy and practice in herbal medicine

Philosophy interests itself in asking the right questions rather than providing convenient answers: although it might hope for resolution, it acts against self-satisfaction and complacency. During training and when teaching, I have often heard that herbal medicine needs a Philosophy. This may have been a call not so much for philosophy as for articles of faith: the yearning seemed more a quest for answers than formulating the right questions, a search for a schedule of principles, of assertions.

A reasonable request, surely, for a practical enterprise with important ethical and social consequences and one which has as many "how does it work…" as "what should I do when …" questions. Doesn't it also depend upon local conditions? Medicine in all its forms has an anthropological pre-history. Some traditions are revered, others marginalised depending upon the time and culture.

Even the notion of a tradition depends upon the speaker. When patients mention their "traditional doctor" to me, they are referring to their GP. I point out that she or he practices modern medicine whereas I practise traditional medicine.

You may be impatient with these distinctions but the subject is morally serious, given that people will be entrusting you with their health. From clinical experience and from reflecting upon what has taken place with every one of my thousands of cases, I warmly recommend that you develop some kind of model of phytotherapy, even some provisional "theory of cure" just so that you can act effectively and convincingly. A model is not an ideology. Constant revision and reexamination provides a due corrective to complacency.

The model

If you leave a training course with a bag of very promising tools, convincing because "validated" by prestigious published research, it will be helpful if you have some idea how they are to be put into practice; you will need to develop some kind of modus operandi. Case studies seemed so illustrative at the time of your training but manage not to resemble the cases that present themselves to you. The confidence of ideas can slip away when faced with having to make a living from them. This is the alleged dichotomy between theory and practice. Philosophers take a primary interest in theory while those with an empirical bent want to know "just what works".

In many spheres, including the market place and the clinic, it would not suit one to practice if one were solely a philosopher. Yet the practitioner with the most prag- matic outlook would develop (or even start with) some assortment of heuristics, some rules-of-thumb. If she or he became successful, they might post-rationalise their heuris- tics into some kind of method. They would have become by so doing, against their incli- nation, somewhat philosophical. This alleged distinction between theory and practice is demonstrably false and just part of human snobbery: the tendency to sneer at people who approach a problem from the opposite end than we do. So, we could contrast a "nuts and bolts" approach against one that is "airy-fairy", the latter exhibited by some- one who is fastidious against blundering, the former impatient to "just get on with it". Both caricatures result mainly from disposition; best not to make too much of it.[278]

There may be a gap between what one claims to be the source of one's practice, what one believes to be the case, and the multitudinous elements of one's formation and expe- rience. These are inseparable from one's beliefs and therefore the way one operates both consciously and from the deeper undertow that sways into view from hidden depths when least expected.

Modelling may turn out to be how memory and learning operate: in order to act effec- tively we need a simple, consolidated mental framework into which new information can be placed. Intuition may actually always be at work—what feels right—in a model, but beware those who elevate this unseen player into some kind of justification for what they do or how they profess to practice.

One could argue that herbalists who prescribe only from a schedule of plants for which modern evidence has demonstrated a positive influence on physiology are fol- lowing a model, and a strict verifiable one at that. But, given the narrow focus research must employ, this model of restless empiricism will shift constantly and rests on the assumption that the questions researchers posed were realistic and did edit out the com- plexities. A model should not be resistant to change and qualification but if inherently unstable, it is a poor model. Galen could have done with some updating during the long periods when his ideas held sway.

Galen's prodigious output included many disparaging references to the Empiricists— those who considered experience to be the only guide, rejecting all medical theorising. My experience of working strictly to a schedule of plants linked to their medical appli- cation has been that whether it works well turns out to be the luck of the draw. Success shows up less than half the time and you never know which portion you'll get and where you go from there. Probably this arises from the reductionist nature of the research being followed. Asking limited questions can only provide limited answers. You don't have to be a medical scientist to be capable of naive reductionism. The several schedules I will

---

[278] Herbalism is a composite affair: pharmacognosy provides all the benefits of observation (never idle) over idle speculation and should be the foundational subject for anyone wishing to call themselves a herbalist.

present in Section 3.6 are derived from a theoretical model which relies on measures but does not actually measure anything but is designed to express relations between things that can be measured.

A physical model can be taken apart and its components viewed but a conceptual model is a representation of a system. It consists of concepts used to help us know, understand, or draw from a subject the model represents. When operating and learning from any model, its limitations should remain in peripheral vision and every possibility of fallacy confronted. The most important point to understand is that the model does not measure anything. Rather it points to relationships and tropisms. When we speak of a patient's response to cortisol, we make a judgement according to the clinical model and have no idea what their serum levels might be.[279]

Opinion

Ideas and opinions—about how the world is or should be—are cheap. They should not (here comes an opinion) be lightly expressed. Yet here I am about to commit one towards (I hope not against) the reader so I had better come out with it without further ado.

Reconciling the empirical and the theoretical will happen automatically because, as mentioned above, it is virtually impossible to act without some heuristic, some rule-of-thumb. The theoretician will look at an outcome (say in the clinic, with a case) and see that it does not quite match the forethought idea that framed the therapeutic intention, the prescription. He (especially he) could rearrange and re-model the ideas and post-rationalise the narrative so that the outcome, though an outlier, was not a mistake. She (especially she) will spot a cock-up and admit the error. Gender stereotypes aside, the theoretician will have altered their model for next time, just like an empiricist!

The best path for a herbalist of either disposition is not to come down too hard on one side or other but to adopt a model consciously. When I started in my herbal studies, there were a number of floating ideas but they did not cohere into any recognisable theory of cure. Physiomedicalism that had provided previous generations of anglophone herbalists with a clinical model was taught with somewhat faint praise though many of the actions with which herbs were credited were retained without much question.[280]

Instead of a distinct model, a miscellany of findings was provided which scientific evidence suggested were true and so could be applied rationally as suggested or dictated by the case. Some of our teachers were doctors so we were always in the shadow of modern medicine, even while finding ways to disparage it. Some of my colleagues apparently felt the lack of a coherent approach and corpus of beliefs and gravitated to TCM, taking up acupuncture or Ayurveda. I had spent four years in the Americas seeking (and not

---

[279] Even if we knew them, we could not evaluate their significance from the measurement alone.

[280] The quality of diaphoretic applied to, say, *Sambucus nigra*, seemed not to explain much beyond managing a fever. I take it often and seem not perspire when doing so, nor have any patients for whom I have prescribed it made mention of it, though they have mentioned many other responses. Further I have never found out how to be sure I have discriminated effectively between trophic states. It was not for lack of exposition: the writings of Priest are eminently clear (Priest & Priest 1983) but they do sound as if delivered from on high and impervious to change. Perhaps the invocation of the vital force that encumbers rather than illuminates biology was the real stumbling block.

finding) a path and so was not about to once again jump ship. But for the first years in practice, I had to rely on my previous good experiences in France to feel I had some idea of what I was doing.[281] Then on a trip to Paris, I came across the work of Drs Duraffourd, Lapraz and others which set me on another phase of learning, this time in the neuroendocrine theory of terrain (now known as Endobiogenic medicine). I knew I had come upon a suitable model even as I barely understood it.

> The model does not measure things but conceives how they are arranged and describes how they function. Things are just a stand-in for relations. The model is an illuminative device for thoughtful action, to shed light on the myriad of alternative explanations. It stabilises thought and action to prevent stumbling in the dark but with critical and sceptical lamplight switched on. Unlike belief, it does not claim infallibility but, in good faith, allows us to operate with open minds and hearts alert to, and adapting to, countervailing evidence and able to be revisionist without prematurely jumping ship. The latter remark implies loyalty and adherence; yes, but to a decent helpful way of doing things, not to a blind creed.

Evidence

Theories, notably medical theories, that lead to intervention or acts of omission are reprehensible if their claims are based upon flimsy thinking or the opposite: hard-baked thinking—seemingly solid—but based on misguided notions. I underwent a needless tonsillectomy when a young infant and may still be suffering its adverse effects. My mother thought she had no choice in the face of the opinion of doctors. My younger brother suffered as a baby a decade after me from other medical opinions. These explanations for his distress sounded implausible to me as an eleven-year-old. He died in his fifties from a misdiagnosed illness. The history of medicine chronicles much outrageous harm.[282] All this might sound like a call for evidence-based medicine.

We as herbalists certainly need an evidential direction, as well as time, for careful thought and feeling before intervening or dissuading people from a medical intervention when our opinion is sought. One way of avoiding harm is to monitor your treatments very carefully so that if no good is coming from them, they can be stopped or suspended. If you persist, it suggests that your ideas are more important than the evidence of experience. Galen was a physician and surgeon with an extraordinary breadth of experience. He was perhaps too autocratic to accept evidence that failed to conform to preconceived conceptions, working with the conviction of theory rather than a flexible model.[283]

---

[281] This was *Cahiers de Phytothérapie Clinique* in five volumes Paris: Masson 1983. As recounted in *Herbal Exchanges* pp. 111–117, a NIMH Publication 2014 Eds Brice-Ytsma H & Watkins F.

[282] See Wootton, David *Bad Medicine ~ Doctors Doing Harm Since Hippocrates* Oxford 2006.

[283] A patient of mine returned to her native America where she consulted a herbalist who insisted on a year long treatment with Wormwood to rid her of her parasites: this is ancient medicine with a vengeance. Modern medicine had to come to her rescue with a liver transplant. Anecdotal evidence, so the story goes, tell us nothing.

Clamour for evidence has become an instrument of aggression in some quarters of modern discourse. The call for it may be occasioned by a good motive such as the prevention of harm from bad ideas but may also come because vested interests—reputation, cognitive allegiance, money, the ego of conviction—are threatened. Or simply because the seeker of evidence wishes to preserve a closed worldview and discredit any group (such as ours) that does not entirely share it or has grave and principled reservations. There is always some bias in wanting to know.

This is where the scientific method discriminates against limitations to accepted wisdom, such as hindsight bias, overconfidence in judgements and intuitions with the human tendency to perceive patterns in random phenomena. One verifiable truth is that all human societies and some animals make some use of plants in food and medicine. The clamour for evidence in competitive societies may operate as a desire to be right rather than thoughtfully kind, which differs entirely from becoming sentimental about suffering.

Surely learning means always ready to change our minds; should we not be glad if evidence suggests that we modify our opinions? Galen cited the evidence of his experiments but they were flawed and he drew erroneous conclusions from them: his experimentation on animals served to confirm his preconceptions and had to fit in with humoral theory.[284] His ideas were never seriously tested and his anatomical errors misled physicians for over a millennium.[285] As for anatomical fantasy, Descartes invented a role for the pineal gland but fortunately he was not a medic nor was his anatomical thought treated seriously even by his contemporaries.

Let's agree that we need enough evidence to prevent falling for false beliefs as these may lead to false practice. Let's also get along with empirical heuristics until they begin to look as respectable as a theory.

Citations

A piece of prose can be blistered by citations. These pustules lay claim for the text to be taken seriously but can result in being overly self-serious. The idea is to pin every assertion to a source which has in some arena been validated. They may provide an excellent corrective to wild and mutable ideas with no grounding except in the mind that created them but they place their readers forever in the examination hall, within an ambit of mistrust.

They also make assumptions about the worthiness of the sources cited. When you can be bothered to read them, the ideas appear sometimes more provisional and biased than might have been expected. So, I have cited only those works that I have read carefully and digested and which support or challenge my worldview, with all its bias and limitation. Physiology is one attempt to explain the reality of human consciousness but could become narrow if restricted to citable, experimental evidence. Other attempts, such as poetical, meditative thought, contribute greatly and sit very comfortably alongside the science.

---

[284] Claude Bernard some sixteen centuries later experimented on animals in much the same way but these at least did lead to discoveries which were testable and durable, such as the discovery of glucagon.

[285] In her Prologue to her biography of Galen (cited previously), Susan Mattern reminds us that his ideas are distributed across 150 titles in twenty-two volumes in modern editions.

Science

Science—or knowledge, from *scientia*—is the collection of axioms that have been derived from our sensory physical experiences and found to be true generalisations, at least so far: an axiom of the scientific project says that all axioms are provisional. They may be highly abstract but are so uniformly applicable that we can use them to create tools, engines and devices. We accept these applications to the extent that they form the texture of our daily lives. If I understand correctly, the position taken by the Amish in their repudiation of modern technology, it is not that science is untrue but that its applications are ungodly. The rest of us rely upon this technology even if we don't know the science that gave rise to it. With the tools of perception, the infant learns that things fall to the ground, that force produces effects, that one sees less in the dark. That science seems to be faithful to our physical experience—so called common sense—gives it power and acceptance. Science is as much observational as experimental.

Even so, the axiomatic descriptions of ultimate reality are fraught with contradictions; phenomena at very small scale defy common sense and divide the communities of physicists. Geologists and marine biologists meanwhile get along with their own observations and measurements without, presumably, being too troubled by the dilemmas facing physics. A question of scale. The scientific enterprise encounters problems when it tries to tackle the phenomena of complex systems; these that might conflict with the beliefs or experience of people, and that may include some herbalists, at least some of the time.

As for the studies that are held to "show" that such and such an intervention or previously held notion turns out to be mistaken or that a previously held intuition turns out to be "actually" the case, the assumptions to be tested may be banal or trivial (ooh, who would have thought?) or the methodologies (preclinical (typically rodent) and clinical studies, in vivo and in vitro) lead one to think that any conclusions reached have the same kind of authority for the faithful as had the medieval Doctors of the Church. Talk about stretching a point, and doing so piously! Research can look for truth but can also be used for partisan purposes, to support an academic bureaucracy or, more menacingly, to silence cultural voices.

By contrast, large scale studies in public health over an extended period produce immense benefits to knowledge and society. These are the kinds I have thought worth citing.

The scientific method has given humans the most complete and coherent understanding of physical systems, but it is not so well adapted to discover and reproduce truths in complex systems whose component parts are meaningless except in association. It is even more poorly adapted to make good sense out of the human psyche and social relations because experiments are based mostly on scoring rather than counting reproducible events.

In medicine, some variant of the scientific method can, when applied to populations, bring a good statistical understanding of whether an intervention obtained real effects or not but is poorly equipped to know how well it will do in any particular case. Besides, there is a limit to the extent to which one can randomise events or control for all confounding variables. When a patient consults a herbalist they are of course expressing their own bias, and then to a physician who by vocation and almost by definition will stand for a particular approach to therapeutic efficacy. The bias is the point.

We have to accept that our personalised intervention is an experiment, a unique experience with outcomes that could later be analysed and quantified beyond crude scoring. Testimonials are evidence of a life that has been touched and altered for the better. Unlike the flawed process of questionnaires which suits the questioner but not the responder, they indicate a qualitative general outcome even if they do not in any way *prove* the efficacy of any plant or recipe. That was not the intention.

In fairness to those seeking evidence, a proper audit should equally monitor one's failures and assess the whole practice, if one is going to be holistic. This is not as straightforward as it might sound. I have had patients return twenty or even thirty years later. When, surprised at their return, I mention that my previous treatment had not been very effective, they graciously accept that it may have been a difficult case, they thought I had done my best, and now want to present something different. They remember the witnessing of their previous problem positively and want to repeat the process. So, the 'failure' was not remembered as negatively as the audit might assume. The scientific method is unlikely to discover and record the value of an even-handed medical conversation.

Speculations provide us valuable means towards learning and must remain provisional until alternative explanations seem more plausible. Rushing to seize on any seemingly positive evidence for medicinal plants is not always the thoughtful approach. The immense thought of Aristotle, as great an observer and biologist as he was, was hampered by the social and cultural norms that prevented the testing of ideas. At least he wasn't a medic and so did not harm individual people. Galen and Paracelsus (who infamously burnt Galenical writing in public) promoted observation over theory but created theories which stubbornly refused to die. The observations of Hahnemann led to another, a perfect example of overextension.[286] His principle dictum that names the theory—"Like cures Like"—is analogic and presumably true in certain circumstances. In the phase transitions at very low doses of complex mixtures, paradoxical effects can certainly be observed but it is a large jump to assert that these unusual conditions amount to the "magic of the minimum dose" in all cases.[287]

These men were all touchy autocrats who bristled at opposition or dissent. The triumph of being right should never be at the expense of patients. Beware lack of humour in the modern (and usually also in the ancient) sense. Beware of any over-riding sense of conviction which harbours no scepticism or self-doubt.

Axioms are those ideas that seem so correct or usable that they are not worth further testing. Nor would accepting that they are true lead to harm. Axioms on which I base my poise hypothesis include the laws of thermodynamics and information.[288]

---

[286] He was a gifted chemist and very accurately described the phase shifts of sulphur and made many astute dose correlations.

[287] For instance, in extremely dilute solutions of extracts of *Rheum palmatum* L as taught to us by Professor Peter Hylands. Discussed also in Harborne JB & Swain, T (Eds) *Perspectives in Phytochemistry* London: Academic Press (1980).

[288] While accepting entirely the postmodern view that the scientific enterprise cannot be separated from the social and cultural environment in which it operates, its discoveries can escape being so bound. Just as a baby in any culture learns about gravity by the practice of seeing things fall rather than being told it.

Only in the field of health is there an inverse relation between the commonsensical, pragmatic and empirical, and overarching theory: we hold on to theories mostly about things we cannot know.

I was once asked by an astrologer whether I was a rationalist. I replied that when it comes to the concrete, we are all rationalists: we do not confuse a container with a sieve. An alternative plumber who did not believe in pipes would be unlikely to do well. I think it self-evident that heavenly bodies intimately affect our lives but only so far as the sun and moon interact with the earth. The month of our birth does influence the prospects in cultures where the data has been collected: the effect is not huge but statistically significant. The hour of our birth may bear upon our tendency to wake with the larks or drowse late and stay up late evening like owls.

When it comes to survival, we are all empirical: the primary senses of smell and taste tend to savour things as they are. Hearing is more interpretive, vision even more so. Sight and sound give us ideas. We develop ideas of how life might be better—how healthy we might be—once food, water and shelter are assured.

Ancient elements are wonderfully descriptive of the way we live physically: feet on earth, breathing air warmed by the sun, eating solar power transduced by plants, largely composed of water and dependent upon it as are all other creatures. Metaphorically, too, we flow through our lives like a sailing boat through changeable waters. Wind in our sails coming from sun and air.

Functional medicine

Over the years, a number of patients have arrived lugging hefty dossiers of blood tests and intricate analyses of body fluids and the results of many other uncustomary examinations. These were accompanied by prescriptions of very many supplements and other compounds, sometimes including medicinal plants. They came to me as no longer able (or prepared) to withstand the heavy costs of test and medical interventions without attendant benefits. Many of these dossiers seemed hyper-rational in that they came to conclusions that seemed to make sense only if you think that all you have to do is follow a number of trails and you will eventually come to the required result. As if the map already exists! I bought the text-book in an attempt to find out what these practitioners thought it was all about.[289] I did not want my frustration and sceptical instincts to be uninformed.[290] Functional medicine looks to me like an attempt to take the guesswork out of diagnosis, to remove arbitrariness; but in being hyper-literal it may have replaced guesswork with literal fictions. A charitable estimation might view it to be a sincere attempt to find *the* root cause of illness but this is treating the human body as if it were complicated rather than what it is: complex. In a complicated system, however intricate and however many finite parts it contains, you can take it apart and examine each part or subsidiary sets of parts in turn to understand the working of the system. You wouldn't

---

[289] *Textbook of Functional Medicine* Ed David S Jones MD, Institute for Functional Medicine Gig Harbor WA 2010.

[290] Nor to dismiss it out of hand as has Wikipedia entry (viewed December 2022) which describes it as "pseudoscience … that encompasses a number of unproven and disproven methods and treatments".

be able to mend a watch or other machine without doing so. But in a complex system, isolating any part loses sense of the whole from which it has been extracted.[291]

Positive thinking has its heroes such as those who have conquered terminal illness but positivity as a creed (like meritocracy) has its victims: those who are not positive enough to survive or those who clearly had not enough merit to thrive.

n = one

Randomised controlled trials aim to discern whether an intervention has delivered a desired effect on a group of people. By trawling huge amounts of data ($n=many$) the trial of the compound to be tested discerns by statistical methods a true signal from highly variable idiosyncratic noise. For the trial to be useful, the effect has to have been precisely and narrowly circumscribed. The other task must observe what other effects the intervention has occasioned and whether these unsought effects are damaging and would present an unacceptable risk to people. The controls are there to dilute the artificiality of the trial, to reduce the effect of noise and be more true to life.

When a drug has been shown to be effective, its benefits to outweigh its unwanted effects, and it has been used in diverse populations for many years, unintended effects that did not show up in the original trials may gradually emerge, as would be expected as the recipient population widens over time.[292] Neither should it come as a surprise to scientists like ourselves who take a systems approach to cause and effect.

Our personal lives are idiosyncratic and are lived without the benefit of a control: we do not know what would have happened had we behaved other than we did, took an opposite decision, turned right at the fork instead of left. When we become ill, what should we do? Follow advice, take a medicine, desist from this, deny ourselves that? In mild but irritating complaints, you could say it hardly matters, but it always matters to the complaining one.

We come to recognise what works well as first aid and what does not, but in severe illness or when a pathological state arises or strikes us down, the question becomes urgent. The scientific method—originally applied to physical phenomena—has been repurposed to investigate the messy and idiosyncratic business of human life. For good reason: medical practitioners have for millennia poured dangerous, toxic and useless substances into patients desperate for relief or a cure. Mistaken beliefs and the unwarranted confidence of medics down the ages have caused humankind untold harm.[293] Plagues and pestilences have scourged all historical ages and societies, accelerated by trade even when the cargo will have helped those who could afford the precious spices. These did not prevent losses of half a population though they had plenty of medicinal plants to hand.

We do have only one life, n=1, though it is of necessity a social, and therefore plural one. Interaction with others, with our extended family—an extension into past history—with

---

[291] Surgeons may have to isolate parts temporarily before allowing them to rejoin the community.

[292] Postmarket Safety Events Among Novel Therapeutics Approved by the US Food and Drug Administration Between 2001 and 2010: Nicholas S.Downing,MD; Nilay D Shah, PhD; Jenerius A. Aminawung, MD, MPH; et al. JAMA. 2017; 317(18):1854–1863.

[293] Ancient wisdoms have sought to mitigate disastrous approaches but of these: "know thyself" from the non-medical Socrates is the most pertinent.

our mate and our mates or on our own lead us always to question our trajectory, our choices and to interpret how our current state of health might have arisen. Clear signals may become obscured by the amount of noise, the clutter of innumerable possibilities. And what do we do to improve our health? Here is the nub of the therapeutic problem: what really helps without doing harm.

People reasonably ask of herbalists "will it help me?" The truthful answer—"I cannot know for sure"—recognises that life without uncertainty is not life. If you have applied medicinal plants in as particular way as possible in the past and will do for them, then to invest in you is sound and as good a risk as they can find. The richness of medicinal plants releases the herbalist to give undivided attention, to relinquish self-importance for the other. As the psychotherapist Adam Phillips remarks: experimentation is a noble undertaking when done with the full assent and collaboration of the patient.[294]

One thing you can say to the patient with some confidence: herbs will complexify your life and that reconfiguration will make you better able to withstand shocks and even improve your future prospects in a way that we cannot know. A life that is daring without being reckless opens to the most of possibilities.

Themes of the strength in vulnerability of human existence were explored in a tender and subtle film made in 1973 by Terence Donovan and written by the great Shinobu Hashimoto (who had everything to do with the classic film *Rashomon* and nothing to do with thyroid disease). The story is about a Japanese detective sent to England on a special mission. In the course of this mission, he meets with an attractive woman. Intimacy grows between them in spite of the language barrier.[295] Dining together at a restaurant, he picks up a flower from its vase on the table and says:

"Flowers are so *daring*".

To her quizzical but affectionate expression he explains:

"They don't ask themselves 'Will I be beautiful, will I be admired, will I do well in the wind, *they just open* ...'".[296]

Herbal medicine as general practice

There are two tiers in herbalism (both opens to first aid requests):

1. Domestic and daily
2. Professional when needed

---

[294] Paraphrasing him from *Terrors and Experts* about the psychoanalyst D.W. Winnicott Faber 1997.

[295] The film could be said to elaborate themes explored by the anthropologist Ruth Benedict in her 1946 book *The Chrysanthemum and the Sword: Patterns of Japanese Culture.*

[296] A year after being involved with this film, I embarked upon my quest for herbal medicine. Perhaps this expression of the daring of nature was one of the triggers to my literal journey as well as a modest change of orientation.

I see it as my duty as a herbalist to encourage the first so as to forestall or reduce the need for my services. Herbs taken with food and drink daily may allow a person to escape the attentions of the physician, not always positive even if not as negative as that scorned by Petrarch:

> Life is short enough, but the physicians with their art, know to their amusement, how to make it shorter.

Materia medica is—like cooking and reading recipes—easily learnt. Its application, on the other hand, needs experience with the benefit of learning from patients, peers, teachers and, at a greater stretch, books like this one. A relaxed and positive manner from the confidence that experience brings will help. The real benefit of experience is being able to discern the signal within the patient's constellated history from the noise of all the symptoms and even some of the signs. It helps to know when the patient's symptom is standing in for a completely different discussion they wish to have.

We want our prescribing to be based upon well observed clinical situations and a well-reasoned therapeutic strategy, but if you are contending with the notion of a reproducible formula, the very awkward truth that faces herbal medicine practitioners is that there must (if we are to treat the individual not the generalised condition that afflicts them) an experimental element to each and every occasion of treatment. It requires trust in yourself and in the knowledge you have acquired (mostly from others) with a sense of certainty almost defused by a countervailing sense of the provisional.

The ANS provides perhaps the most reliable landmark or even a beacon. Each of us has an external world to which we have to respond but simultaneously to our inner historical minds. While the primary response may come from the ANS, the settings are provided by endogenous signals, inherent capacities and learnt knowledge. Many of these internal informatic structures can be modified by longer-term herbal medication but the autonomic patterns of response are modifiable within hours, days or very few weeks by appropriate prescription of medicinal plants.

Relief or resolution

The itch, the sore, the ache and pain, let alone the cough and constipation and other chronic complaints, surely these call out for relief, for balm. Pain is wearisome and aching reduces the spirit. Isn't the role of the physician to alleviate suffering where possible? Relief is in the moment and the moment matters to the sufferer. Resolution looks to a better future but in the moment may seem too ambitious, almost abstract.

I would suggest that the context decides and that one remains nimble so that you can offer either course of therapy and keep both in mind as the relationship develops. Herbalists can indeed choose from a wide repertoire of symptomatic remedies for all manner of ailments but, perhaps uniquely, they can modify the terrain and bring about resolution. Resolving one problem provides an ending but endings engender new beginnings. Resolution of an illness means it no longer preoccupies a life whose course has changed.

Resolution may seem to take too long—perhaps many months—though it can be quicker in the long run in the sense that relief may need to be provided for years.

Very often it is the patient who decides. They have arrived at the conclusion that something needs to change otherwise why would they invest in a lengthy consultation and personalised medicine? In this way, they have made the choice for the practitioner.

Enough

If illness is a loss of capacitance from a failure of adaptation,[297] its resolution can be provided by increasing the person's adaptive capacity or by reducing their load, or preferably both. Depletion or surfeit produce similar burdens, in spite of being opposites. One thing that the nutritional supplement industry chooses to overlook is that humans are opportunistic feeders who have had to adapt to famine and this adaptation is built into our metabolism. Overlooking this element means ignoring an important midpoint for health: our biological capacitance. Acquisitiveness in the absence of famine belongs to a craving for insurance which, mistrusting the future, becomes more difficult to treat than current hardship. In some measure, though, objects can be talismanic and speak of human yearning: the photo, the love letter. Acquisitiveness on a grander scale may conceal a sense of loss, the disappointment behind much depression.

Happiness is probably achieved most easily by those who have enough with ample reserve. Isn't that what we call being comfortable? Much of this lies within the realm of politics and economics but then that is where in great part health resides. It lives also within cultural norms where an ecological sense of medicine can help: to find the therapeutic spot that feels just right, then enhance it with a generous surplus. Ideas of hearth and home give us the *eco* (in ecology and economy, from the Greek οικοσ). Not every eventuality has to be covered by acquiring an abundance of remedies, fuelled by anxiety. Both the assessment and the herbal prescription that follows will be comprehensive but economical.

The elixir of life is life itself.

---

[297] As I have argued in *Illness as a failure of adaptation* The Hein Zeylstra Memorial Lecture to NIMH Conference 2012.

Sensory priming and the pharmakon

How would you conduct a trial on tea and coffee or on chamomile tea? Could you separate the taste and flavour from their effects, and what would be the point? When you imbibe any liquid, your consciousness changes so what can "no effect" mean? Perhaps a "desired effect" is meant, but who desires, the researcher or the subject?

The pharmakon

Life forms develop in parallel, interdependent within their shared environment. Evolution by natural selection means that information fits the situation until it doesn't: when there is a change, altered sequences start to fit better; additionally random changes are sometimes more suited to the environment. Plants don't intend alkaloids for our use but because they and their predators are coeval with ourselves, we have learnt to appropriate them for what seems like our benefit.

So, pharmacology is born and humans evolve as even more opportunistically medicinal than other species, as discussed in the Introduction. Leaving aside material for tools, vehicles, building and shelter, parallel streams of exploitation proceed from our use of plants for food and for better digesting food: we found plants, fungi and ferments that alter consciousness in singular ways. The potency of such phenomena has produced much good and much harm.

Learning methodically to separate single compounds from their source material in recent centuries has provided insights and reduced some of the uncertainty but not eliminated it, as the important work of Peter Hylands and others have shown.[298]

---

[298] I drew attention to this work in the Preface.

Folk medicine has always thrived in all cultures under the elevated strata of apothecaries and physicians in mercantile classes, aristocracies, and all manner of religious and clerical systems in all civilisations. What we now call Ayurveda and TCM (traditional Chinese medicine) are derived from more diverse traditions than the terms imply. Modern clinical phytotherapy, likewise, is a broad umbrella term for practices and ideas that are diverse and sometimes at odds with each other. Some phytotherapists use models, others a schedule of empirical findings, some subscribe to vitalist notions, yet others to eclectic modes of thought and varieties of practice.

What they could all be said to have in common is that medicinal plants are central (though not exclusive) to their practice.[299] My own approach focuses on the practice of medicine independently of the pharmacons, though it would be odd to call yourself a herbalist unless in most clinical circumstances you actually prescribed herbs. At the centre of practice is the ill person not a named illness: the human phenotype rather than a category. You might call it phenotypic individualised medicine if that did not sound absurdly pretentious. I mean it sincerely, though: I do not have any "herbs for eczema" though of course there will be a few common principles when treating its many manifestations.

Impurities

The elemental operations of matter in the biosphere: earth, air, fire and water are all compounds and mixtures for which purity has no meaning. These ancient elements combined in different ways to create totality. Only the atomists sought unity underneath the combinatorial. Alchemists at a later age pursued purity as a condensation of base matter. Their successors, chemists, are also of course refiners and purifiers but life remains resolutely impure.

Pharmacists want to remove impurities and standardise and homogenise so that you know exactly what you get. Just as well, given the potent effects of powerful compounds, to know exactly what you are receiving. Herbalists want to remove adulterants from their plant material, of course, along with any undeclared admixture but conceive the whole plant in all its compound multiplicity as the therapeutic entity.

Most benign effects are mixed effects.[300] As the 18th century proverb would have it: "we must all eat a peck of dirt before we die".[301]

Hormesis

Why should a peck of dirt be beneficial? It seems that in stable biological systems, the introduction of a minute amount of toxin increases the stability of a homeostatic fixed point, somewhat akin to a buffer (Section 1.8). No doubt this is what Hahnemann

---

[299] The use of parts of endangered species of animals shows that in the past a very wide trawl was made of nature.

[300] Tenner (1996) spends two chapters on medicine and health. See p. 91 for the perils of purification.

[301] I have heard it and thought it always a contemporary saying until I looked it up in the Oxford Dictionary of Quotations (8th Edition).

perceived as the minimum dose. It is no surprise (if unfortunate) that he extended it in 18th century essentialist thinking by insisting on the "law" of similars. If a toxin is a compound that has no nutritive value (and even water and nutrients have a toxic dose) then culinary and medicinal plants are toxic (as many pharmacologists might assert). To suggest that all our remedies are hormetic may overstate our case, which is just the position taken by Paracelsus. The herbalist king (or Eupator)[302] Mithradates VI of Pontus is perhaps the most famous historical exponent of hormesis: he took minute doses of poisons all his life to benefit from their protective effect.[303] Hormesis is a Greek word cognate with hormone, indicating an impulse to motion or effect. It refers to the adaptive benefits afforded by exposure to small amounts of toxins or stress.

In an age devoted to avoiding stress, the distinction between toxic unproductive stress and beneficial stress is not often made except by those justifying their choice of poison. The whole point about hormesis is that the dosage is minute. My experience as a patient in France where the liquid preparations are often mother tinctures were even more positive than with my own, but the alcohol levels were higher and small doses of alcohol are hormetic.

Stochastic resonance is a form of hormesis where adding a little noise to a system improves the clarity of the signal.

Focus on oxidative stress as a cause of ageing now appears to have been misplaced and a little beneficial mischief and disturbance might be just the ticket to stave off the harms of an entirely uneventful old age. Unlike antioxidants, it would give the health food industry nothing to sell.

Hormetic benefit has always been ascribed to 'a little of what you fancy' and it is through the sensory allure of culinary plants that can lead to a gently medicinal way of life.

The primary senses

Touch is primal, taste is a form of discriminatory touch. Smell (patent nasal passages permitting) gives us access to quality over quantity. These primary senses suffuse our limbic systems. Sensory priming coupled with stochastic resonance gives a lift to our lives with saving rather than expenditure of energy, facilitating poise.[304]

Pathology, process and constitution

I personally found the study of clinical medicine interesting in its own way and did have occasion to put the knowledge to good clinical use, but not that often. It is a descriptive, classificatory subject in the main with occasional deep insights to biology. So, and this

---

[302] Commemorated in *Eupatorium, Agrimonia eupatoria*. Pontus, the ancient name for the Black Sea gives us *Rheum rhaponticum* (rhubarb), Rha being its old name.

[303] The ingestion of the tiny amounts of cyanide in apple seeds provides an example of what is still known as mithridatism.

[304] See Section 1.4.

might come across as a rather facile observation, you can learn about pathology in rather a summary fashion (unless you are going to be a surgeon) providing you are committed to refreshing your knowledge from time to time and, then, you can always look things up. But how and where would you look up a patient's constitution? The notion of an inborn disposition itself, cannot easily be formalised. You cannot look up and revise the subject. Such a reference book does not exist in the definitive kind of way you expect of a pathology textbook.

Surgical practice depends upon a close and continuous reading of pathology but otherwise it describes developments you are not in a strong position to remedy. Fascinating as the study may be, and it is good if herbalists understand the territory, it hardly helps the patient to dwell on things we are not well placed to alter but rather on modifying the terrain to better manage the disease process. Of course, an understanding of the procession towards disorder is necessary, particularly in autoimmune conditions. You must also understand what part of physiology has been disrupted (for instance in multiple slerosis) to know how and where to direct any treatment. In other words, you have to know as much as you can of the itinerary but not focus on the destination.

Feeling unwell does not indicate disease but it is disheartening for a person who feels unwell very often to be told that "there is nothing wrong with you". At the other end of this spectrum, people with well-managed disease can be surprisingly cheerful.

An emphasis on pathology to the exclusion of all else may deflect our attention and compassion from the appreciation that a sizeable source of illness arises from fear and loneliness.

Infectious disease

When relations change within an ecosystem, the system changes. People crowded together with large stores of food create the conditions for epidemics. Mass movements between populations (war and trade) along with opportunistic rodents and attendant microbes deliver one crowded ecosystem into another.[305] The result is human misery and a vast number of deaths.[306]

Hygiene plays a part in prevention but throughout human history medical interventions of any sort have played the smallest of bit parts. The rise of the antibiotic age altered that gloomy picture in that some people alive and well today survived infantile disease that would previously have incapacitated or killed them. Still, tuberculosis, malaria, measles, syphilis and others continue to cause devastation in many parts of the world. Only smallpox has been removed from that list but AIDS from HIV has been added and other infections and infestations are on the rise.

Given the scale of the problem, it is just as easy to devalue and dismiss herbal medicine from the discussion as it is for us to exaggerate its importance. Dietary and culinary plants are important for prevention, for improving resistance and for quicker, more permanent recuperation. These are huge effects and deserve to be celebrated.

---

[305] See for instance: *Global Burden of Disease* published annually by Institute for Health Metrics and evaluation; WHO 2004 *GLOBAL BURDEN OF DISEASE AND INJURY SERIES VOLUME IV*.

[306] The numbers compounded by injury on the road, interpersonal violence and self-harm.

That Artemisinin was extracted from *Artemisia annua* is of course good news but that converts Artemisinin to a commodifiable drug and not part of the habitual dispensing habits of a medical herbalist. Epidemics aside, herbs help people recover from common infections and when these are severe, essential oils from plants and various oxymels can be very effective and herbal antiviral remedies are nearly always the best thing, remembering that bed rest and remedial fluids take pride of place. Medicines should not be in competition for supremacy and acute infectious illness can bring out the heroic when what is needed is the sensible.

The discovery of penicillin brought an insight into ecology: fungal spores drifting on air currents mature when they come into contact with a nutrient-rich environment. In commodifying and manufacturing antibiotics for the good of all, the ecological message became lost and resistance organisms have become endemic. Just as the lessons of history are never learnt, the consequences of packaging a system into a box is that the elements cease to behave as a system.

Recurrent infections

Proneness to repeated "infections" over a short while, often complained of as a tendency to catch a series of "colds" throughout the year has often to do with mucous membranes of the ear, nose, and throat rendered susceptible to inflammation (and perhaps a flare of commensal organisms) by overwork and stress.

These debilitating bouts are often transient or cyclical responses to a loss of poise and mediated to a great extent by histamine (in tandem with serotonin and cortisol). I hope that it will now be clear that the obvious strategy is to sustain poise rather than just offer herbs that reduce histamine though, of course, given the polyvalent nature of medicinal plants, it might be difficult not to be doing both at the same time if, for example, *Glycyrrhiza*, *Agrimonia* and *Matricaria* come to mind.

The laryngitis and catarrh is real enough but emphasis should be on restoring HPA balance, good digestive function and restorative sleep rather than focus on resistance to a virus though, again, with plants like *Inula*, *Hyssopus* and *Olea* the distinction is a shallow one.

Such cases are common and respond well to treatment. When I ask, in the course of a systemic review whether the person suffers from hay-fever, I hear the common response, "Usually no, but in recent years I have". In other words, the patient at a critical age or after a period of stress or overwork or both has succumbed to the impedance against loss of poise supplied by histamine. Don't blame the pollen.

The dispensary

How many plants should you keep in your dispensary? Should you stock only those you grow in your garden? Should you stock only those for which the research literature shows significant effects? In which case let's hope clients show up with the designated indications.

As a very rough guide, although one might remember 600 or more botanical names, it would surprise me if anyone could nimbly entertain such a large number and bring them to bear therapeutically on any one patient. How many could you realistically recall when faced with a patient in need of a prescription? NIMH used to offer a specialised course to GPs who wanted to extend their practice to herbal medicine. I well remember one of these—an experienced naval doctor—who had come to visit me for clinical training. I left him briefly to study the prescription and returned to find his head slumped on his hands on the dispensary bench. "*How*," he wailed despairingly "do you keep up with all this lot?" Not to mention the cost.

I have tried over the years to suggest to those in charge of courses in herbal medicine that they steer student dissertations away from nebulous topics or practitioner-questionnaires[307] towards an audit of those plants actually stocked and dispensed by herbalists with long continuous practices, but to no avail. Such studies would provide invaluable historic information.

As the first cohort to graduate from the School of Herbal Medicine, we had got used to the very wide range of materials that Hein Zeylstra stocked for his own practice and, by consequence, for his training clinic. He generously offered us eighty different tinctures in half-litre bottles on credit from his own manufactory (where I was fortunate to have

---

[307] Asking unrealistic questions in unhelpful ways.

worked for a couple of years).[308] He reckoned that number should cover most eventualities. Years later, John Hyde suggested we reduce the number of herbs to those we really could keep in clear focus and learn from. I think he whittled that number down to twenty-seven plant preparations, just one short of the number of herbs one of my teachers would sometimes put in a single prescription.

I suspect that whittling down is how the dispensing mind works until you wake up and realise again that nature is not that narrow and you remember of a sudden that you have not used or thought of a plant that has stood neglected upon the shelf a year or more. Also, unless you are a staunch empiricist or bend with the fashion, your choice of plants will be influenced if not dictated by the therapeutic model by which you operate.[309]

Necessary and almost sufficient

Simon Mills would tell his students that it is no bad thing from time to time to run out of a herb you rely upon because it affords you the opportunity to re-evaluate the parts of your materia medica that you have neglected. I have found that to be good advice but have a number of plants for which no substitution genuinely suggests itself. So here is my list of plants that are necessary and almost sufficient to run a full herbal medical practice, grouped by roughly botanical affiliation as they are in my dispensary.

Ruscus	Calluna	Salvia
Zingiber	Vaccinium	Thymus
Ribes	Borago	Menyanthes
Glycyrrhiza	Olea	Achillea
Galega	Vitex	Arctium
Melilotus	Ballota	Calendula
Agrimonia	Lamium	Matricaria
Alchemilla	Lavandula	Inula
Rubus idaeus	Leonurus	Echinacea
Crataegus	Lycopus	Sambucus
Humulus	Marrubium	Valeriana
Urtica	Melissa	Angelica
Hypericum	Marjorana	Foeniculum
Tilia	Rosmarinus	Levisticum

With these forty-two plants I could just about manage most movements of most terrains but I would be sorely pressed to do without the following plants; they are almost (to make a weak play on words) indispensable to my dispensary:

---

[308] From the point of view of experience not from that of comfort—an unheated converted cowshed with a concrete floor and corrugated roof in midwinter made us martyrs to our craft!

[309] See Model in Section 3.2.

Agropyron	Ulmus	Stachys/Betonica
Alliums	Damiana	Hyssopus
Zea	Salix	Mentha
Fumaria	Citrus aurantium	Ocimum
Medicago	Capsella	Salvia sclarea
Trigonella	Vinca	Satureja
Prunus	Dulcamara	Taraxacum
Filipendula	Fraxinus	Artemisia
Poterium/Sanguisorba	Plantago	Eupatorium
Rosa	Verbena	Solidago

And then to have dried buchu, eyebright and chervil always in stock. You will see that I use mostly aerial parts as potentially more sustainable than barks or roots. Leaves have the added benefit of folic acid. Trees and shrubs are slower than most herbaceous plants to reach sexual maturity so I tend to use the more replaceable leaves of woody plants.

There are so many more that I have used and still use from time to time but if you stock them all at the same time, it is more difficult to bring the necessary focus to bear in order to learn and develop your knowledge.

From botany to dispensary and dinner table

If the philosopher Aristotle was the first biologist in the modern sense, his younger colleague, Theophrastus was the first botanist.[310] His two major surviving works *Enquiries into Plants* and *Causes of Plants* examine plant physiology and comparative morphologies. He was the first to attempt a taxonomy of the plant kingdom. His description of these 'natural orders' survived into the twentieth century.[311] They are 'natural' in the sense of belonging together by their observed characters. While the use of Theophrastean names are becoming phased out, they are recognisable and still commonly used by gardeners and horticulturalists. He describes and classifies the following: coniferae, cruciferae guttiferae, leguminosae, umbelliferae, labiatae, compositae, palmae, graminae.[312] I would find difficult to know how to practice herbal medicine without including several medicinal and a good many culinary plants from the following 'natural orders'.

---

[310] For an excellent account of his life and work, see Morton (1981).

[311] The abbreviation N.O. is unaltered in the ninth edition of Potter's Cyclopaedia. We would now call them plant families.

[312] The names were revived in the early modern period. Theophrastus make a good start in his overview of the plant world but herbalists might wonder that he did not include Rosaceae (given their wide distribution and economic importance then as now) or at least treat Prunoideae or Maloideae separately in their own right (as some modern authorities do). But it is a huge and diverse group of species that hybridise and clone so confusingly, and contemporary taxonomists continue to wrestle with their classification and to understand their biology.

1. Plants in Coniferae give us the wonderfully sustaining pine kernels, that protect against disease, augment resistance, reduce hypersensitivity and sustain beta–adrenergic energy. Oil of pine or an infusion of the needle-like leaves provide sympathomimetic support in upper and lower respiratory tract conditions.
2. Crucifers are an obvious group from their cruciform corolla and the taste of mustard oils with their liver-sparing properties. *Capsella* is most useful for its haemostatic and anti-oxytocic properties.
3. Guttiferae (a source of many useful timbers) give us Hypericum.
4. Leguminosae provide staple foods for most populations. They, and a number of medicinal plants are not only anti-hyperglycaemic with uses in diabetes but offer many neuroendocrine benefits.
5. Umbelliferae—a major source of culinary herbs and spices. In most cases, no sharp distinction between dispensary and dinner table can be made.
6. The aromatic plants in Labiatae prime us to the good things to eat. As they are indispensable to good eating and digestion, they provide us with aromatic bitters, anti-microbial and anti-spasmodic medicines. These and many plants in these nine taxa will also modify the terrain.
7. We rely on the huge and diverse Compositae for bitters and other complex hepatics, diuretics and other agents for digestive and metabolic assistance, as well as some vegetables and seed oils.
8. Plants in Palmae offer a wide range of dietary and medicinal cultigens.
9. Grasslands, like humans, evolved relatively recently, replacing woodland in most cases. Graminae provide us with cereals and fodder for the herbivores we have exploited. As the botany is complex, I devoted several pages with illustrations as overview for the botanic herbalist to this group. Zea would not, of course, have been known to Theophrastus.

Elements of the prescription

T he prescription calls for focus and precision. You need to select from the great mass of material absorbed during the consultation with all its complex counter-currents, even contradictions, to make up something that is physical and definite. You don't need to worry about missing some of the complexity because even a single plant is manifestly complex. Unless you can extract simple ideas from the data, you are at risk of drowning in a morass of detail.

It is also important to simplify, not just for your own head-space but to answer the question that you will ask yourself and others may ask of you. What is it that I am trying to do?

And in this book: What is it that I am trying to say? Time to simplify and follow the advice of the great music teacher Nadia Boulanger: "Never strain to avoid the obvious."[313]

When it comes to writing the prescription, all the sections of the book—notably those (like Section 1.8 and others) that try to answer that question—converge upon this simple idea:

Life expresses both the particular and the waveform nature of matter as dual aspects of the same process
Waves
in physics and physiology
exhibit sequences of peaks and troughs:
What goes up must come down

---

[313] (1887–1979) She also maintained that you cannot teach anyone anything but you can and should try to sustain their interests and drives. Music unites the horizontal and vertical in physics and physiology.

With your prescription you intercept the waves in the following manner:

	Finding:	Prescribe to:
Peaks	Too high	Reduce
Midpoint	Too fluctuant	Sustain and temper
Troughs	Too low	Augment

Sustain is the important word here. We need always to have a two-handed approach: you hold a baby with one hand below and one hand above to contain it: its comfort is as important as preventing its fall.

We are all bipolar: that is how life is made—night and day. But most people manage the transitions more or less well by ballast for the upswing and buffers to the down-swing.[314] Herbs have the wonderful benefit of both buffering and ballasting at the same time so that a beta-reducing herb can be combined with a beta-agonist and ditto for the parasympathetic. That is why I prescribe in a bipolar fashion: putting more ballast in the morning mix and more buffer in the evening. Sometimes the effects are too much and too little especially for cyclothymics who benefit from a single prescription.

> You will have emerged from the consultation, with all its exceptions and contradictions, and will have fulfilled the first imperative in listing what exactly you wish your prescription to achieve.
>
> Now we need to work backwards to explore in physiological terms how those decisions were reached. We need to identify the waves that need to be tempered and sustained so that we can bring our patients to a comfortable median space, buffered and ballasted against fluctuations from their current situation and from all their pasts.
>
> In Section 3.6 that follows we will analyse the scope for physiological change amenable to modification by nurture and medicinal plants and so generate the principal therapeutic strategies.
>
> Whatever model of herbal medicine you operate, the medicinal plants you prescribe will affect most or all of these physiological systems whether or not you intended them to.

---

[314] Manic-depressive disorder is a major psychopathy, which has been renamed bipolar disorder, to no good purpose, in my view, as bipolarity is part of the architecture of life.

Therapeutics herbal treatment strategies by levels

A s medicinal plants operate at different levels, some simultaneously, others in stages, the herbalist needs to consider all the potential levels when writing the treatment plan ready for the dispenser. By combining plants you will be combining levels.

Here are the main therapeutic levels:

1. Autonomic nervous system: constitutional dominance and current expression
2. Supporting digestive organ deficiencies, gut motility and bile flow Organ management of metabolism and the circadian systems
3. The H-P vertical axes and, consequently:
4. Metabolic outcomes (anabolic/catabolic)
5. The horizontal flow within the pituitary gland through the H-P axes: dominances and deficits
6. Constitutional and acquired biases in the posterior pituitary (oxytocin and ADH)
7. Current and historical expression of the autocoid hormones and adrenaline: histamine, noradrenaline, dopamine, serotonin throughout the systems, including the ocular-hypothalamic-pineal pathway, with especial relevance to digestion, sleep and skin
8. Interplay between prolactin and dopamine
9. Idiosyncratic
   NOTE: Aspects of level 2 really proceed the whole list because enhanced enzymatic function applies to all succeeding functions.

Within the bounds of a linear scheme to denote cyclical complexity, the levels are in order of time and necessity—autonomic functions operate from moment to moment so must always be considered first, while endocrine loops always take more than a day, while metabolic drives operate within weeks and months.[315] Even within these times-cales, there are immediate and relatively delayed effects and novel and accustomed signals as expressed in the following figure.

Immediate signals	Level	Relatively delayed signals
Sensory effects, habituated or novel		
Endothelia, coagulability of blood		Cellular elements of blood
Reflexes, such as cough		
Gastric and pancreatic deficiency		Gut motility and bile flow
	1	Autonomic nervous system
	3	Organ management of metabolism and the circadian systems
	4	The H-P axes vertically to periphery
	5	Catabolic or anabolic dominance
	6	Dominances between the H-P axes in the horizontal flow through the pituitary gland
	7	Constitutional and acquired biases in the posterior pituitary (oxytocin and ADH)
Adrenaline	8	Autocoid hormones and the systems
	9	Interplay between prolactin and dopamine

Figure 19: Signal levels

Immediate signals

This table precedes the other levels because of their rapid and important effects, especially on small blood vessels and mucosae. Antispasmodic plants are included because of their strong effects on smooth muscle.

---

[315] See Figures 6, 12 and 13 for more integrative pictures.

Table 2: Plants with effects both rapid and cumulative on small blood vessels and mucosae

Therapeutic name	Influence	Therapeutic notes
Achillea	Antispasmodic	Most versatile aromatic bitter
Agrimonia	Anti-allergic	Reduces histamine & serotonin; ↓viral and bacterial load
Agropyron	Anti-inflammatory	
Anemone pulsatilla	Antispasmodic	Helps in tobacco withdrawal
Arctium	Reduces blood sugar, ↓viral & bacterial load	
Calendula	Antispasmodic	Especially uterine
Calluna	Anti-inflammatory	Buccal, uterine and urinary
Chrysanthemum parthenium	Antispasmodic	Especially uterine reducing serotonin
Citrus aurantium (dulce)	Anti-coagulant	
Crataegus	Antispasmodic	Although takes longterm use to reach plateau
Echinacea	First aid	
Fraxinus	Anti-platelet aggregation	
Fumaria	Anti-allergic	Reducing histamine
Glycyrrhiza	Anti-allergic	Not always appropriate to use longterm
Hibiscus	Anti-inflammatory	Cumulative: taken daily late afternoon
Hyssopus	Anti-allergic	
Inula	Anti-allergic	↓Viral load
Lamium album	Anti-metrorrhagic	
Levisticum	Antispasmodic	Uterine and urinary
Marjorana	Emotional first aid	
Melilotus	Antispasmodic	Anti-coagulant
Origanum	Antispasmodic	In connective tissue and digestive tract
Phaseolus	Anti-inflammatory	Important food to counter auto-immunity
Plantago	Anti-allergic	
Ribes nigrum	Anti-allergic	
Rubus fruticosus	Anti-inflammatory	Combats strep sore throat
Ruscus	Anti-haemorrhagic	
Salix	Antispasmodic	Neuro-muscular

(Continued)

Table 2: Plants with effects both rapid and cumulative on small blood vessels and mucosae (Continued)

Therapeutic name	Influence	Therapeutic notes
Thymus	Antispasmodic	
Tilia	Antispasmodic	Digestive, vascular and uterine
Trigonella	Anti-coagulant	
Urtica	Anti-allergic	
Vaccinium	Vasculo-protector	Anti-bacterial. Anti-fungal
Viburnum prunifolium	Antispasmodic	
Vinca	Antispasmodic	Neuro-muscular; capillary protector
Zingiber	Anti-platelet aggregation	

Level one: autonomic nervous system constitutional dominance and current expression[316]

Although its importance is primary, the ANS is an output disposition, not an agent. It is autonomic in the sense of automatic and self-adjusting from moment to moment. It operates the critical alternation between dilation and constriction of blood vessels of all sizes. It manifests the states of the endocrine drivers and other elements of the municipality (Figure 12) further down in this artificial list of levels.

There is an obvious correlation between temperament (Section 1.9) with autonomic dominance showing up strongly in modes of thought, patterns of activity, and capacities for sleep and digestion. Metabolic outcomes do tend to show up in the overall physical makeup of a person but correlating them with temperament is a temptation to be resisted. To denote that your patient is vagotonic tells of a tropism that might be modified for the benefit of their health. It is not a classification.

Parasympathetic

As the main cranial outflow of parasympathetic fibres is via the tenth nerve, the vagus; vagotonia refers to a relative dominance and therefore a potential delay in the diurnal cycling because the vagus slows things down. Congestive states are the dominant feature because the purpose of the parasympathetic is to increase and retain trophic elements in the cavities of the axial skeleton. High levels of interiority in the mental state and introversion are characteristic. Fungal overgrowth commonly occurs in skin folds and on congested mucosae.[317] When there is a good ratio between parasympathetic and orthosympathetic, few if any of the problems listed in the figure below occur in adult

---

[316] This device is no more than a way of organising prescriptions, roughly temporal but not a physiological hierarchy. See Figures 4 and 6 for interconnectivities.

[317] Avoiding yeasts may help a little but consumption of mushrooms and seafood which compete with yeasts will positively reduce infection of the mycotic terrain.

life although the alpha branch of the sympathetic complicates the picture greatly. If congestion from high parasympathetic tone is unrelieved, the following states are likely to ensue:

Location	Common manifestations of high vagal tone	Notes
CNS	Vertigo, nausea, vomiting easily	
Cranial cavity	Headache, sinusitis, otitis, laryngitis	1
Thoracic cavity	Asthma	2
Abdomen	Gastric and pancreatic insufficiency, slow gut motility	3
Pelvic cavity	Proctitis, diverticulosis and other signs of high luminal pressure internal reproductive organs primed for growth	4
Skin	Dermatitis signals a strong parasympathetic	5

Nightmares and sleep terrors are associated with *low* parasympathetic tone

Figure 20: Vagal tone

Notes to figure
1. Children are more parasympathetic, contain relatively more fluid and so bouts of inflammation and infections of the upper respiratory tract are to be expected
2. Asthma requires in addition strong alpha-sympathetic tone
3. The autocoid associated with vagotonia is serotonin (see Bile and Gut motility in Section 2.5b)
4. The influence of oestrogens and androgens on prostatic hypertrophy depends upon priming by the parasympathetic and/or sympathetic, as is the case for uterine fibroids
5. Psoriasis requires in addition strong alpha-sympathetic tone as does acne.

Alpha branch of the orthosympathetic

The alpha-sympathetic can be seen as a transition from the congestive drowsy state of the parasympathetic (mediated by acetylcholine) to the outright musculoskeletal activity of the beta-sympathetic with its dopamine and adrenaline from the adrenal medulla. By analogy with the sequence that sets off an athletic race—ready, *steady*, GO!—The 'steady' is supposed to be the briefest phase before the starter's gun, but a person whose alpha-sympathetic receptors are over-taxed lives in a constant state of steady-ness. In physiological terms, their sphincters are tightly closed under the influence of noradrenaline.

This state of heightened and prolonged vigilance blocks the normal transmission of waves and sends them back just as a sea wall blocks an ocean current and sends it back to sea. All counter-currents, then, such as acid reflux, biliary colic, ureteric colic, middle insomnia, and tonic constipation can usually be ascribed to high alpha-sympathetic tone.

Those with high tone in both parasympathetic and alpha-sympathetic phases of the ANS are particularly susceptible to asthma and migraine. The difference between these two disorders reflects the autocoid hormones that mediate them. In asthma, histamine congests and delays while migrainous states are attenuated by serotonin. This led Dr Duraffourd in his private teachings to call migraine "the asthma of the brain".[318] Parasympathetic states are deepened by serotonin, alpha-sympathetic states by histamine.

In the autonomic sequence, alpha dominance will cause delay in the launch of the beta-sympathetic. In such cases, but notably in asthma, beta-mimetics will restore the faltering cycle. Pharmaceutical beta-blockers will stall this resolution and so are contra-indicated. In migraine, if they work at all, they may temporarily lower a highly charged anxious mood but are a poor choice of therapy. Fortunately, many anti-hypertensive herbs like *Tilia, Lavandula, Crataegus* modify beta gently and reduce alpha tone at the same time so, even in asthma, some gentle reduction of beta-sympathetic tone by herbs will be offset by the gains in alpha-sympathetic reduction. (See Table 3) Such herbs will also modify endocrine circuits to induce harmonies in parallel.

Stress requests, requires and demands (as British passports used to declare) energy to be provided swiftly which, to supplement glucocorticoids (when they prove inadequate), is found in the hypothalamic driver to the thyroid axis: TRH is a short message of a mere three amino acids so is cooked up in a trice. This is what Dr Hedayat in his lectures has called central-beta and is conveniently modified by an infusion of *Lamium album*. Oestrogens and TRH are potent stimulants of prolactin in the adjacent axis.

Chronic stress causes and perpetuates hyper-vigilant states in people who are startled by the slightest noise. This is a clear sign of alpha-sympathetic dominance. Chronic depression in combination with high alpha is the usual cause of hyperacusis and, like tinnitus, has little to do with the ears.

> We treat the surfeits and deficiencies that arise from the our patients' struggle to adapt to their personal challenges. In most cases, their difficulties manifest in the alpha-sympathetic zone. As we have the means, modifying alpha should be at the centre of our therapeutic intention.

Voluntary muscle and drive

The parasympathetic and beta-sympathetic are structurally opposed, contrasting the different needs of the axial and appendicular skeletons, contrasting smooth muscle and organs with voluntary muscle. Needing beta to find food, para to digest it and anabolise in sleep. Section 1.3 was dedicated to movement and the nurtures (in Section 2.2) to rest or a harmonious balance between the two.

The spring is slowly coiled during the parasympathetic, fastened tight, braced for release by the alpha-sympathetic and let fly by the beta-sympathetic.

While alpha-sympathetic receptors respond to noradrenaline, beta-sympathetic receptors respond to dopamine and adrenaline. Beta-dominant individuals transition more easily from sleep to a waking state. Nearly all medicinal plants influence the autonomic nervous system. A small selection appears in Table 3.

---

[318] He alludes to it in the *Traité* (2002) p. 508.

Table 3: Plants with effects upon branches of the ANS

Therapeutic name	Para–	Alpha–	Beta–	Additional therapeutic levels and notes
Achillea	↓↓↓			2,4,6
Allium cepa	↓↓			
Allium sativum			↓↓↓	
Angelica	↓↓	↓↓	↓↓	2,4,6
Ballota	++		↓↓	Unique balance helps nausea and migraine
Capsella	+		↓	7 and haemostasis
Centaurium	↓↓		++	2,5
Cinammomum			++	
Citrus aurantium (dulce)		↓	↓	Primes the senses!
Citrus limon			+++	
Crataegus		↓	↓↓	Benefits from longterm use
Fumaria	+		↓	2
Gentiana	↓↓↓			2
Hypericum	++			2 very complex effects
Hyssopus	↓		++	
Lactuca	↓			
Lavandula	↓↓	↓↓↓	↓↓	
Leonurus		↓↓	↓↓	
Levisticum	↓↓		↓↓	Anxiolytic
Marrubium	++			
Matricaria	↓	↓	↓	
Melaleuca	↓		↓	
Melilotus		↓↓↓		Anti-coagulant
Melissa		↓↓		
Mentha piperita	+		↓	
Menyanthes	↓↓	↓	+++	
Ocimum	↓		↓	
Pinus			++	Anti-osteoporotic
Ribes nigrum			+++	
Rosmarinus	+			
Salvia officinalis			+++	
Salvia sclarea		↓↓		Hyperoestrogenising
Satureja			+++	
Silybum			mild lytic	

(Continued)

Table 3: Plants with effects upon branches of the ANS (Continued)

Therapeutic name	Para–	Alpha–	Beta–	Additional therapeutic levels and notes
Solanum dulcamara	↓↓			
Stachys betonica	++			
Thymus	↓↓↓			
Tilia		↓↓	↓↓	
Trigonella	++			
Urtica	++			
Valeriana	↓		↓↓	
Verbena	+++			
Viburnum opulus	+		↓	
Viburnum prunifolium	↓			
Vinca	↓		↓	Increases FSH
Vitex		↓↓↓		
Zingiber			++	

Level two: supporting digestive organ deficiencies, gut motility and bile flow

Organ support leads to better management of circadian metabolism. The ANS can only operate within the enzymatic matrices and their cofactors, so cannot be considered in isolation. I give these therapeutic levels for ease of reference, but they are of course artificial demarcations. They do, however, collect together some of the more definite repeatable effects. A small selection from a vast repertoire is given in Table 4. The plant effects are demarcated by organs to provide emphasis, not sharp boundaries. Protective effects on the small intestine are too numerous to mention.

Table 4: Plants supporting digestive organs, gut motility and bile flow

Stomach	Liver	Gallbladder	Pancreas	Therapeutic notes
Achillea	Achillea			One of the finest aromatic bitters
	Agrimonia			Protector of GALT and the caecum
Angelica				
			Arctium	One of many anti-hyperglycaemic plants
	Calendula	Calendula		
	Centaurium			
	Citrus limon			
			Eucalyptus	

(Continued)

Table 4: Plants supporting digestive organs, gut motility and bile flow (Continued)

Stomach	Liver	Gallbladder	Pancreas	Therapeutic notes
	Fumaria		Fumaria	
	Gentiana			
	Hypericum			Very complex actions
	Lactuca			
Leonurus				
Levisticum				Anxiolytic
	Marrubium			
Matricaria				
Melissa				Probably indirect from endocrine effects
Mentha				
	Menyanthes			
	Olea		Olea	Protects the kidney
			Pinus	
		Rosmarinus		
			Rubus fruticosus	
			Salvia officinalis	
			Sambucus nigra	
			Scrophularia nodosa	
	Silybum			
S. dulcamara				
	Stachys betonica			
Thymus				Relaxes and protects the whole tract
			Trigonella	
			Vinca	Increases FSH
Zingiber				

Level three: the H-P vertical axes

Refer to Figure 6 in section 1.5a for an overview of these axes. The corticotrophic and gonadotrophic axes are yoked on account of their products being steroid molecules. The plants that I have found indispensable for modifying hormones and receptors (as per Section 3.5) are given in Table 5 below where corticotropic and gonadotropic stand for the two steroid axes on the left.[319]

---

[319] –trophic means 'feeding', tropic 'turning towards'. I consider them synonymous but Dr Hedeyat prefers the latter version.

Thyroid and Somatotrophic axes are proteinaceous, not steroids and their entries constitute the two righthand columns. Some plants inhibit prolactin without a commensurate reduction in growth hormone.

Table 5: Plant at level three: the H-P vertical axes

Therapeutic name	Corticotropic	Gonadotropic	Thyroid	Somato
Achillea		Luteotrophic		*They help regulate the prolactin/dopamine cycle*
Alchemilla		Luteotrophic		
Allium sativum			Stimulates	
Angelica		Oestrogenic		
Avena sativa		Oestrogenic	Stimulates	
Borago	↓Mineralocorticoid	Inhibits	Inhibits	
Calendula	Supports	Oestrogenic		
Convallaria			Inhibits	
Foeniculum		Oestrog +++	Stimulates	Stimulates
Galega				Stimulates
Glycyrrhiza	↑Mineralocorticoid	Oestrogenic		
Hedera		Oestrogenic		
Humulus		Oestro+ ↓Androgens		
Inula		Trophic		
Lamium album				↑peripheral↓CNS-beta
Leonurus			Inhibits	
Lycopus	Inhibits	Inhibits	Inhibits	
Levisticum		Oestrogenic		
Malus		↓Oes ↑LH		
Marrubium		Oes ↓LH+Andro		
Medicago		Oes ↓LH+Andro		↑indirectly
Menyanthes		Oestrogenic		
Ocimum		Trophic		
Pimpinella		Oestrogenic		Stimulates
Poterium	Supports			Inhibits
Ribes nigrum	Supports			
Rosmarinus	Supports			
Rubus idaeus	Supports indirectly			Inhibits
Salix		Oestrogenic	Stimulates	
Salvia officinalis		Oes ↓FSH	Stimulates	
Salvia sclarea		Oes+++ ↓FSH	?	

(Continued)

Table 5: Plant at level three: the H-P vertical axes

Therapeutic name	Corticotropic	Gonadotropic	Thyroid	Somato
Sambucus				↑periph↓Central-Dopa
Thymus	Supports			
Trigonella		Complex		Complex
Vib prunifolium				Inhibits
Vinca		↑FSH		Inhibits
Vitex	Inhibits	↓Peripheral oes	↑t4>t3	Stimulates
Zingiber	Supports	↑Androgens	↑t4	

Crucial to remember that the cyclicity of the H-P axes are circadian. Transitions, of season, year and heptade alter their relationships dramatically precipitating sudden illness and worsening chronic conditions. Transitions in time affect all physiological levels are the commonest source of illness, an understanding to be shared during the consultation. Intrauterine and early life disruptions in the corticotrophic axis will influence development and may underlie lifelong alterations in immune responsiveness.

Level four: metabolic outcomes of relations within the H-P axes: balance between anabolic and catabolic drives

Disease of the vertical axes are relatively rare if we exclude the contemporary increase in diabetes mellitus. But disorders within them are so common that they are the major source of illness in clinical practice. As Hans Selye was the first to register methodically, these are the axes that each of us mobilises to adapt to our daily and seasonal lives.

Each of the four H-P axes has a vertical relation as it directs peripheral organs or tissues but they operate interdependently. They are connected in the hypothalamus and in sequence—like falling dominoes—along a horizontal axis within the pituitary gland.[320]

The axes alternate between catabolic and anabolic drives. Catabolism (breaking down) liberates the materials, which will build (anabolise) bodily structures and enzymatic material without which no physiological process can proceed. Overall, the parasympathetic is anabolic and the orthosympathetic catabolic, with day favouring the release of materials and night their incorporation but the demarcation is relative and metabolism (combining the two) goes on all the time. The H-P axes calibrate both arms of metabolism to respond to current and episodic demand. Hyper-catabolism does not allow for storage.

---

[320] It seems scarcely credible that endocrinologists pay scant if any attention to this integration and that Doctors Duraffourd, Lapraz and Hedayat seem to be voices in the wilderness. The circadian physiology (starting with the daily surge of cortisol) has been known and accepted for a long time but seems to go no further than the timing of cortisol testing.

Hypothalamus	CRF	GnRH		TRH	GH-RH	Dopamine
Pituitary	MSH ACTH	FSH	LH	TSH	GH	Prolactin
Products of peripheral organs and tissues	Gluco- & mineralo-corticoids, compensatory and rogens	Oestrogens, progestogens, androgens		Thyroid hormones	Long bones	Most tissues, especially skin and breast
Overall outcome	CATABOLISM	ANABOLISM	ANABOLISM	CATABOLISM	ANABOLISM	ANABOLISM

Figure 21: Hypothalamic Vertical Pulses and Pituitary Horizontal Tides
(after Duraffourd, Lapraz & Hedayat)

Your patient will present with some overall balance and may even complain of an imbalance: failure to put on or lose weight, most commonly. Whatever their complaint, endocrine and metabolic balance will form an essential part of your assessment, from their birth weight, childhood morphology and adolescent growth spurts as discussed in Part Two.

Anabolism has to be supported with care: you need to be careful what kind of tissue you are advancing. Treatment will consider each axis in turn and not favour one over the other too strongly so as to avoid reactivity in the untreated axes. Refer back to Table 5.

Level five: the horizontal flow within the pituitary gland through the H-P axes—dominances and deficits

As well as the metabolic balance just considered, there are considerable endocrine effects from potential imbalance between the axes. The three glycoprotein hormones TSH, FSH and LH are structurally similar and generated by the same gene so it is better to think of similarity rather than difference: all are cooperating to maintain the organism. The most abundant cells of the pituitary are somatotrophic producing GH and prolactin; both are required for adult maturity. As we are mammals, the predominance of prolactin should not surprise but as prolactin is secreted throughout life in both sexes, it must serve global needs, probably to calm and dampen rampant immunity. Prolactin rises greatly during sleep and with stress. GH, prolactin and insulin need to be considered together as does the inhibitory effect of dopamine. I suspect that insulin-like growth factors will bridge the many unresolved physiological puzzles that beset researchers.

ACTH (like MSH) is a polypeptide that has circadian activity corroborating the notion that the adrenal gland is our wake-up call. As it seems to support osteoblastic activity, its relationship with sunlight in the metabolism of vitamin D (and the effect of MSH) comes as no surprise in a diurnal species. CRH stimulates ACTH but seems also to initiate horizontal integration between each of the hypothalamic releasing hormones. Their pulsatile harmonies may resonate within the pituitary then amplify throughout the body.

Given all this complexity and interconnectedness, complex organic molecules such as those found in plants might be just the best thing to comfort the whole rather than throw a spanner into the works and expect a harmonious outcome.

The pituitary hormones are proliferative, so in conditions of unwanted cellular proliferation, dampening with *Vitex agnus-castus* and members of Boraginaceae might be a place to start. Acne and psoriasis have been discussed in section 2.5b. Colitis and Crohn's disease need FSH to be dampened (as if one were helping with the oestropause). LH needs to be restrained in cases of uterine fibroids. Reducing excessive catabolism lowers the risk of providing elements for the building of unwanted tissues: obvious when facing a present tumour, benign or malignant, but the risk of promoting cancer must always be at the back of one's mind, especially with highly oestrogenising herbs such as *Foeniculum, Salvia* (especially *S. sclarea*) and *Humulus*. Dosage and duration of treatment should be carefully considered rather than avoiding them altogether. There are more than enough endocrine disruptors in our modern environment; Rinsing detergents from dishes and avoiding cling film being the most obvious ones.

Disorders of the thyroid axis are commoner than disorders of the thyroid gland itself. Over-diagnosis of the latter leading to inappropriate and longterm hormone replacement therapy (HRT) with levothyroxine can be helped gradually with herbal restraint of hyper states and support for real or supposed hypothyroidism. As endobiogenic medicine has taught, estimation by blood test of creatine phosphokinase (CPK) and lactate dehydrogenase (LDH) give a truer report of thyroid yield. CPK represents the phosphate reservoir for the fundamental energetic cycling of ATP in mitochondria. Also, the ratio between neutrophils and lymphocytes indicates the efficiency of the thyroid, whatever the levels of TSH might suggest.[321] No single measure will tell the whole story which is recounted more effectively by a complex model.

I have found that reducing the intensity of the hormonal landscape magnifies the benefits of other therapeutic strategies. The intensifiers are secreted rapidly by the posterior pituitary. Their expression often points to a lifelong disposition and correlates probably with the mother's experience of pregnancy, childbirth and the post-partum period. Let's turn next to the plants that have great therapeutic potential for this therapeutic level.

Level six: hormones of the posterior lobe of the pituitary gland

As these hormones are stored in termini of neurones, direct neural connections make their effects rapid and targeted. Oxytocin levels are greatly increased by oestrogen and levels in the brain have been found to far exceed those in the periphery, perhaps explaining its occasional paradoxical effects. In the emoticon version of endocrinology, oxytocin favours bonding and attachment but these are context driven and may

---

[321] This ratio generates the second index in the Biology of Functions (the Genito-Thyroid index) and should normally fall between 1.5 and 2.5.

include fixations and attachments in psychopaths. Oxytocin, a hormone with a good press, intensifies the current state—whether happy or not—and tends to amplify a person's current social orientation, which may or may not be typical for them. Its peripheral activity is gonadic in both sexes with powerful effects on smooth muscle invoked in childbirth, letting milk down and, in the ovulation on which these situations would have been predicated, and possibly on attendant orgasm. Of course, receptors need to be present and proliferated for which oestrogen seems to be the prime driver though olfactory cues are also potent up-regulators in certain primed situations. Hormones do not operate on their own just as a key is just a lump of metal until it is inserted into a receptive lock.

According to Dr Duraffourd, in his private teachings, melatonin stimulates ADH to inhibit nocturnal micturition; ADH and serotonin liberate oxytocin which, I speculate, may promote dreaming. The fall of predawn ADH signals the morning surge of ACTH and MSH. This is facilitated by prolactin if high (and can be lowered by *Mercurialis annua*).

Oxytocin amplifies pleasure and dampens acoustic sensitivity. Biosynthesis may be dependent on vitamin C. As an intensifier of experience you might expect it to be associated with responsiveness and emotivity but—and this seems to be influenced by early experience—it can deepen anxious attachments, and give rise to anxiety and even protective detachment: the opposite to its reputation.

Levels of oxytocin are higher in the brain than in peripheral tissues and this differential may explain its deep role in social dispositions like trust and honesty, and the paradoxes of social context. Being ticklish is another indicator of intensity, and how pleasure and pain are thinly demarcated and depend upon acquiescence and other social markers.

I have found the plants in Table 6 that reduce oxytocic anxiety reduce other types of negative affect. Those that stimulate it may do so by their oestrogenising properties.

Table 6: Plants with strong effects upon the posterior lobe of the pituitary gland

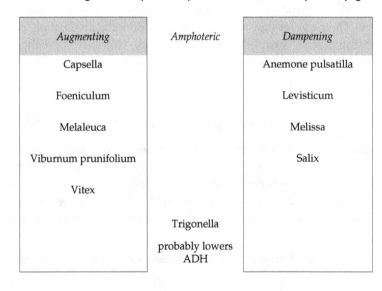

Augmenting	Amphoteric	Dampening
Capsella		Anemone pulsatilla
Foeniculum		Levisticum
Melaleuca		Melissa
Viburnum prunifolium		Salix
Vitex		
	Trigonella probably lowers ADH	

Level seven: the autocoid hormones—histamine, noradrenaline, dopamine, serotonin

Below poise, three levels of active braking impedes any impulse to overspend energy. Restoring reserves liberates energy for future use.[322] Spasm in smooth or voluntary muscle provides the first drag on spending. The second level of impedance provokes histamine release from mast cells and tissues in the alimentary tract. Supporting all dissipations of energy will be more holistic a therapeutic approach rather than automatically reaching for plants that reduce the histamine response though these may be also useful depending upon the case. My selection of these is to be found within Tables 2, 3, 4. It is most important to assess the patient's autonomic disposition so as not to frustrate the effort of the terrain to restore poise by histaminic impedance.

Any of the plants that reduce alpha-sympathetic drive in Table 3 will reduce noradrenaline and also reduce dopamine and adrenaline from the adrenal medulla.

Serotonin deepens and lengthens parasympathetic activity. Just reducing vagal tone with a morning mixture may relax the bowel but the digestive organs need to be supported and paradoxically mild vagomimetic plants given in the same prescription will normalise bowel serotonin.

Translocation of serotonin from the retinae to the pineal gland where melatonin is metabolised has profound physiological and protective effects and is linked to restorative sleep. Like the terrain itself, these pathways are imprinted early in life.[323]

Hypericum is usually best mixed with *Melissa* and then prescribed to be taken on an occasional basis. If treating cyclothymia or moderate depression, I prescribe a phased regime where the mixture is taken then suspended for consecutive unequal periods. This may be alternating days of four days on, three off or, most usually, eleven on, six off or days eight to twenty-one of a menstrual cycle.

Phasing might in theory optimise all therapeutics. To repurpose Heraclitus: because a body is in constant movement and as the treatment changes the terrain, the treatment itself does not remain the same, nor does the person. Although we cannot step in the same river twice, a constantly changing approach would be impracticable in most circumstances. Besides, there are treatments (for instance lowering blood pressure) where you want to gain the cumulative benefits of, say, Hawthorn and not keep chopping and changing.

Level eight: prolactin and dopamine oscillation

As discussed in Level Five, over 60% of cells in the pituitary gland secrete growth hormone and prolactin so their roles in anabolism are probably complementary. As the more specialised function of lactation requires osmotic control and lipid conservation, these effects no doubt transpose onto all people of all ages.

---

[322] As illustrated in Figure 2 in Section 1.2. See also Appendix II.

[323] During pregnancy, the maternal melatonin circadian rhythm provides cues for the SCN of the foetus to recognise time-of-day and time-of-year (Reppert *Maternal entrainment of the developing circadian system*) Annals NY Academy of Sciences February 1985 453:162-9.

Dopamine drives the discharge sought by desire and, being catabolic, can only be temporary. As we saw in Level Four, anabolism has a greater number of drivers because accumulation is slower and more complex than catabolism.[324] Prolactin is quantitatively the major anabolic driver. The capacity to delay gratification has been shown to confer great adaptive advantages for which we may thank the anticipatory judgement to the foresight of prolactin. While the evolutionary benefits may be clear, when gratification is too long delayed, it fails to gratify. Prolactin infused personalities contrast with impulsive presentists.[325]

The opposition between majestic Apollonian order and chaotic Bacchanalian disregard for constraint (mixing Greek and Roman metaphors) was expressed in classical times (and with greater bias in biblical times). Prolactin resists the dopaminergic drive towards pleasure and discharge. Craving order, it may become dictatorial in its demands for rigid process and structure. Ritual reduces mayhem. But the cost is huge: it is very stressful to create a world which excludes stress.[326] So, while we can enjoy silence in libraries we can frolic in festivals. Retention and discharge are equally central to physiological and social lives.

Prolactin with oestrogens, FSH (and probably oxytocin) builds the areola so if you can inspect or ask about its shape and size, hormonal information is offered you. Oxytocin contributes to the erection and size of the nipple which is low when inverted, though a strong parasympathetic can dampen it further.

The complex interactions between prolactin, the pituitary and hypothalamic stimulating hormones mean that reducing prolactin—as one may do with infusions of raspberry leaf[327] may provide short-term benefits but may induce unwanted knock-on effects downstream.

For instance, if you wanted to shrink the size of fibroids, you would want to reduce anabolic hormones, primarily androgens (because the endometrium is muscle) but also prolactin. However, this will gradually allow LH to reassert itself with another pulse of prognenolone promoting resurgence of androgens rather than be aromatised in a susceptible patient to oestrogen.

The overall point is that prolactin dominance is pervasive and that only dopamine is capable of inhibiting it without triggering a cascade of unwanted hormones. Dopamine dominance has problems of its own but these are less likely to come your way and would respond to *Galega, Foeniculum* and *Lamium album*. This prolactin and dopamine oscillation cycle has most profound effects in development and behaviour. Flowers of *Sambucus nigra* provide the most reliable stabilisation of the rhythm without rebound effects or relaunching hormonal axes that are unwanted.

---

[324] See also Ageing in Section 2.7.

[325] As discussed in Section 1.9, the situation is not binary. Nuances in the necessity for living presently is expressed by the Sufi saying: "if not for me, then for whom? If not now, when?"

[326] Sapolsky (2017) 63.

[327] And greater burnet and chervil when you can get them.

Level nine: idiosyncratic

I do not want this to seem like an offhand postscript, trivialising and sentimentalising our practice and I would also like to avoid going to the other extreme and sounding too earnest.

Not only is personalised medicine idiosyncratic by definition but each plant species has a particular idiosyncrasy that cannot be generalised, even though they may share common features with other members of their genus and to a much lesser extent in the family and larger taxa.

So rather than rehearsing repeated schedules from the herbals and the many excellent books and monographs,[328] the greatest recommendation I would urge upon the herbal apprentice is to live among plants and visit often those ones that do not grow near where you live. Going further, I recommend resisting the temptation to prescribe plants you have not seen in the wild or in cultivation, however alluring reports of their powers might be. Consulting the reference literature will be good confirmation of your practice but is no substitute for the gathering of primary knowledge from the plants themselves. This is not mystical immersion, just using the extraordinary perceptive powers open to all of us. All knowledge is practical because as we apply it, what we know changes us in the subtlest of ways.

---

[328] Especially those produced by the European Scientific Cooperative on Phytotherapy which number over 100. Unfortunately, the acronym ESCOP is shared by other unrelated organisations.

Mixed messages

All plant extracts are complex mixtures and we add further complexity when we make up prescriptions of more than one plant. Contemporary practice rightly frowns on the extreme polypharmacy that was common, at least in Britain, before the 1980s, a practice that we questioned as students. One of my tutors put into her mixtures as many plants as the number of actions she wished to achieve. In a mixture containing twenty-six plants to which Dandelion leaf contributed two–and–a–half percent "for its diuretic effect", it was easy to calculate that this would amount to only a tiny piece of a single leaf, a portion you could tear off on the lawn and chew in a moment or two. Besides which, wanting to achieve twenty-six separate actions, seemed implausibly lavish. This additive, almost agglutinative, approach to prescribing seemed to be hedging an improbable number of bets. Tokenism is as ineffective as offering plants of poor quality. Our teachers, especially Simon Mills and Hein Zeylstra, were already moving towards simplified therapeutics, away from the uncritical many to the chosen few.

Even so, we do mix plants in the way that a meal is made of more than a single ingredient. Herbal medicine may not be the same as cooking, but there are some parallels between the two. Apart from the number of actions, there are synergistic effects to consider, and sometimes a blending of flavours and textures, especially when it comes to tisanes. We do not have to be as extravagant as the Theriac of Venice (with its purported 104 ingredients) or even as lavish as my former tutor to recognise that, even with a single plant, or three or four, we are bringing to bear a large number of factors on a person's physiological state, itself unknowable in its full entirety. Faced with this imprecision, pharmaceutical science sought and continues to seek and find key components so as to isolate (in theory) one effect from another, removing each element from its mixed context. That approach can produce known and repeatable effects, certainly as well as unwanted effects that also are unknowable. Barbara Griggs positions the birth of this approach onto the introduction of foxglove (*Digitalis purpurea*) by a Welsh herbalist in eighteenth century England in that chapter of her *Green Pharmacy*.[329]

The polyvalence of plants provides us with their efficacy in treating the complexity of human physiology but, as with theriacs and polypharmacy, the notion can be extended too far. Even with the parsimonious approach that has become commonplace and which I firmly endorse, mixtures will inevitably convey mixed messages. There will be paradoxes, even opposition between desirable actions and less wanted consequences. For instance, *Zingiber* reduces platelet clumping and has anti-inflammatory effects with beneficial benefits for endothelia, but also is sympathomimetic and supports peripheral thyroid activity along with androgenic properties. There are circumstances when you would want most of these effects, but would like to exclude the male hormone effects. Well, you can't. But you can minimise them or balance them out with other plants or achieve mostly the wanted effects by:

1. Dosage
2. Mixture with other plants (which will also modify dosage)
3. Choose another plant with the effects that you want that lacks those you would like to avoid

The third option is of course the easiest. Even when the contradictory actions are not so marked, before making any prescription the first task for the herbalist, following a first consultation (or a follow-up consultation that imposes some review of the previous treatment) requires an analysis of the clinical data and the formulation of a therapeutic strategy. For your list of requirements, you will need a sense of the different physiological levels at which plants can operate, which I summarise here:

1. Autonomic nervous system
2. Neuro-hormones & hormones from posterior pituitary
3. Hormones from the four axes of the anterior pituitary
4. Tonic mutual inhibition between dopamine and prolactin in the 4th axis
5. Circadian regulators via pulsatile hypothalamic drivers of the anterior pituitary
6. Organ function, which coordinates all of these inputs and manages outputs and excretions.
7. Endothelia, coagulability and cellular elements of blood

As a general rule of thumb (and this most definitely must be taken as a heuristic and not as a rule), you may incorporate different actions by adjusting levels of dosage in the following way when using tinctures:

1. Use high doses or proportions when you want to influence the autonomic nervous system or the posterior pituitary hormones
2. Low doses or proportions when you want to influence the anterior pituitary hormones
3. Intermediate doses or proportions when you want to favour organ function

---

[329] See bibliography.

By "doses" above I mean the therapeutic emphasis you wish to place upon the patient's terrain and can be achieved by:

1. Limiting the number of plants in a mixture. A range of between two and five plants per prescription means that the contribution of each plant is likely to be adequate.
2. Adjusting the prescribed dosage of a mixture of tinctures where 2.5 ml would be a low dose, 7.5–10 ml a high dose and 5 ml intermediate. Occasionally doses can be higher but in my own practice, don't recall prescribing doses greater than 20 ml though these are routinely appropriate for plant juices and aromatic waters.
3. The proportion of the plant in a mixture so that a "low dose" can be achieved by making it contribute, say, 10% towards the mixture and a high dose by at least 40%. Low doses might be chosen for plants potent in taste of effect, or to minimise a high percentage of alcohol. Doses that contribute less than 10% would be unusual unless they provide realistic therapeutic benefits.
4. Using contrasting contributions: giving a smaller dose of a potent plant (as anyway you must) with a much larger contribution from one or two others. For example, *Anemone pulsatilla*, with its narrow therapeutic window, would be unlikely to have much therapeutic effect if it made up less than 20% of a mixture (assuming dosage at 5 ml) but where a greater percentage would be undesirable. You could, however, double that contribution to 40% by halving the spoon dose to 2.5 ml, leaving you with 60% for the rest of the mixture. This makes best sense if you limit yourself to a single additional plant (giving 40:60) or at most two so as to maximise the plants that do best at a relatively high dose and minimise the potent plants that nonetheless require an adequate dose.

You can see that by juggling the elements of the prescription in various ways, you are matching effects with plants and playing out your strategy with simple arithmetic.

Blending, after all, is a common practice in the commercial presentation of plant products for consumption, such as coffee, tea, and for applying to the skin and hair. These are generalised to sell to a population whereas our blending is to particularise a blend to an individual patient. With the diffuse nature of the plants we give, where there are many "inert" buffers such as chlorophyll, pectins and gums, it is not uncommon to find a beta-mimetic plant in a prescription for, say, asthma with a strong alpha-lytic plant that, in apparent contradiction, cannot avoid being mildly beta-lytic. It justifies putting the strongly parasympathetico-lytic *Thymus* together with the weakly parasympathetico-mimetic *Rosmarinus* in a mixture on account of the corticotrophic activity of both plants. this apparently contradictory mixture will also provide the relaxant activity to the intestines of the thyme with the beneficial effects on liver and gall-bladder of the rosemary, but you will need to adjust the ratio between the two to adapt to the individual patient whose adrenal state you are trying to help. There are other situations, such as asthma, where opposite strands of the therapeutic drive are to be expected: you would combine strong parasympathetico-lytic remedies like *Thymus* and *Achillea* with beta-mimetic plants like *Salvia*, *Pinus*, *Hyssopus* and *Zingiber*, adding possibly one of any number of alpha-sympathetico-lytic plants such as *Lavandula* which is also parasympathetico-lytic, as is *Hyssopus*. All in all, the treatment of asthma and migraine and other conditions relies on plants which operate at the same time at opposite poles of the ANS to great therapeutic effect. Not in a crisis so much but to reduce the occurrence of crises and to lessen their severity.

Speaking of crises, occasionally I use a heroic dosage on myself to try to abort or modify an acute infection at its onset.

Last thoughts on materia medica and the elements of practice

The materia medica that was presented in Section 3.7 and throughout this book is gathered in the light of experience that does not run counter to any evidence and hopes to add collaboratively with existing ideas. My own clinical experience validates the endobiogenic repertoire of endobiogenic medicine and saw it replicated in the consulting rooms of Drs Duraffourd and Lapraz. The 'actions' of the plants represent physiological tropisms that practice validates and are consonant with what is known of phytochemistry. They are observations rather than claims but need to be monitored by the phytotherapist who is applying them in practice.

There are many encyclopaedias of herbal medicine and I relied on them as a student and in the first few years of practice but soon the lists of plants grow tedious as the friends in your dispensary seem to be up to the mark most of the time. Even when the list of plants is narrowed down to those I chose in Section 3.4, there remains a wealth of material. It would be difficult to practice as a herbalist without good knowledge of the range of plants in the following families.

- Rosaceae
- Malvaceae
- Lamiaceae (Labiatae)
- Rutaceae
- Apiaceae (Umbelliferae)
- Solanaceae
- Myrtaceae

Although rural rambles and gardening give the daily insights, making a day of it at the Order Beds at Kew or another botanic garden counts as the best kind of continual professional development.

Case studies

I think they are popular but I have never liked them. They illustrate an individual and their condition but how do you extend those insights into other individuals and other conditions in personalised medicine? They frustrate me because they always seem to imply generalities but, when questioned, such extensions are elusive and slip away. The attraction, no doubt, is to hear of someone with a grave problem getting much better.

I must have written many thousands of prescriptions, as have my colleagues, so could fill a book with them. But to what end? If a student sits with me, we of course discuss the case and the prescriptions. That is how we all learn, but to write them down is to fossilise them which would render them worthless, or, much worse, templates. The tables I have given in Section 3.6 give ample scope to match quite a wide range of plants to conditions seen in practice and to amplify them with plants from the same genus or family.

Even so, one generalisation I can make is to match the elements of herbal prescriptions to circadian rhythms.

An approach to prescription

The qualities of morning physiology are in great contrast to those of the afternoon and evening. Accordingly, one would want to match those changes so that a morning mixture would, for example, help a vagotonic shrug off the congestion of sleep. Herbs like lavender that diminish concentration would better suit the evening while rosemary would give focus to the morning. Occasionally I do prescribe a single mixture to be taken twice or even four times a day, according to levels of stress, for overwrought people. Usually, my therapy consists of three preparations: a tincture to be taken after breakfast and a different one to be taken after the evening meal. A tisane provides a hydrating bridge between them and might be specified as before or after noon, depending upon the herbs. Thyroid yield peaks at eleven and slumps between two and four in the afternoon. Inflammation peaks from five to six pm. The prescription tries to map along the curve of the circadian day. For tinctures, I recommend putting the dose (usually 2.5–7.5ml) into a mug to which boiling water is added, drinking when warm. This has the benefit of burning off the alcohol and gives the patient a long hot toddy which itself has a diffusing effect. The small amount of remaining alcohol may be hormetic.

Here is an example of such a scheme, with variant months given in Roman numerals, the tisane remaining the same:

Post Jentaculum	V	VIII
Salvia off.	30	
Salvia rosmarinus		20
Menyanthes	20	
Glycyrrhiza	30	
Ballota	20	
Calendula		20
Angelica		30
Thymus		30

TISANE	
Lavandula	25
Lamium	25
Sambucus	25
Tilia	25

Post Cena	V	VIII
Lavandula	25	
Vitex	25	
Melissa	25	30
Tilia	25	
Melilotus		30
Anemone		20
Levisticum		20

The other approach to differential prescription recognises the variations of the menstrual cycle so that a woman might have different remedies for the menstrual phase, the ovulatory phase (nominally from day 8 until day 19) and the pre-menstrual phase. Epileptic sufferers of menstruating age need very specialised measures.

I tend to change all prescriptions in recognition of the seasonal midpoints as discussed in Section 1.5b.

Acute attacks

I so enjoy not feeling ill to the point that I overreact if threatened. If I sense an impending viral attack in the evening, I let an *Echinacea* tablet dissolve over a few minutes in my mouth before swallowing and repeat once or twice near bedtime. Usually this does the trick and, if I may add a property to the list, it gives me very good sleep.

If the following morning, the *Echinacea* trick had failed to remove a persistent sense of illness, I take 100 ml of a tisane from a dessertspoonful of Agrimony and then, separately, pour 150 ml of boiling water onto a cup of 5 ml of each of the following tinctures: *Echinacea, Hyssopus, Inula, Glycyrrhiza, Thymus, Zingiber, Fumaria*. I drink a third of the tisane and then the hot mixture of tinctures to which I add several drops of each of the following volatile oils: *Pinus, Lavandula, Eucalyptus, Melaleuca, Thymus* getting it all down me within an hour or two.[330] My personal experience suggests that the usefulness of this approach does not persist much after the third day of an infectious illness so after this initial approach to the acute attack, I ply myself with tisanes for the following days or weeks until I feel quite recovered.

This approach is quite at odds with the idea of hormesis (Section 3.3) and to explain away my hypocrisy, I could claim that the hormetins I take regularly and the eustress I build into my life makes these viral attacks quite rare. I should perhaps pay more attention to Hein Zeylstra who, though not averse to heroic doses on occasion, would advise not drenching a patient with medicine when unsettled by illness: "Don't blow too hard on sputtering candle".

---

[330] When it comes to volatile oils, neat Tea-tree oil clears many annoying minor skin irritations and sebaceous eruptions.

Part Three Résumé

- Plants figure as primary articles of all human cultures. Knowledge of them provisions us with advantages for well-being, cultural capital and even survival.
- For those of us who prescribe them, medicinal plants offer more than a mere inventory of therapeutic agents. Most herbalists have struck up a relationship with living plants in their natural habitat.
- Two parallel approaches run alongside one another in herbal therapeutics. Herbalists may apply plants as remedies to presenting complaints or may apply plants to shift the patient's terrain so that the complaint is edged out of existence. This distinction is more one of emphasis than absolute partition. Very often, the nurture given by a plant remedy will speak for itself in its own way in a particular situation. Just as geneticists tell us that there is no *gene for* anything so herbalists should remind themselves that there no *herb for* anything Actually, the distinction hinges on whether the patient as much as the herbalist seeks a commodity to fix their problems without expecting to understand how that problem arose and without expecting to have to alter their behaviour.
- Personalised Medicine: holistic in the best sense means personalised and it really does mean, unless we are merely paying lip service and trading on a brand, that each person gets their own medication and that you neither possess nor stock any formulae. In these matters there can be a lot of faith-talk but not enough fidelity.
- The message of the book, sandwiched between physiology and botany, is that to practise herbal medicine is to practise medicine in the fullest and broadest sense.
- Relational: there is no essence because single elements do not exist in the world. An essential oil consists of a nexus of interrelated compounds that express the relation of a plant with its environment. Even a physical element requires two charges and at least two particles. A drug interaction involves conformation between drug and receptor.

- In herbal therapeutics, with sensory priming, the effects experienced are often physiological rather than pharmacological and offer long-term preventative care. Herbs are adjuncts, not supplemental, to diet. Supplements imply some deficiency state. You cannot have a deficiency of, say, silymarin!
- Properties of medicinal plants do not belong to them or to us but to the relationship between us.

POSTSCRIPT

We are the beneficiaries of the scientific and industrial revolutions but it has come at great cost to the natural world and, apart from being founded upon forced labour, may have enslaved us all.

The industrial medical complex is a double-headed monster: its benign face has led us to better understand disordered physiology and to identify the vectors of communicable disease. It has reduced pain and suffering and, along with public health and hygiene measures, has made previously common killers—like cholera, typhus and many others—rare or better managed. But medicine coupled with industrialisation has led to biodiversity loss with untold ecological damage and has financialised the whole world.

To emphasise the effects of the work ethic on the issues raised under the second nurture—balance of work, rest and recreation—in Section 2.2, I append the text of Benjamin Franklin's approach to work and the conception of limitless growth as benign:

> Remember, that time is money. He that can earn ten shillings a day by his labor, and goes abroad, or sits idle, one half of that day, though he spends but sixpence during his diversion or idleness, ought not to reckon that the only expense; he has really spent, or rather thrown away, five shillings besides. […] Remember, that money is the prolific, generating nature. Money can beget money, and its offspring can beget more, and so on. Five shillings turned is six, turned again is seven and threepence, and so on, till it becomes a hundred pounds. The more there is of it, the more it produces every turning, so that the profits rise quicker and quicker. He that kills a breeding-sow, destroys all her offspring to the thousandth generation. He that murders a crown, destroys all that it might have produced, even scores of pounds.[331]

---

[331] Weber (*see* bibliography) points out that this is not mere greed but a morality of growth.

The notion of the spiritual has, I believe, falsely divided physics from metaphysics. If one means it to refer to the undivided totality, there is no reason to exclude physicalism or materialism from the spiritual. On a physical note, though, textures (such as hard and soft) do contrast. In France, herbal medicine is advertised in pharmacies as *La médicine douce*. But soft medicine, beyond advertising trope, need not be a romantic notion for the affluent. It is a refuge, often a last resort, for those whose state of unwellness cannot be labelled and commodified. The following quotation, almost certainly apocryphal, was claimed to be an address to the US Congress by a delegation from the Cree nation.[332]

> Only when you have felled the last tree, killed the last animal, caught the last fish and poisoned the last river, will you realise that you cannot eat money.

As well as obeying the Hippocratic injunction 'At least do no harm,' plant medicine offers enormous potential for herbalists to do good.

---

[332] I have searched the US National Archive online and all reputed Native American utterances (including the famous one by Chief Seattle) have been disputed as genuine. Whatever the case, the poetic force and finality of this statement is undeniable, and less adorned than that of Franklin. For testament to the catastrophic ecological and cultural damage perpetrated on the North American continent, Teri McLuhan's *Touch The Earth* (*Abacus* 1973) is highly recommended.

A LIST OF PLANTS MENTIONED IN THE TEXT MATCHING THERAPEUTIC SHORTHAND NAMES WITH SCIENTIFIC BINOMIALS

Shorthand therapeutic name	Parts used	Scientific binomial	Common names
Achillea	Flowering tops; Leaves	*Achillea millefolium* L	Yarrow
Agnus-castus	See Vitex		
Agrimonia	Dried aerial parts	*Agrimonia eupatoria* L	Agrimony
Agropyron	Rhizome	*Agropyron* is the name still used by herbalists. This grass has been classed in several genera, some defunct, such as *Triticum, Elytrigia, Elymus.*	Couch Grass
Alchemilla	Dried aerial parts	*Alchemilla vulgaris* L agg. [an aggregate name for populations of agamospecies]	Lady's Mantle
Alliums	Bulbs and leaves	Onions, chives, leeks and garlic	
Anemone pulsatilla	Dried aerial parts	*Pulsatilla vulgaris* Miller (Anemone pulsatilla L)	Pasqueflower
Angelica		*Angelica archangelica* L	Garden Angelica
	Parts used in order of clincal importance: Root and Rhizome Fruits; Leaf; Fresh Stems		

(Continued)

(Continued)

Shorthand therapeutic name	Parts used	Scientific binomial	Common names
Apium	Fruits, fresh or dreid. Fresh aerial parts	*Apium graveolens* L	Wild celery
Arctium		*Arctium lappa* L	Burdock
	1. Root, best fresh from mature plants. 2. Leaf, best fresh, eaten raw or as tisane or light decoction. 3. Infructescence with seeds, harvested when ripe, fresh or dried, best decocted.		
Arnica	Ligulate florets (or inflorescence with involucral bracts for ease of harvest)	*Arnica montana* L	Mountain Arnica, mountain tobacco
Artemisia	Dried aerial parts, fresh or dried Many other species are used medicinally	*Artemisia vulgaris* L *A. absinthium* L *A. dracununculus* L var *sativa* *A. dracunculoides* L *A. abrotnum* L	Mugwort Wormwood French Tarragon Russian Tarragon Southernwood
Ballota	Aerial parts	*Ballota nigra* L	Black Horehound
Betonica	See Stachys		
Borago	Flowers and upper leaves	*Borago officinalis* L	Borage
Boswellia	Resin	*Boswellia serrata* Roxb. and related species	Frankincence
buchu	Leaves	*Agathosma betulina* (Bergius) Pill.	
Calendula	Inflorescence with involucral bracts; leaves have been used	*Calendula officinalis* L	Calendula, Pot Marigold

(Continued)

(Continued)

Shorthand therapeutic name	Parts used	Scientific binomial	Common names
Calluna	Flowering tops, fresh or dried	*Calluna vulgaris* (L) Hull	Heather
Capsella	Aerial parts	*Capsella bursa-pastoris* (L) Medicus	Shepherd's-purse
chervil	Leaves	*Anthriscus cerefolium* (L) Hoffm	Garden Chervil
Chrysanthemum parthenium	Fresh leaf or dried and powdered	*Tanccetum parthenium* (L) Shultz Bip	Feverfew
Citrus aurantium	Flowers; Leaves	*Citrus aurantium* L var. *dulce* *Citrus aurantium* L var. *amarum*	Orange
Crataegus	Fruit; Leaves; Flowers	*Crataegus* laevigata (Poiret) DC and *C.* monogyna Jacq	Hawthorns
Daisy	Inflorescence with involucral bracts; leaves have been used	*Bellis perennis* L	
Damiana	Dried Leaves	*Turnera diffusa* Willd. var *aphrodisiaca*	Damiana
Dulcamara	2–3 yr old dried Stems	*Solanum dulcamara* L	Bittersweet, Woody Nightshade
Echinacea	Roots; aerial parts	*Echinacea purpurea* (L) Moench, *E. angustifolia* (DC) Heller *E. pallida* (Nutt) Britt	
Eupatorium	Leaves; Inflorescence with involucral bracts; Root	*Eupatorium perfoliatum* *E. cannabinum* *E. purpureum* [moved to *Eutrochium*]	Boneset Hemp Agrimony Sweet Joe-Pye

(Continued)

(Continued)

Shorthand therapeutic name	Parts used	Scientific binomial	Common names
Euphrasia	Aerial parts, usually dried	*Euphrasia* belongs to a conglomerate of hemiparasitic microspecies and apomicts	Eyebright
Filipendula	Flowering tops (best fresh); upper leaves dried or fresh	*Filipendula ulmaria* (L) Maxim (*Spiraea ulmaria* L)	Meadowsweet
Foeniculum	Parts used in order of clincal importance:	*Foeniculum vulgare* Miller	Fennel
	Fruits with seeds; Leaf; Fresh Stems; Root		
Fraxinus	Leaflets, stripped from stalks	*Fraxinus excelsior* L	Ash
Fumaria	Aerial parts	*Fumaria officinalis* L	Fumitory
Galega	Flowers; herb; seeds	*Galega officinalis* L	Goat's-rue, French lilac
Glycyrrhiza	Root and stolon	*Glycyrrhiza glabra* L	Liquorice
Guaicaum	Resin	*Guaicaum officinale* L (also *G.sanctum* L)	Lignum-vitae
Harpagophytum	Roots and tubers	*Harpagophytum procumbens* DC ex Meissner	Devil's Claw
Hedera	Younger leaves, preferably fresh	*Hedera helix* L	Ivy
Humulus	Strobiles (female cone-like inflorescences)	*Humulus lupulus* L	Hops
Hypericum	Flowers; herb	*Hypericum perforatum* L	St John's-Wort
Hyssopus	Aerial parts	*Hyssopus officinalis* L	Hyssop
Inula	Root and rhizomes (preferably fresh)	*Inula helenium* L	Elecampane
Lamium	Aerial parts	*Lamium album* L	White Deadnettle

(Continued)

(Continued)

Shorthand therapeutic name	Parts used	Scientific binomial	Common names
Lavandula	Flowers and flowering spikes with upper leaves	*Lavandula angustifolia* Miller (*L. officinalis* Chaix *L. vera*) DC For a review of names, cultivars and species, see The Genus Lavandula Upson & Andrews Royal Botanic Gardens Kew (2004)	Lavender
Leonurus	Dried leaves or fresh flowering tops	*Leonurus cardiaca* L	Motherwort
Levisticum	Parts used in order of clincal importance:	*Levisticum officinale* Koch	Lovage
	Root and Rhizome; Leaf; Fruits with seeds		
Lycopus	Aerial parts, fresh or dried	*Lycopus europaeus* L	Gipsywort
Marjorana	Aerial parts, fresh or dried	*Marjorana hortensis* Moench or *Origanum marjorana* L differs from Wild Marjoram *Origanum vulgare* L	Sweet Marjoram, Pot Marjoram
Marrubium	Dried leaves or fresh flowering tops	*Marrubium vulgare* L	White Horehound
Matricaria	Inflorescence with involucral bracts	*Matricaria recutita* L (previously removed to *Chamomilla*, now reinstated but subject to review)	Chamomile, German Chamomile
Medicago	Fresh or dried leaf; seed and sprouted seeds	*Medicago sativa* L	Alfalfa, Lucerne
Melaleuca	See Tea-tree oil		
Melilotus	Flowers; dried aerial parts	*Melilotus officinalis* (L) Pallas	Melilot
Melissa	Leaves	*Melissa officinalis* L	Lemon Balm, Balm

(Continued)

(Continued)

Shorthand therapeutic name	Parts used	Scientific binomial	Common names
Mentha pip	Leaves	*Mentha x piperita* L (a cross between *M. aquatica* & *M. spicata*)	Peppermint. Many other mints are used therapeutically and domestically
Menyanthes	Leaflets, preferably dry, after flowering	*Menyanthes trifoliata* L	Bogbean, Buckbean
Ocimum	Herb	*Ocimum basilicum* L	Basil
Olea	Dried leaves	*Olea europaea* L var *europaea*	Olive
Plantago	Leaves fresh (or dried, carefully excluding blackened material) Seeds (rarely separated in practice from the semi-ripe fruits)	*Plantago major* L *Plantago lanceolata* L Psyllium seeds or husks are from *Plantago ovata* Forsk.	Plantain, Greater Plantain, Waybread Ribwort Plantain Psyllium, Isphagula
Poterium	Aerial parts, fresh or dried; dried root	The therapeutic Burnets: *Sanguisorba officinalis* L (*Poterium officinale* (L) A. Gray) Great Burnet; *S. minor* Scop. (*Poterium sanguisorba* L) *S. minor Ssp minor* Scop.	Salad Burnet; Greater Burnet
Pinus	Buds; Leaves; Seeds	*Pinus sylvestris* L	Pine, Scots Pine
Prunus	Almonds and apricots and other seeds and fleshy fruits of species in this genus, should be recommended for daily consumption by most patients.		
Ribes	Buds; Leaves; Fruit	*Ribes nigrum* L	Black Currant

(Continued)

(Continued)

Shorthand therapeutic name	Parts used	Scientific binomial	Common names
Rosa	Petals	A complex genus of crop plants of long standing with a multitude of hybrids in the wild as well as countless cultivars.	Rose
Rosmarinus	Leaves and young twigs	NAME CHANGE from *Rosmarinus officinalis* L to: *Salvia rosmarinus* Spenn.	Rosemary
Rubus idaeus	Leaf, best dried	*Rubus idaeus* L	Raspberry
Ruscus	Roots and rhizomes [**Caution:** all aerial parts are toxic]	*Ruscus aculeatus* L	Butcher's Broom
Salix	Dried bark of at least 2 years old branches	From species of *Salix* A complex genus of hybrids	Willows
Salvia	Leaves	*Salvia officinalis* L	Sage
Salvia sclarea	Leaves and flowering tops	*Salvia sclarea* L	Clary Sage
Sambucus	Flowers	*Sambucus nigra* L	Elder
Sanguisorba	See Poterium	The variant therapeutic names reflect the uncertain utilisation, mainly in France, of obsolete botanic nomenclature (*Sanguisorba* is the modern genus name which includes former *Poterium*)	Burnets
		Sarcopoterium spinoaum (L) Spach, a spiny shrub from the dry shores of the Adriatic and Aegean is anti-hypoglycaemic	Thorny Burnet
Satureja	Aerial parts	*Satureja montana* L *Satureja hortensis* L	Winter Savory Summer Savory

(Continued)

(Continued)

Shorthand therapeutic name	Parts used	Scientific binomial	Common names
Silybum	Fruits	*Silybum marianum* (L) Gaertner	Milk Thistle, Marian Thistle
Solidago	Flowering tops; Leaves	*Solidago virgaurea* L *Solidago canadensis* L	Golden Rod Garden Golden Rod
Stachys	Aerial parts with flowers	*Stachys officinalis* (L) Trevisan (*S. betonica* Bentham *Betonica officinalis* L)	Betony, Wood Betony
Taraxacum	Leaf Root Florets	*Taraxacum* is a large critical genus of apomicts, delimited into sections and micro-species. By convention, the medicinal plant is assigned to the *Taraxacum officinale* group.	Dandelion
Tea-tree oil	Volatile Oil from Leaves	*Melaleuca alternifolia* (Maiden & Betche) Cheel and several other species in the genus	Also: cajuput
Thymus	Aerial parts	*Thymus vulgaris* L	Common or Garden Thyme
Tilia	Inflorescence with bracts; Sapwood	The medicinal benefits of species and hybrids in the genus *Tilia* are interchangeable.	Linden or Lime-trees
Trigonella	Seeds. Leaves	*Trigonella foenum-graecum* L	Fenugreek
Ulmus	Powdered bark	*Ulmus rubra* Mühlenb (*U. fulva* Michx)	Slippery Elm
Urtica	Leaves	*Urtica dioica* L	Stinging Nettle
Vaccinium	Leaf; Bud; Fruit	*Vaccinium myrtillus* L and similar species such as Cowberry *V. vitis-idaea* L, Cranberry *V. oxycoccos* L	Bilberry; Blueberry (Cranberry)

(Continued)

(Continued)

Shorthand therapeutic name	Parts used	Scientific binomial	Common names
Valeriana	Rhizome and root	*Valeriana officinalis* L	Valerian
Verbena	Herb; flowering spikes	*Verbena officinalis* L	Vervain; 'Verbena' a name also given to Lemon Verbena
Vib op	Barks	*Viburnum opulus* L	Cramp bark
Vib prunifolium		*Viburnum prunifolium* L	Black Haw bark
Vinca	Leaves	*Vinca minor* L	Lesser Periwinkle
		Vinca major L (*V. herbacea* auct. non Waldst. & Kit.)	Greater Periwinkle
		[Other subspecies from the Mediterranean and Balkans also in use]	
Vitex	Fruit; (flowering tops)	*Vitex agnus-castus* L	Chaste tree; known better as Vitex or Agnus-castus
Zea	Stigmas and styles	*Zea mays* L	Maize, Corn
Zingiber	Rhizome, fresh or dried	*Zingiber officinale* Roscoe a cultigen of probably Indian origin.	Ginger

A LIST OF PLANTS MENTIONED IN THE TEXT ARRANGED BY BOTANIC FAMILY ACCORDING TO RECENT PHYLOGENETIC RESEARCH (APG IV 2016)

In the table below, Families are numbered according to Angiosperm Phylogeny Group (APG IV 2016).

Number following some Family names denotes their rank in top 20 of largest vascular plant families. See Christenhusz et al and Judd et al in bibliography.

TAXON	Binomial
Gymnosperms	
31 Pinaceae	*Pinus sylvestris* L
MONOCOTS	
109 Amaryllidaceae	*Alliums, Ruscus aculeatus* L
125 Zingiberaceae	*Zingiber officinale* Roscoe
139 Poaceae (Gramineae) (5th)	*Agropyron, Zea mays* L
EUDICOTS	
142 Papaveraceae	*Fumaria officinalis* L
147 Ranunculaceae	*Pulsatilla vulgaris* Miller (*Anemone pulsatilla* L)
164 Grossulariaceae	*Ribes nigrum* L
174 Zygophyllaceae	*Guaicaum officinale* L (also *G. sanctum* L). Also *Tribulus*

(Continued)

(Continued)

TAXON	Binomial
LEGUMINOSAE	
176 Fabaceae (3rd)	*Glycyrrhiza glabra* L, *Galega officinalis* L, *Medicago sativa* L, *Melilotus officinalis* (L) Pallas, *Trigonella foenum-graecum* L
179 Rosaceae	*Agrimonia eupatoria* L, *Alchemilla vulgaris* L agg., *Filipendula ulmaria* (L) Maxim (*Spiraea ulmaria* L), Prunus, *Rubus idaeus* L, *Sanguisorba officinalis* L (*Poterium officinale* (L) A. Gray) Great Burnet; *S. minor* Scop. (*Poterium sanguisorba* L) *S. minor* Ssp *minor* Scop., *Crataegus laevigata* (Poiret) DC and *C. monogyna* Jacq., Rosa
184 Ulmaceae	*Ulmus rubra* Mühlenb (*U. fulva* Michx)
185 Cannabaceae	*Humulus lupulus* L
187 Urticaceae	*Urtica dioica* L
222 Hypericaceae	*Hypericum perforatum* L
238 Passifloraceae	*Turnera diffusa* Willd. var *aphrodisiaca*
240 Salicaceae	*Salix* spp.
254 Myrtaceae (8th)	*Melaleuca alternifolia* (Maiden & Betche) Cheel and others
270 Burseraceae	*Boswellia serrata* Roxb et al. Also *Commiphora*
273 Rutaceae	*Citrus aurantium* L
283 Malvaceae (13th)	Species and hybrids in the genus *Tilia*. Hibiscus, cocoa and cotton are also found in this large family.
306 Brassicaceae (Cruciferae) (18th)	*Capsella bursa-pastoris* (L) Medicus
381 Ericaceae (12th)	*Calluna vulgaris* (L) Hull, *Vaccinium myrtillus* L Bilberry Cowberry *V. vitis-idaea* L, Cranberry *V. oxycoccos* L
392 Apocynaceae	*Vinca minor* L, *Vinca major* L (*V. herbacea* auct. non Waldst. & Kit.) [Also *V. major* var. *oxyloba* Stearn (*ssp. hirsuta* auct. non (Boiss.)) Stearn]
393 Boraginaceae	*Borago officinalis* L
396 Solanaceae	*Solanum dulcamara* L
402 Oleaceae	*Fraxinus excelsior* L, *Olea europaea* L var *europaea*

(*Continued*)

(Continued)

TAXON	Binomial
405 Plantaginaceae	*Plantago major* L, *Plantago lanceolata* L
411 Pedaliaceae	*Harpagophytum procumbens* DC ex Meissner
417 Verbenaceae	*Verbena officinalis* L
418 Lamiaceae (Labiatae) (6th)	*Vitex agnus-castus* L, *Ballota nigra* L, *Hyssopus officinalis* L, *Lamium album* L, *Lavandula angustifolia* Miller (*L. officinalis* Chaix *L. vera*) DC, *Leonurus cardiaca* L, *Lycopus europaeus* L, *Marrubium vulgare* L, *Melissa officinalis* L, *Mentha x piperita* L, *Ocimum basilicum* L, *Marjorana hortensis* Moench, *Origanum marjorana* L, *Salvia rosmarinus* Spenn. (*Rosmarinus officinalis* L), *Salvia officinalis* L, *Salvia sclarea* L, *Satureja montana* L, *Satureja hortensis* L, *Stachys officinalis* (L) Trevisan (*S. betonica* Bentham *Betonica officinalis* L), *Thymus vulgaris* L
422 Orobanchaceae	*Euphrasia* collective of microspecies and apomicts
435 Menyanthaceae	*Menyanthes trifoliata* L
438 Asteraceae (COMPOSITAE) (2nd)	*Achillea millefolium* L, *Bellis perennis* L, *Arnica montana* L, *Tanccetum parthenium* (L) Shultz Bip, *Arctium lappa* L, *Calendula officinalis* L, *Matricaria recutita* L (*Chamomilla*), *Inula helenium* L, *Silybum marianum* (L) Gaertner, *Taraxacum officinale* group, *Artemisia* spp., *Eupatorium perfoliatum, E. cannabinum, E. perforatum, Solidago virgaurea* L, *S. canadensis* L, *Echinacea purpurea* (L) Moench, *E. angustifolia* (DC) Heller *E. pallida* (Nutt) Britt
443 Adoxaceae	*Sambucus nigra* L, *Valeriana officinalis* L *Viburnum opulus* L, *Viburnum prunifolium* L
449 Araliaceae	*Hedera helix* L
451 Apiaceae (Umbelliferae) (19th)	*Apium graveolens* L, *Angelica archangelica* L, *Anthriscus cerefolium* (L) Hoffm., *Foeniculum vulgare* L, *Levisticum officinale* Koch

Dietary prescriptions and sleep regime

An example of an anti-inflammatory diet

Foods	Frequency
Sardines or salmon or tuna or anchovies or herring	2–5 times per week
Black unpitted olives (at least half a dozen, preferably more)	Daily
Tomatoes	Daily
Green beans (frozen if need be)	3–7 times per week
Puy lentils	3–7 times per week
Carrots	More or less daily
Potatoes as resistant starch	More or less daily
Turmeric and paprika in food	More or less daily
Dried basil and fresh or dried parsley in food	More or less daily
Sweet potatoes cooked in the oven with parsley and butter	2–3 times per week
Basmati rice is probably neutral to inflammation	So as liked
Butter [high heat only in French omelettes, otherwise cold or baked in oven]	Daily
Olive oil [cold or baked in oven; avoiding high heat]	Daily
Lamb's liver	Once a fortnight
Tongue	Once a week or fortnight
Carcass meat: lamb or beef	Once a week or fortnight

(Continued)

(Continued)

Foods	Frequency
Carcass meat: chicken or turkey or rabbit	2–3 times per week, if liked
Carcass meat: game	Best avoided
Processed meats: sausages, bacon, pâté, etc	Avoid altogether
Yoghurt	As liked
Cheese: from high altitude herds grazed on herby meadows	As liked
Parmesan	As liked
Milk	Very little or none
Chocolate 90–100%	As liked
Chocolate Less than 80%	Avoid altogether
Added sugar	Avoid altogether
Slow proved sourdough bread unsliced	As liked
Flour and other flour products	Best avoided

Resistant starch

This is starch that resists digestion in the small intestine and so enters, undigested, into the colon or large intestine where it will be welcomed by the good hungry bacteria of our microbiome. Resistant starch will contribute considerably to anyone's health but especially to those who suffer from abdominal bloating after eating, which may stem from bacterial overgrowth in their small intestine. Though the bloating will subside, there may be some odourless flatulence but this will decrease quite soon when resistant starch becomes part of the diet. The additional benefits from an improved microbiome will be better than medicine and almost as good as an expensive probiotic.

Potatoes provide one of the best sources of resistant starch and has the benefit of being solanaceous. Never put them in water but steam them. Then let them go cold. The starch becomes resistant once cold which remains when reheated.

Resistant starch has been added to processed food and sold as a supplement on the assumption that because such starch reduces the glycaemic index of carbohydrates. The research for such claims is not very substantial.

Liver sparing diet and herbal treatment

These measures are recommended in cases of acute hepatitis. If very jaundiced and itchy, do not eat but take instead on its own a course of *Aubier du Tilleul* for up to a fortnight. These are small flat pieces of sapwood of wild Lime-trees (one patient with liver disease referred to them as "my planks"). Place three or four small batons (about forty grams) in a litre of cold water; bring to the boil and simmer gently until the volume is reduced by about a quarter. The resultant liquid is drunk hot or cold, the bulk of it preferably first thing in the morning, consuming the rest within 24 hours.

When ready to eat anything, proceed with the following fourteen-day regime which combines maintenance of protein, calories and a little fat with a light metabolic and allergenic load.

1, 3, 5	Break the fast with a hot drink made from boiling water on a few slices of lemon and drinking with a little honey. Perhaps afterwards or later eat a little soaked oats with yoghurt and/or a rice cake or a thin slice of bread or a buckwheat pancake with a smear of blackcurrant or quince or blackberry or blueberry conserve.
	Have a light lunch at eleven or twelve o'clock of a slice of ox tongue on a leaf of lettuce on pumpernickel or thin sourdough bread, lightly buttered or smeared with cold-pressed olive oil accompanied by a couple of radishes and a black unpitted olive or two. Finish with a tisane of orange leaves infused for a few minutes.
	Between five and six o'clock drink a large cup of hibiscus tea.
	In the evening, take a slice of braised veal with some potatoes from the fridge (see Appendix II), which you can reheat by steaming and serving with a little unsalted butter and chives and or chervil.
	About an hour after the meal, drink a cup of chamomile or lime-flower tea.
2, 4, 6	Repeat yesterday's breakfast.
	Repeat yesterday's lunch with steamed breast of chicken in place of the tongue. Instead of yesterday's tisane, follow the meal with olive leaves lightly decocted for twenty minutes.
	Between five and six o'clock drink a large cup of hibiscus tea.
	In the evening, take a slice of braised veal with some potatoes from the fridge (see Appendix II) which you can reheat by steaming and serving with a little unsalted butter and chives and or chervil.
	About an hour after the meal, drink a cup of chamomile or lime-flower tea.
Day 7	almost a fast day with a reduced diet of wholemeal rice and some fruit and water as the only drink, with lemon and no honey.
8, 10, 12	As for days 1, 3, 5
9, 11, 13	As for days 2, 4, 6
Day 14	Repeat Day 7

This therapeutic fortnight may be followed by a course of *Aubier du Tilleul* for a further six consecutive days.

Mono-diets

If your digestion is upset seasonally or apparently out of the blue, respond by doing *one* of the following:

1. an absolute fast in which you take nothing by mouth except water despite pangs of hunger for at least six hours [but not longer than 18 hours without taking further advice]

2. a Mono-diet for an indeterminate length but never more than twenty-one days
3. a Mono-diet for a length of time [usually three, five, eleven, or twenty-one days]

A mono-diet consists of restricting your intake to one food only; usually the choice is made from one of the following:

a. Rice
b. Grapes [best between mid–August and late October]
c. Melon [best between late June and late October]
d. Dried fruit
e. Lemons

The restriction is only on the type of food; the amount is entirely unrestricted, as is the amount of plain water taken, but salt must be monitored, and flavourings entirely excluded. As an alternative to the mono-diet, elaborate protocols have been developed, especially for grapes, melons and what is known as The Lemon Cure, but they are not as simple and easy as the mono-diet.

[Advise patients never to delay eating when exhausted, angry, anxious, upset or dehydrated]

Sleep hygiene: ten techniques to help better sleep

Sleeping tablets, except for short temporary courses, actually make sleep more difficult and entrench insomnia. The following may or may not be practical in your case, but after extensive research into all kinds of insomnia, studies from the Karolinska Institute in Stockholm and elsewhere make the following recommendations:[333]

1. Be in bed without any lights visible from the bed from 10 until 6 from November until March, and use a black-out for the rest of the year. If you have to go to the toilet in the night, try to do so in the dark. If this is tricky, employ children's night lights in the way to the bathroom.
2. Don't have a television or a computer in your bedroom. Don't watch television or use the computer after 9.30 which is the time to switch off the router.
3. Wear bed-socks at night.
4. Keep the bedroom temperature between 15°C and 18°C and ventilated if that is consistent with noise reduction and stable temperature.
5. Keep electrical equipment and alarm clocks well away from your bed.
6. Don't read or work or watch television in bed. Use it only for sleeping or for intimacy.

7. Take regular moderate physical exercise for 6 days out of 7. But do not exercise in the half-hour before bedtime.
8. Try to avoid bright lights in the half-hour before bedtime.

---

[333] These and other references will be found in Walker (2017) in bibliography.

9. Don't eat anything sweet before bed except for yoghurt or ripe banana. The evening meal should contain some fat and protein with a complex carbohydrate such as rice.
10. Go to sleep always at the same time.

APPENDIX II

Poise—a developmental model of human health

Maintaining health is fundamentally energetic: it can be denoted by the capacity of the organism to distribute its energy so as to reconcile inevitable stresses and strains with creating and maintaining its trajectory. This distribution depends upon capacitance: the ability to maintain a reserve of energy in a stable proportion to available energy within a field of unending flux. This continual fluctuation strives towards maintaining a constant distribution, tending to converge towards the golden mean: **1.618** of reserve to the unit equivalent of available energy. So, it enmeshes the dynamic of life in time and space: as if we are forever jumping off or back onto a moving vehicle.

The ratio is not obtained arbitrarily: its prevalence in biological structures points to it being a space-saving, time-saving and therefore an energy-saving proportion. Energy is mobilised and shuttles constantly between these two unequal compartments (like a seesaw with a moveable pivot) as we strive to match our internal circadian clock with the daily alternation from light to dark that regulates the lives of all organisms. Lunar, seasonal and annual cycles enmesh with this rhythm, creating turbulence in our cease-less movement.

In our movement back from the exercise of the day or days towards this pivotal point, we will often experience a time-lag and delay. This impedance will create temporary strain and transient un-wellness during the catch-up period. The range and intensity of experience, translating into symptoms, will depend upon the individual terrain as modified by life's eventualities. After fatigue, the body's primary lever against a fall in reserves is *spasm*, giving ionic and macromolecular reservoirs the chance to replenish. Over-riding fatigue and spasm will lead inevitably to a longer, steeper climb back to health as an index of energetic capacitance.

Reserve (or an obligatory redundancy) is an absolute requirement of the energetics of any biological system according to Shannon's Theory of Information, just as entropy is to the Laws of Thermodynamics, as discussed in Section 1.4.

I give the name Poise to this conserved ratio between available energy and reserve.

In the first place, to maintain poise will depend upon the successful calibration of internal regulation with circadian and other periodic rhythms. This calibration is a signal-processing operation distributed between all the systemic components of the body and all the cumulative developmental modifiers of the terrain. These offer locations for herbal therapeutics.

This pressure can be reduced by: the application of the nurtures with the aid of medicinal plants, leading to the good management of sleep, digestion, immunity and the circadian organisation by the organs. These interventions gain their leverage over the energetic management of the system by augmenting and improving ballast and buffering systems within tissues and between all organs. They apply positive pressure but are not enforcers in the way that pharmaceutical drugs and drug plants are.

Disease, with all its signs, must be inevitable given that the capacity for adaptive modification of the biosphere by any organism can only be limited and finite in a random physical world: the need to extract information, material and energy is equally urgent for all life-forms. Perfect adaptability is as nonsensical as a perpetual motion machine. As we restrict the predation on us by other organisms and the physical environment, we eliminate all infectious disease at the peril to the planet, as has been documented in recent decades by environmental scientists but has yet to penetrate medical thinking. Hippocrates said: "at least do no harm" and did not say: "perpetuate human life at all costs".

The influence of disease in humans can be minimised ecologically by the management of our internal and immediate environment, which is all Hippocratic medicine intended. Buffering and ballast provide us with reserves of strength and control.

Here is a graphic comparison between Poise achieved & compromised:

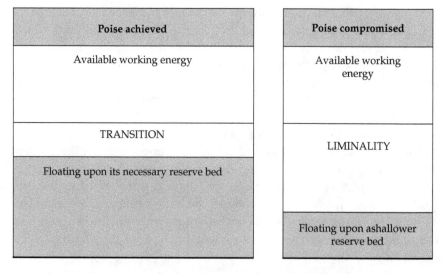

Figure 22: Contrast between Poise achieved and compromised

Many migrainous, vestibular, inflammatory occur in the liminal zone, often the site of spasm and inflammation where the biological stress correlates strongly with psychic distress.

The concept of impedance as a systemic drag on expending energy that was not matched by adequate reserves was introduced in Section 1.1 and revisited in the segment on Diagnosis in Section 2.3 and again in Level 7 in Section 3.6. Here is a graphic depiction of the levels of impedance to poise:

Poise, when impeded	Manifests as:	
First stage of impedance	Spasmophilia	High disturbance; 'noisy', symptom-rich, fluctuant
Second stage of impedance	Histaminic states	Skin, digestion, mood irritable. Often recurrent 'colds'
Third stage of impedance	Arthritic states	Movement and proprioception impaired

You will notice that the initial response to loss of poise is rich in highly distributed symptoms, while the ultimate response tends to be settled, localised and more entrenched.

Each case history and systems review will direct you to where attention is needed and the likely duration of treatment.

* * *

APPENDIX III

A Model of a Consultation Sheet: This is intended to be printed as a single double-sided A3 folded allowing for A4 reports, notes and prescription sheets to be enfolded without clips or staples

F	dob	

Psych	sleep	1
Drive		2
energy libido		3

NECK	headache	
nausea	migraine	
balance	eyes	
	ear nose throat sinus	
immunity	Lungs	
allergies		
tobacco	Heart	
appetite cooks	peri-oral	
Food Choice	*reflus*	
	abdomen	
alcohol	bowels	
	stools & peri-anal	
oedema	renal	
thirst	U-G	
itch	Skin	
pets	Hair	

COLD	Circulation	*venous*
HEAT	hands feet	

Exercise	myalgia	
	arthralgia	
	knees	
cramp	BACK	
	sensorimotor	
blood group	Haem	
ethnicity	bruises easily?	
Seasonal	endocrine/metabolic	

Age at fv	dob	
%		

Broody?   *fertile?*

Menstruation

Cycle

ov

amen   epimen

PMS

mastosis   areola   nipple

Menopause

Contraceptive Pill

Pregnancies   T

To term   Misc

Labour

Lact

21	Surgery	
	Weight	
	ideal ?	
acne	Height	*Spurt ?*
menarche		
Childhood	*Sporty ?*	
Infancy	**Morph**	
Breastfed ?	**Birth Weight**	M F
Term		
pregnancy		of by

Mother	/	Father	/
GM	gf	Gm	gF

brothers		sisters	

Children   spouse

sons		daughters	

Occupation   Religious   Resemblances

recommendation :   referral :   continued...

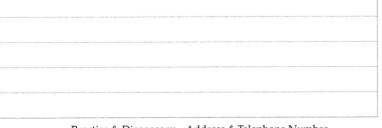

A   dob   f

CONFIDENTIAL MEDICAL RECORDS

Practice & Dispensary   Address & Telephone Number

A LIST OF FIGURES AND TABLES

ACKNOWLEDGEMENTS

When Dr Lapraz read my draft of Human Health, he commented "You want to give something to the world" so I took that as implicit acceptance that I had not bungled too much. In this current attempt to impose myself on the world, which perhaps ought to be my last, I must thank my son Reuben for his unflinching encouragement to my practice, my thought and my writing. Likewise, I have been sustained while writing by Josephine Munday and thank her warmly for her support. That Jonathan Treasure understood what I was getting at was a great boon, so I thank him warmly.

I also owe much to those whose message I resisted: there is no seminar so tedious that one fails to learn something new and important. Many of my insights, such as they are, have come from being startled out of boredom by an arresting notion, often unintended and out of context but one that flies to the correct place, like a dove entering its cote.

By great contrast, my teachers provided me with the opportunity to understand the texture of the field of study. They provided for stable learning with a steady flow of interesting material and novel applications. They are: Hein Zeylstra, Simon Mills and Robin Royston at the School of Herbal Medicine, and Dr Jalal Sharif, at the time a senior registrar seconded from Guy's to Farnborough hospital, near Orpington. There I was able, along with Kerry Bone and other students to witness ward rounds, routines and the nitty-gritty of the operation of orthodox medicine.[334]

Then, after some years in practice, my learning started again with the teachings of Dr Christian Duraffourd in Paris and, more especially, with Dr Jean-Claude Lapraz in Paris, London and in my own clinic and in his. I owe the trajectory my practice took almost entirely to him. Then from 2016 until 2019, came consolidation and new learning from Dr Kamyar Hedayat at Kaunas University in Lithuania, generously funded and supported by Nicolas Ortiz and his brothers. During this time, I was privileged to be

---

[334] We never saw the consultant, even from a distance.

invited to translate the work of Dr Jean-Claude Lapraz. Aeon Books brought this out in 2020 as *Personalized Medicine: Regaining and Maintaining Health*. We all hope that it will introduce readers to the Endobiogenic approach and extend the anglophone repertoire into new territory. I did much of this writing on the Baltic Sea and on trans-European buses and trains, so it was as much adventure as work!

I have relied on my cherished library along with new books to remind me of the details of research ideas and results and have helped keep me on track with the evidence.

I am grateful to Oliver Rathbone for taking another punt on my work and must thank all at Aeon Books for making the production experience so smooth. Alice Rathbone oversaw the gestation of the book with the patience and kindness of a midwife. Eve Brazil combed the text with a fine tooth and I am greatly in debt to her recommendations for making many opaque passages readable and generally expanding what was over-compressed, lightening what was heavy. Her suggestions improved the text considerably, but I must take responsibility for what remains after her handiwork.

The real impetus to the writing comes from working with patients over four decades and more. The ever-varied experience of witnessing the terrain unfold its constellation has inspired me to reflect and try to understand the structures beneath presentation of their signs and symptoms. The matching of medicinal plants with people has led me to celebrate their unique value in preventing illness and maintaining health. I hope all fellow apprentices will share my enthusiasm and hope these expressions of my thought will find some resonance with their own work with their own patients.

BIBLIOGRAPHY

Herbal, phytotherapeutic and botanical sources and references

Barker, Julian *The Medicinal Flora: Field Guide to the Medicinal Plants of Britain & Northwestern Europe* Winter Press 2001

Barker, Julian *History, Philosophy and Medicine: Phytotherapy in Context* West Wickham, Winter Press in association with University of East London, 2007

Barker, Julian. *From Solstice to Equinox and Back Again: The influence of the midpoint on human health and the use of plants to modify such effects.* Order of Bards Ovates & Druids online 2011; in print Lewes, Order of Bards Ovates & Druids, 2016

Barker, Julian *The Photic Calendar: a circannual approach to health: text with calendar* published online by Philip Carr-Gomm 2020

Barker, Julian *Personalised Medicine* Aeon 2020 (Translation) *see* Lapraz

Barker, Julian *Human Health and its maintenance with the aid of medicinal plants* Aeon 2020

Barnes, Joanna; Anderson, Linda A; Phillipson, J David *Herbal Medicines* 2nd Edn Pharmaceutical Press 2002

Cazin, Francois-Joseph *Traite Pratique Et Raisonné de L'Emploi Des Plantes Medicinales Indigènes* Boulogne & Paris 1850

Chardenon, Ludo *In Praise of Wild Herbs—Remedies & Recipes from Old Provence* London: Capra 1984

Christenhusz, Maarten JM; Fay, Michael F; Chase, Mark W *PLANTS OF THE WORLD—An Illustrated Encyclopedia of Vascular Plants* Kew Publishing with UP Chicago 2017

Duraffourd C & Lapraz JC *Traité de phytothérapie clinique* Paris 2002

Durrell, Lawrence *The Plant Magic Man* Yes! Capra Chapbook 5, Santa Barbara 1973

Francia, Susan & Stobart, Anne Eds *Critical Approaches to the History of Western Herbal Medicine —From Classical Antiquity to the Early Modern Period* Bloomsbury 2014

Griggs, Barbara *Green pharmacy—The history and evolution of western herbal medicine* Rochester, 1996 & 97

Hedayat, Kamyar; Lapraz, Jean-Claude et al. *A novel approach to modeling tissue-level activity of cortisol levels according to the theory of Endobiogeny, applied to chronic heart failure* 2018. DOI https://doi.org/10.21595/chs.2018.19954

Hedayat, M. Kamyar; Lapraz, Jean Claude; Schuff, M. Benjamin; Barsotti Tiffany; Golshan, Shahrokh; Hong, Suzi; Greenberg, H. Barry; Mills, J Paul A novel approach to modeling tissue-level activity of cortisol levels according to the theory of Endobiogeny, applied to chronic heart failure Journal of Complexity in Health Sciences June 2018

Hedayat, KM; Lapraz, JC The Theory of Endobiogeny Volume 1 *Global Systems Thinking and Biological Modeling for Clinical Medicine* Elsevier 2019

Hedayat, KM; Lapraz, JC The Theory of Endobiogeny Volume 2 *Foundational Concepts for Treatment of Common Clinical Conditions* Elsevier 2019

Hedayat, KM; Lapraz, JC The Theory of Endobiogeny Volume 3 *Advanced Concepts for the Treatment of Complex Clinical Conditions* Elsevier 2019

Hedayat, KM; Lapraz, JC; Scuff, B. The Theory of Endobiogeny Volume 4 *Bedside Handbook* Elsevier 2020

Heinrich M, Barnes J, Gibbons S, Williamson EM *Fundamentals of Pharmacognosy & Phytotherapy* Churchill Livingstone 2004

Hooper's *Physician's Vade Mecum: A Manual of the Principles and Practice of Physic* 10th Edn 1882

Judd et al *Plant Systematics—A Phylogenetic Approach* 4th Edn Sunderland MA: Sinauer 2016

Keen, Barbara & Armstrong, Jean *Herb Gathering* Brome & Schimmer 1941

Lauterborn D *Mémoires d'un herboriste* Equinox France 2004

Lapraz, Jean-Claude; Hedayat, Kamyar; Pauly, Patrice Endobiogeny: *A Global Approach to Systems Biology* in Global Advances in Health and Medicine 2013

Lapraz, Jean-Claude & Carillon, Alain (Supervisory Editors): Charrié, Jean-Christophe; Hedayat, Kamyar; Chastel, Bernadette; Cieur, Christine et al Plantes Médicinales—Phytothérapie clinique intégrative et médecine endobiogénique Paris, Lavoisier 2017

Lapraz, Jean-Claude; de Clermont-Tonnerre, Marie-Laure *La Médicine Personalisée: Retrouver et garder la santé* Odile Jacob Paris 2012
Personalized Medicine: Regaining and Maintaining Health English Translation Barker, Julian Aeon 2020

Lis-Balchin, Maria *The Chemistry & Bioactivity of Essential Oils* East Horsley 1995

Lis-Balchin, Maria *Aromatherapy Science A guide for healthcare professionals* Pharmaceutical Press 2006

Lorrain, Eric *Grand manuel de phytothérapie* Dunod 2019

Mulot, Marie–Antoinettte *Secrets d'une Herboriste* Paris 1984

Pendell, Dale *The Pharmako Trilogy: Pharmako Poeia* 1995 *Pharmako Dynamics* 2002 *Pharmako Gnosis* 2004 all by North Atlantic Books

Priest, AW & Priest LR *Herbal Medication–a Clinical and Dispensary Handbook* UK CW Daniel 2000 (1983)

Schauenberg, Paul & Paris, Ferdinand *Guide to Medicinal Plants* Lutterworth 1977

Tetau, Max & Bergeret, Claude *La Phytothérapie Rénovée* Paris 1979

Valnet J, Duraffourd C, Lapraz J–Cl *Une Medicine Nouvelle: Phytothérapie et Aromathérapie: comment guérir les maladies infectieuses par les plantes* Paris 1978

Other sources and references

Alon, U *An Introduction to Systems Biology* Chapman & Hall/CRC, Boca Raton 2007

Balint, M *The Doctor, his Patient and the Illness* Pitman Medical 2nd Edn, 1964

Balint, M & Balint E *Psychotherapeutic techniques in Medicine* London 1961

Barker, David *Mothers, babies, and health in later life* Churchill Livingstone 1998

Barker, David *The fetal origins of adult disease* The Wellcome Foundation Lecture, 1994

Barrett, Louise; Dunbar, Robin *Oxford Handbook of Evolutionary Psychology* 2007

Barrow John *Pi in the Sky: counting thinking and being* London 1992

Bateson, Gregory *Steps to an Ecology of Mind* San Francisco & Chicago 1972

Bateson, Gregory *Mind and Nature: A Necessary Unity (Advances in Systems Theory, Complexity, and the Human Sciences)* Hampton Press 1979

Bronk, J Ramsey. *Human Metabolism: Functional Diversity and Integration* Addison Wesley Longman 1999

Capra, Fritjof *The Web of Life: a new synthesis of mind and matter* Flamingo 1996

Damasio, António How the brain creates the mind Scientific American 281 (6): 74–79 (1999)

Damasio, António *Descartes' Error: Emotion, Reason, and the Human Brain* (Putnam 1994) Penguin 2005

Damasio, António *Self Comes to Mind: Constructing the Conscious Brain* Random House 2011

Damasio, António *Feeling & Knowing: Making Minds Conscious* Robinson, London 2021

Douglas, Mary *Purity and Danger* Routledge, London 1966

Ekirch, A.Roger *At Day's Close: Night in Times Past* Norton 2005, 2006

Foster, Russell & Kreitzman L *Rhythms of Life—the biological clocks that control the daily lives of every living thing* Profile Books 2004

Foster, Russell & Kreitzman L *Seasons of Life—the biological rhythms that enable living things to thrive and survive* Profile Books 2009

Foster, Russell *Life Time: the New Science of the Body Clock, and how it can revolutionize your Sleep and Health* Penguin Life 2022

Francis, Gavin *Recovery: The Lost Art of Convalescence* Profile Books in association with Wellcome Collection London 2022

Frankl, Viktor E. *Man's Search for Meaning* (1959) 2004

Gibson, JJ *The Theory of Affordances: the Ecological Approach to Visual Perception* Boulder, Taylor & Francis 1979

Gibson, JJ *The Ecological Approach to Visual Perception* Boston: Houghton Mifflin 1986

Goffman, Erving *The Presentation of Self in Everyday Life* Allen Lane UK 1969 (New Jersey 1959)

Goffman, Erving *STIGMA—Notes on the Management of Spoiled Identity* Pelican UK 1968 (New Jersey 1963)

Graeber, David & Wengrow, David *The Dawn of Everything: A New History of Humanity* Penguin 2021

Grünbaum, T; Christensen, MS (Eds) *Sensation of Movement* Routledge 2018

Guillaume AC *Vagotonies, Sympatheticotonies, Neurotonies—Les états de désequilibre du système nerveux organo–vegetatif* Paris 1928

HIPPOCRATES see Lloyd

Kahneman, Daniel *Thinking Fast and Slow* Penguin 2011

Kahneman, Daniel; Sibony, Olivier; Sunstein, Cass R *NOISE: A Flaw in Human Judgement* William Collins, London 2021

Lane, Nick *The Vital Question: Why is Life the way it is?* Profile Books 2016

Leader, Darian *Why Can't We Sleep?* Hamish Hamilton 2019

Levitt, Theresa *Elixir: a Story of Perfume, Science and the Search for the Secret of Life* Basic Books 2023

Lieberman, Daniel *Exercised: The Science of Physical Activity, Rest and Health* Allen Lane 2020

Lloyd, Sir Geoffrey (ed); (trans Chadwick, Mann et al) *HIPPOCRATES: Hippocratic Writings* in Penguin Modern Classics Harmondsworth 1978 (1983)

McDonald, Roger B. *Biology of Aging* Garland Science, Taylor and Francis, 2014

McGilchrist, Iain *The Master and his Emissary: the Divided Brain and the Making of the Western World* Yale, New Haven and London (2009) New expanded edition 2019

McGilchrist, Iain *The Matter with Things: Our Brains, Our Delusions, and the Unmaking of the World* Perspectiva Press 2021

McLuhan, Marshal *The Gutenberg Galaxy—the making of Typographic Man* London, Routledge & Kegan Paul 1962

Maturana, Humberto; Varela, Francisco *Autopoiesis and Cognition: The Realization of the Living* Boston 1980

Milo, Ron; Phillips, Rob (illus: Orme, Nigel) *Cell Biology by the Numbers* Garland Science 2016

Minsky, Marvin *The Society of Mind* New York 1986

Money, Nicholas *Nature Fast and Nature Slow* Reaktion Books 2023

Montague, Jules *The Imaginary Patient: How Diagnosis gets us Wrong* Granta Books 2022

Morton, AG *History of Botanical Science* London 1981

Nutton, Vivian *Ancient Medicine* 2nd Edn Routledge 2013

Odling-Smee, F. John; Laland, Kevin; Feldman, Marcus W. *Niche Construction: The Neglected Process in Evolution* Princeton UP 2003

Refinetti, Roberto *Circadian Physiology* Boca Raton CRC Press 2006

Rovelli, Carlo *Seven Brief Lessons on Physics* Penguin Random House 2015

Rovelli, Carlo *Reality Is Not What It Seems: The Journey to Quantum Gravity* Penguin 2016

Rovelli, Carlo *The Order of Time* Allen Lane London 2018 [*L'ordine del tempo* 2017]

Rovelli, Carlo *Anaximander and the Nature of Science* Allen Lane London (2016) 2023

Reich, Wilhelm *The Function of the Orgasm: Sex–Economic Problems of Biological Energy* Farrar, Strauss & Giroux New York 1961

Ribeiro, Sidarta *The Oracle of Night: the History and Science of Dreams* trans Robert Hahn Bantam/Transworld, 2021

Sapolsky, Robert *Stress, The Aging Brain and the Mechanisms of Neuron Death* MIT Press, Cambridge, MA 1992

Sapolsky, Robert (video course) *Biology and Human Behavior: The Neurological Origins of Individuality*

Sapolsky, Robert *Behave: The Biology of Humans at Our Best and Worst* Penguin 2017

Scarr, Graham *Biotensegrity: The Structural Basis of Life* Handspring Publishing 2018

Shannon, Claude E; Weaver, Warren *The Mathematical Theory of Communication* University of Illinois Press 1998

Smith, Pamela H *From Lived Experience to the Written Word* Chicago 2022

Swanson RL (2013) Biotensegrity: A unifying theory of biological architecture with applications to osteopathic practice, education, and research—a review and analysis. *J Am Osteopathic Assoc* **113**: 34–52

Taleb, Nassim Nicholas *The Bed of Procrustes: Philosophical and Practical Aphorisms* Random House 2010

Taleb, Nassim Nicholas *Antifragile: Things That Gain From Disorder* Random House 2012

Taylor, Charles *The Explanation of Behaviour* Routledge 2021

Tenner, Edward *Why Things Bite Back: Technology and the Revenge of Unintended Consequences* Knopf: New York 1996

Tenner, Edward *The Efficiency Paradox: What Big Data Can't Do* Knopf: New York 2018

Thompson, William *The World of Tides* London, Quercus 2017

Vaihinger, Hans *The Philosophy of 'As If'* Routledge 2021

Varela, Francisco J; Thompson, Evan; Rosch, Eleanor *The Embodied Mind: Cognitive Science and Human Experience* MIT Press (1991) 2017

Vignale, Giovanni *The Beautiful Invisible: creativity, imagination and theoretical physics* Oxford UP 2011

von Baeyer, Hans Christian *Information: The New Language of Science* Weidenfield London 2003

Walker, Matthew *Why We Sleep—the new science of sleep and dreams* Allen Lane 2017

Weber, Max *The Protestant Ethic and the Spirit of Capitalism* Routledge Classics 2001

Williams, Peter L., Warwick, Roger (Eds) *GRAY'S ANATOMY* Thirty-Seventh Edition, Longmans Churchill Livingstone 1989

Winearls, Jane *Choreography: The Art of the Body* London: Dance Books 1990

Wolff, JE *The Metaphysics of Quantities* Oxford 2020

Yudkin, John *Pure, White and Deadly: How Sugar Is Killing Us and What We Can Do to Stop It* Penguin (1972) (1986) 2012

INDEX

9 781801 521352